THE
RIGHT
TEST

Carl E. Speicher, M.D.

Director, Clinical Laboratories
The Ohio State University Hospitals
Professor and Vice-Chairman
Department of Pathology
The Ohio State University
Columbus, Ohio

3RD EDITION

THE RIGHT TEST

A Physician's Guide to Laboratory Medicine

W.B. SAUNDERS COMPANY
A *Harcourt Health Sciences Company*

Philadelphia   London   New York   St. Louis   Sydney   Toronto

W. B. SAUNDERS COMPANY
A *Harcourt Health Sciences Company*
The Curtis Center
Independence Square West
Philadelphia, PA 19106

Library of Congress Cataloging-in-Publication Data

Speicher, Carl E.

The right test: a physician's guide to laboratory medicine / Carl E. Speicher.—3rd ed.

p.   cm.

Includes bibliographical references and index.

ISBN 0–7216–5123–2

1. Diagnosis, Laboratory—Handbooks, manuals, etc.   I. Title.
   [DNLM: 1. Diagnosis, Laboratory—handbooks.   QY 39 S742r 1998]

RB38.2.S64 1998   616.07′56—dc21

DNLM/DLC   97–43314

THE RIGHT TEST:
A Physician's Guide to Laboratory Medicine   ISBN 0–7216–5123–2

Printed in the United States of America.

Last digit is the print number: 9   8   7   6   5   4   3

To Our Patients

Preface

My long interest in medical decision-making by laboratory tests is reflected in a book I coauthored in 1983 with Jack W. Smith, M.D., Ph.D., called *Choosing Effective Laboratory Tests*. This book explored the theoretical aspects of medical decision-making by laboratory tests. In 1990, it was followed by the first edition of *The Right Test* in which I tried to make practical recommendations for the use of laboratory tests for common patient care problems and their component medical decisions. In 1993, in the second edition of *The Right Test*, I expanded these recommendations.

As I wrote the third edition of *The Right Test*, a wave of managed care and capitation was moving across the United States. There was talk about reducing medical laboratory testing by up to 50%. I am concerned about the pendulum swinging from too much laboratory testing to too little laboratory testing.

We need evidence-based practice guidelines for medical laboratory testing; and, in the context of continuous quality improvement, we need to study outcomes to determine what does and does not work. Thus, we can eliminate poor practice and make good practice better.

In this third edition, I tried to find evidence for the recommendations for laboratory testing. Most recommendations come from the opinions of authoritative groups and medical experts. More evidence is needed, but, for now, it's the best we have. For some recommendations there is consensus; for others there is partial or no agreement. At the beginning of each problem, I have provided the reader with the source of the recommendations, and, where possible, a sense of whether there is agreement or disagreement. Then, given these different recommendations, I have suggested a prudent approach that can be taken.

I apologize for errors of commission or omission and welcome comments and suggestions.

CARL E. SPEICHER, M.D.

Acknowledgments

I am grateful to my colleagues and students at The Ohio State University as well as to my associates across the country for their help in formulating the ideas expressed in this book. Special thanks are extended to Tennyson Williams, M.D., Chairman Emeritus of the Department of Family Medicine, The Ohio State University, for his critical reading of the manuscript and his valuable comments and suggestions. I am deeply indebted to Chris Anderson for her meticulous typing and her many hours of research in support of this work. Finally, I wish to thank Ray Kersey and John Dyson of the W.B. Saunders Company who saw the merit of this book and guided me through this and previous editions.

CARL E. SPEICHER, M.D.

Contents

CHAPTER **10**

Acid-Base, Fluid Volume, Osmolality, and Electrolyte Diseases 305

Introduction

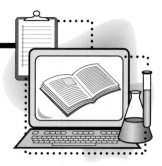

In 1994 the United States spent about $1 trillion on health care—14% of the gross domestic product, a proportion far higher than that of any other nation. And according to the Congressional Budget Office, under current law, the share will grow to 20% in the year 2003. Recently, however, the growth rate has been decreasing. Estimates of the cost of clinical laboratory tests range up to 10% of total health-care costs. No one knows how much of this testing is wasteful, and some boldly predict that in an optimally managed, capitated care system, approximately 50% of tests can be eliminated.

The use of clinical laboratory tests by physicians is a topic of great interest not only because of the cost of such tests but also because laboratory testing has a significant effect on the quality of patient care as well as on total health-care costs; that is, in terms of cost-effectiveness, laboratory test results are often leveraged to include not simply the cost of the tests but how the test results affect the outcomes and costs of the entire episode of care. A good example of this leverage effect is the use of laboratory tests to diagnose acute myocardial infarction (AMI) in the emergency department. Although the cost of these tests is important, it is more important for the testing strategy to have high positive and negative predictive values so that patients without an AMI are not admitted to the coronary care unit and patients with an AMI are not sent home.

The goal of appropriate testing is conceptualized in the following table:

Amount and Kind	Outcomes			
of Testing	*Poor*	*Average*	*Good*	*Excellent*
Too little	A			
About right			C	X (the ideal result)
Too much		B		

Source: Adapted from Robert H. Brook, M.D., Director, Health Sciences Program, Rand Corporation, Santa Monica, California.

The goal is not A, B, or even C. It is X. To achieve the best outcomes, physicians must not only choose the right tests but must also have the tests performed in an accredited laboratory. Moreover, the test results must be properly interpreted, and the correct therapy must be implemented. Through appropriate laboratory testing—not too little, not too much—physicians practice high-quality, cost-conscious medicine, which is philosophically consistent with the concept that good medicine is cost-effective.

Under managed care and capitation, the clinical laboratory changes from a profit center to a cost center. In the pursuit of low-cost testing, the production of test results is undergoing decentralization and regionalization. The use of laboratory tests is being regulated, and laboratory utilization may swing from overtesting to undertesting. Managed care organizations ranked the following factors as important to success in the marketplace:

• Price	69%
• Patient satisfaction	50%
• Access to doctors	31%
• Quality improvement processes	20%
• National network affiliation	11%
• Use of clinical guidelines	10%
• Publishing outcomes	9%

Source: Winslow R: In health care, low cost beats high quality. Wall Street Journal, p B1, January 18, 1994. Reprinted by permission of The Wall Street Journal, © 1994, Dow Jones & Company, Inc., All Rights Reserved Worldwide.

Recently, these managed care organizations have required evidence to support laboratory testing before they pay for it—so-called evidence-based medicine. A problem with this approach is that relatively little evidence exists, and, for the most part, laboratory testing strategies represent expert opinion based on experience and tradition. A concern is that too rigid a requirement for evidence-based testing could result in an overly restrictive laboratory testing environment allowing too little testing.

LABORATORY TESTING BY PHYSICIANS

More than 1000 individual tests are available to physicians each time they face a medical decision that depends on laboratory tests, and the number of new tests continues to grow. The physician's task of learning about tests can be frustrating and time-consuming. It makes sense to organize the approach to laboratory testing in terms of a limited number of common and important medical problems rather than an almost endless list of individual laboratory tests. These problems encompass a wide variety of test-dependent medical decisions.

Because laboratory tests are used to make medical decisions, the decision-making model is a useful framework for characterizing the role of laboratory tests in patient care.

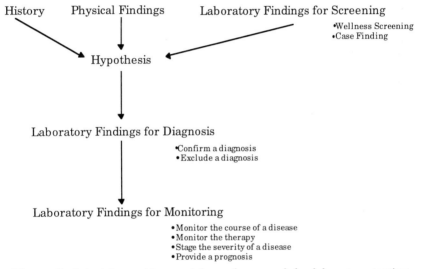

History   Physical Findings   Laboratory Findings for Screening

•Wellness Screening
•Case Finding

Hypothesis

Laboratory Findings for Diagnosis

•Confirm a diagnosis
•Exclude a diagnosis

Laboratory Findings for Monitoring

•Monitor the course of a disease
•Monitor the therapy
•Stage the severity of a disease
•Provide a prognosis

The medical decision-making model as a framework for laboratory testing.

In addition to their use for diagnosis and monitoring, laboratory tests are used for screening. There are two types of screening tests: (1) wellness screening, in which the individuals are asymptomatic and basically healthy, and (2) case finding, in which the individuals are symptomatic or have a disease (i.e., they are patients). In a survey, physicians indicated that they use laboratory tests almost equally for these three reasons: diagnosis, monitoring, and screening.

Wellness screening of everyone for every disorder can lead to false-positive test results and fruitless follow-up testing, with little gain and potential for real harm. One should screen for diseases that are relatively common, that can be detected before clinical findings develop, that are treatable, and that have harmful consequences if left untreated. Case finding, on the other hand, which refers to the additional testing of patients who already have a problem, such as performing a urinalysis in a diabetic patient because diabetics are prone to urinary tract infections, may or may not be appropriate depending on the circumstances.

Diagnosis involves more than just the type of logic that is needed for identifying and ruling out a specific condition. Diagnostic reasoning proceeds from effect to cause, that is, from symptoms, signs, and laboratory data to cause. On the other hand, pathogenetic reasoning (the method by which medical students are usually taught) proceeds from cause to effect, that is, from cause to symptoms, signs, and laboratory findings. Medical students and physicians in training tend to adopt an exhaustive approach to medical diagnosis, relying heavily on the laboratory rather than on clinical testing. In contrast, experienced physicians favor a more pointed and abbreviated approach. They use a minimum number of tests, often clinical, and are parsimonious in requesting laboratory studies; that is, they use a rifle rather than a shotgun approach. It is possible that because experienced physicians have developed a better intuitive sense of the probability of a given diagnosis with fewer data, they are able to function with fewer laboratory measurements. In addition to confirming or excluding a diagnosis, diagnostic reasons for initiating testing strategies include clarifying a diagnosis and providing clues when the diagnosis is unclear.

In some settings, tests are used to make monitoring decisions more often than is commonly realized. In tertiary-care hospitals, over 60% of the most common laboratory tests are performed to monitor therapy rather than to make an initial diagnosis. Primary-care health-care facilities may differ from tertiary-care hospitals and may have tests performed more often for diagnostic than for monitoring purposes. It is in the area of monitoring that good testing strategies are particularly lacking.

MEDICAL DECISION-MAKING APPROACH TO LABORATORY TESTING

The effective use of laboratory tests can be best understood in the context of the medical decisions that the tests influence. The physician's task of managing a patient's problem is composed of a series of medical decisions. Some decisions rely heavily on laboratory tests for their solution; some decisions use test results as ancillary information to clinical, radiographic, or electrocardiographic data; and other decisions do not depend on laboratory tests at all. For example, when caring for a patient with an AMI, physicians are confronted with a number of medical decisions, which vary in their test dependency.

MEDICAL DECISIONS CONCERNING
ACUTE MYOCARDIAL INFARCTION (AMI)

Medical Decision	Dependence on Laboratory Tests
Deciding to admit an emergency department patient with chest pain	**Yes**—using serial CK-MB and troponin I
Estimating the size of an AMI	**Partially**—the higher the abnormal test result, the larger the infarct
Deciding to use thrombolytic therapy in a patient with AMI	**No**—therapy should be initiated before CK-MB and troponin I elevation

CK-MB = creatine kinase-isoenzyme MB.

Source: Adapted from Speicher CE: Decision-oriented test request forms: A system for implementing practice parameters in laboratory medicine. Clin Lab Med 11:255–265, 1991.

In the hospital coronary-care unit, serial measurements of creatine kinase-isoenzyme MB (CK-MB) have been the "gold standard" for diagnosing AMI, whereas in the emergency department setting, the diagnostic sensitivity and specificity of a single measurement of CK-MB for diagnosing AMI are much lower because there is usually time for only one measurement of CK-MB. This emergency department dilemma can be approached by either using better tests for the diagnosis of AMI and/or holding the patient for serial CK-MB determinations. Troponin I is a new and better test for AMI that can be used with CK-MB to improve the diagnostic strategy.

Although in the future this may change, certain medical decisions currently cannot be made using laboratory tests. For example, the decision to use thrombolytic therapy in a patient with probable AMI currently must be made clinically—not by laboratory tests. A test for the earlier diagnosis of AMI needs to be developed and used. Thrombolytic therapy has significant risks, and if an earlier diagnosis of AMI could be made, the medical decision about whether or not this therapy is appropriate for a particular patient could be improved.

CALCULATING THE EFFECTS OF LABORATORY TESTS ON MEDICAL DECISIONS

It is important to understand how the information obtained from the performance of a laboratory test changes the pretest probability of disease to the posttest probability (predictive value) of disease. This is accomplished using Bayes' theorem, likelihood ratios, and odds. Using a receiver operating curve is a way to analyze the overall performance of a test. One of the problems with calculating posttest probability (predictive value) is the requirement for an estimate of pretest probability. This estimate may be obtained by using prevalence data available in the literature for various clinical settings and estimates based on clinicians' experience.

Predictive Value

Several definitions are needed:

- **Predictive value (posttest probability) of a positive test:** probability of a disease being present if the test is positive.
- **Predictive value (posttest probability) of a negative test:** probability of a disease being absent if the test is negative.
- **Prevalence (pretest probability):** the frequency of patients with a certain disease in the group being tested with the measurement.
- **Diagnostic sensitivity:** the percentage of true-positive results in patients with the disease.
- **Diagnostic specificity:** the percentage of true-negative results in healthy patients.

The relationships of these statistical concepts can be summarized in the following table:

PREDICTIVE VALUE TABLE

	No. with Positive Test Result	No. with Negative Test Result	Totals
No. with disease	TP	FN	TP + FN
No. without disease	FP	TN	FP + TN
TOTAL	TP + FP	FN + TN	TP + FP + TN + FN

TP = True positives; the number of sick subjects correctly classified by the test.

FP = False positives; the number of subjects free of the disease who are misclassified by the test.

TN = True negatives; the number of subjects free of the disease who are correctly classified by the test.

FN = False negatives; the number of sick subjects misclassified by the test.

Prevalence = Percent of total subjects examined who are diseased.

$$\text{Sensitivity} = \text{Positivity in disease} = \frac{TP}{TP + FN} \times 100 = \frac{TP}{\text{No. with disease}} \times 100$$

$$\text{Specificity} = \text{Negativity in health} = \frac{TN}{TN + FP} \times 100 = \frac{TN}{\text{No. without disease}} \times 100$$

$$\text{Predictive value of a positive test} = \frac{TP}{TP + FP} \times 100 = \frac{TP}{\text{No. positive}} \times 100$$

$$\text{Predictive value of a negative test} = \frac{TN}{TN + FN} \times 100 = \frac{TN}{\text{No. negative}} \times 100$$

Source: Galen PS, Gambino SR: Beyond Normality: The Predictive Value and Efficiency of Medical Diagnoses. Philadelphia, Churchill Livingstone, 1975, p 124. By permission of WB Saunders.

It is important to appreciate the effect of prevalence (pretest probability) on predictive value as follows:

EFFECT OF PREVALENCE ON PREDICTIVE VALUE

Effect of Prevalence*		Effect of Prevalence†	
Prevalence (%)	Predictive Value of a Positive Test (%)	Prevalence (%)	Predictive Value of a Positive Test (%)
0.1	1.9	0.1	9.0
1.0	16.1	1.0	50.0
2.0	27.9	2.0	66.9
5.0	50.0	5.0	83.9
50.0	95.0	50.0	99.0

*Sensitivity = 95%; specificity = 95%.
†Sensitivity = 99%; specificity = 99%.
Source: Adapted from Galen PS, Gambino SR: Beyond Normality: The Predictive Value and Efficiency of Medical Diagnoses. Philadelphia, Churchill Livingstone, 1975, p 16. By permission of WB Saunders

The predictive value (posttest probability) of a test is simply the a posteriori probability as computed using a mathematical expression, Bayes' theorem. It allows quantification of how the performance of a test changes the pretest probability of a disease to the posttest probability of a disease.

An example of these relationships is illustrated in the following table, for which a pregnancy test of a given sensitivity and specificity was performed on a group of women with a certain prevalence (pretest probability or a priori probability) of pregnancy.

PREDICTIVE VALUE OF PREGNANCY TEST RESULTS

	No. with Positive Result	No. with Negative Result	Total
No. pregnant	90	10	100
No. not pregnant	180	720	900
TOTAL	270	730	1000

Prevalence: 10.0%
Sensitivity: 90.0%
Specificity: 80.0%
Predictive value of a positive: 33.3%
Pedictive value of a negative: 98.6%

Source: Speicher CE, Smith JS: Choosing Effective Laboratory Tests. Philadelphia, WB Saunders, 1983, p 49.

In practice, today's pregnancy tests have higher positive predictive values (posttest probabilities) than the one depicted in the table for two reasons. First, the prevalence (pretest probability) of pregnancy is usually higher than 10% because women who have pregnancy tests have a higher prevalence of pregnancy (i.e., they preselect themselves from nonpregnant women because they have findings of pregnancy such as a missed menstrual period). Second, modern pregnancy tests have higher diagnostic sensitivities and specificities than the one depicted in the table.

Likelihood Ratios and Odds

Likelihood ratios (LR) and odds are other methods that may be used to interpret quantitative test results. These methods are helpful when interpreting sequential tests or single tests with multiple cutoffs. See the discussion of early detection of alcohol abuse in Chapter 1 for the use of LR to interpret the results of the CAGE questionnaire.

Degree of Test Abnormality

The greater posttest probability for disease of markedly abnormal test results than minimally abnormal test results is an important concept that has general applicability, not just for the CAGE questions but for other tests as well. (For example, a markedly high serum cholesterol concentration has a greater positive predictive value for coronary heart disease than a minimally high cholesterol concentration; a markedly high serum glucose concentration has a greater positive predictive value for the diagnosis of diabetes mellitus than a minimally high glucose concentration; a markedly high serum human immunodeficiency virus [HIV] antibody titer has a greater positive predictive value for HIV infection than a minimally high HIV antibody titer; and a markedly high serum prostate-specific antigen [PSA] concentration has a greater positive predictive value for the diagnosis of prostate cancer than a minimally high PSA concentration.)

Decision Analysis

The previously mentioned techniques have been used to structure medical problem-solving in the form of a decision tree, that is, formal decision analysis. In the decision tree the management choices are delineated, allowing calculation of the probability that each clinical outcome will occur if a particular strategy is used. Moreover, the relative worth of each outcome is depicted.

COMMON MEDICAL DECISIONS THAT REQUIRE LABORATORY TESTING

The laboratory request form is like a restaurant menu, but one that is in need of better decision-making choices. At present, it consists of long "a la carte" lists of individual tests together with multitest panels (also called batteries or profiles). These panels or combinations of tests have sometimes been predetermined by instrument manufacturers and often have no pathophysiologic basis. The use of these panels has been criticized as inappropriate and wasteful; however, it is the content of the panel—not the concept of the panel—that has been problematic.

It is possible to describe and categorize the common and costly medical problems and component medical decisions that depend on laboratory testing for their solutions. These decisions entail diagnosis, monitoring, and screening, and a list of them can be used to develop a "dinner" menu for laboratory testing whereby the physician would not only be able to choose from the "a la carte" menu of individual tests but also be able to choose from a "dinner" menu of testing strategies for medical decisions that are both effective for patient care and cost-efficient.

In applying a medical decision-making approach to the use of laboratory tests, sound, scientifically based guidelines for ordering tests in common patient-care situations, although urgently needed, are not always available. Guidelines are useful to describe what should be done, what may be done, and what should not be done.

Because physicians see patients in either an ambulatory-care (outpatient) setting or in a hospital (inpatient) setting, it makes sense to identify common medical problems and component medical decisions in each setting. By concentrating on these common problems, one can reduce the issue of appropriate laboratory test utilization from an endless number of individual laboratory tests to a finite list of medical problems and component medical decisions of manageable proportions.

COMMON MEDICAL PROBLEMS IN THE AMBULATORY (OUTPATIENT) SETTING

Rank	Description	Total	%	Cumulative %
1	Other medical examination for preventive and presymptomatic purposes	43,951	8.4	8.4
2	Benign or unspecified hypertension	30,235	5.7	14.1
3	Lacerations, amputations, contusions, and abrasions	21,137	4.0	18.1

COMMON MEDICAL PROBLEMS IN THE AMBULATORY
(OUTPATIENT) SETTING *Continued*

Rank	Description	Total	%	Cumulative %
4	Pharyngitis (including febrile sore throat and tonsillitis)	20,176	3.8	21.9
5	Bronchitis, acute	13,511	2.6	24.5
6	Sprains and strains	12,830	2.4	26.9
7	Diabetes mellitus	12,435	2.4	29.3
8	Coryza (nonfebrile common cold)	10,951	2.1	31.4
9	Obesity	10,679	2.0	33.4
10	Febrile cold and influenza-like illness	9,366	1.8	35.2

Source: Adapted from Marsland DW, Wood M, Mayo F: Content of family practice. Part I. Rank order of diagnoses by frequency. Part II. Diagnoses by disease category and age/sex distribution. J Fam Pract 3(1): 37–68, 1976. Reprinted by permission of Appleton & Lange.

COMMON MEDICAL PROBLEMS IN THE HOSPITAL
(INPATIENT) SETTING

Rank	Description	Total	%	Cumulative %
1	Normal delivery/live born	4,392,000	14.8	14.8
2	Complications of birth, puerperium	2,265,000	7.6	22.4
3	Ischemic heart disease	1,617,000	5.4	27.8
4	Complications during pregnancy	911,000	3.1	30.9
5	Pneumonia and influenza	879,000	3.0	33.9
6	Cerebrovascular disease	808,000	2.7	36.6
7	Fractures (not hip)	784,000	2.6	39.2
8	Congestive heart failure	685,000	2.3	41.5
9	Respiratory infections (not tuberculosis)	688,000	2.3	43.8
10	Spondylosis, intervertebral disk disorders, cervical disorders, miscellaneous back pain	681,000	2.3	46.1

Source: Adapted from Elixhauser A, Harris DR, Coffey RM: Trends in hospital procedures performed on black patients and white patients: 1980–1987 (AHCPR Publication No 94-0003). Provider Studies Research Note 20, Agency for Health Care Policy and Research. Rockville, MD, Public Health Service, April 1994, pp 202–204.

Because the variety of outpatient and inpatient medical problems may differ from one location to another, the problem lists and component decisions should be individualized for each health-care facility.

RECOMMENDATIONS FOR THE USE OF LABORATORY TESTS

In an attempt to provide scientifically based recommendations for test ordering in common patient-care situations, medical societies, health-care organizations, and other groups and individuals have developed practice guidelines, consensus statements, and other expert advice for appropriate laboratory testing. Of these various kinds of recommendations, practice guidelines have been most prominent. The problem with these recommendations is that few have been subjected to scientific evaluation to measure outcomes and costs. Many are based on expert opinion with few experimental data. Rigorous evaluations need to be conducted.

Among the many available consensus statements, the National Cholesterol Education Program Recommendations for managing patients with elevated blood cholesterol is one of the best known. These recommendations have been recently updated and continue to emphasize low-density lipoprotein cholesterol as the primary target of cholesterol-lowering therapy and to recommend dietary changes as initial therapy, reserving drug therapy for those at high risk for coronary artery disease.

In addition to practice guidelines and consensus statements, the medical literature is full of recommendations about laboratory testing emanating from experts, health-care organizations, and miscellaneous sources.

Practice Guidelines

Practice guidelines are recommendations for patient management that have been developed to assist physicians in medical decision-making. Based on a thorough evaluation of the scientific literature and relevant clinical experience, practice guidelines describe the range of acceptable approaches to diagnose, monitor, prevent, and treat specific diseases or conditions. Practice guidelines are educational tools that enable physicians to (1) obtain the advice of recognized clinical experts; (2) stay abreast of the latest clinical research; and (3) assess the clinical significance of conflicting research findings. Practice guidelines provide a rational foundation for quality assurance, utilization review, facility accreditation, and other review activities.

Consider two examples. Practice guidelines developed by the American College of Cardiology clarified and improved the appropriate use of cardiac pacemakers. These guidelines received widespread acceptance by physicians, and the utilization rates for pacemakers among Medicare patients subsequently declined from 2.44 per 1000

Medicare beneficiaries in 1983 to 1.76 in 1988, an approximate 25% reduction in utilization rates. In another experience, use of the American Society of Anesthesiologists' practice guidelines for basic intraoperative monitoring in Massachusetts was associated with a marked reduction of hypoxic injuries. This allowed the Massachusetts Medical Malpractice Joint Underwriting Association to offer a 20% premium reduction to anesthesiologists who agreed to follow the guidelines.

Implementation of Practice Guidelines

A problem with the national practice guideline effort is that, for the most part, groups and societies that write practice guidelines are working alone. There is little cooperation aimed at producing a single practice guideline on a given topic that represents the consensus recommendations of all parties. This is illustrated by practice guidelines for wellness screening, for which the American College of Physicians, the College of American Pathologists, the Canadian Task Force on the Periodic Health Examination, the U.S. Preventive Services Task Force, and others have developed separate and different recommendations.

Because local physician practices can differ from those of national groups, practice guidelines developed by national societies and groups should be evaluated by local medical experts in the context of local expertise and resources for the purpose of producing local guidelines on specific patient-care problems. Pathologists should participate with other local medical experts to generate guidelines for laboratory testing. This process is used at The Ohio State University Medical Center (OSUMC).

Updating Practice Guidelines

Practice guidelines must be frequently reviewed and updated so that they are consistent with the latest available scientific information. The following figure reviews how laboratory testing for the diagnosis of AMI has changed over the years.

Complete blood count/Erythrocyte sedimentation rate
↓
Aspartate aminotransferase (AST)/Alanine aminotransferase (ALT)
↓
Creatine kinase (CK)/Lactate dehydrogenase (LDH)
↓
Creatine kinase-MB (CK-MB)/Lactate dehydrogenase isoenzymes (LD1:LD2)
↓
Creatine kinase-MB and Troponin I

The evolution of laboratory testing for the diagnosis of acute myocardial infarction.
Source: Adapted from Speicher CE: Laboratory utilization: A discussion of the appropriate use of clinical laboratory tests by physicians. *In* Weinstein RS, Graham AR (eds): Advances in Pathology and Laboratory Medicine. St. Louis, Mosby–Year Book, 1995, Vol 8, pp 3–37.

The lupus erythematosus cell test is an example of an obsolete test that is now superseded by definitive immunologic tests.

EVIDENCE-BASED MEDICINE

Consensus is growing among medical experts that medical decisions and actions should be based on the best possible evidence, and the randomized trial has been suggested as the "gold standard" for establishing the basis for diagnosis, prognosis, and therapeutics. The collective body of evidence that is being incorporated into clinical practice is called evidence-based medicine. The reality is that for many medical decisions and actions, little evidence is available. Thus we are left with practice guidelines that are based on consensus conferences and expert opinion. Groups who are developing practice guidelines have attempted to categorize the quality of the evidence and the strength of the recommendations as follows:

QUALITY OF EVIDENCE

Level of Evidence		Evidence
I	Good	Evidence obtained from at least one properly randomized controlled trial or from well-designed cohort or case-control analytic studies, preferably from more than one center or research group.
II	Fair	Evidence obtained from multiple time series with or without intervention, or dramatic results in uncontrolled experiments.
III	Poor	Opinions of respected authorities, based on clinical experience, descriptive studies, or reports of expert committees.

Source: The Ohio State University Medical Center Leadership Council for Clinical Value Enhancement: Clinical Practice Guidelines, Definitions of Recommendation Levels, 1996.

STRENGTH OF THE RECOMMENDATIONS

Recommendation		Definition
A	It is advised that this be done. . .	in a periodic health examination, or a diagnostic maneuver should be done, or treatment of a medical problem should be given. There is good evidence (Level I) to support the recommendation.

STRENGTH OF THE RECOMMENDATIONS *Continued*

Recommendation		Definition
B	This may be done. . .	in a periodic health examination, or a diagnostic maneuver may be done, or treatment of a medical problem may be given.
B1	It should be done in most cases.	There is fair evidence (Level II) to support the recommendation.
B2	It should **not** be done in most cases.	There is poor evidence (Level III) regarding the recommendation, which may be made on other grounds.
C	It is advised that this **not** be done. . .	in a periodic health examination, or a diagnostic maneuver should not be done, or treatment of a medical problem should not be given. There is good evidence (Level I) to support the recommendation that this not be done.

Source: The Ohio State University Medical Center Leadership Council for Clinical Value Enhancement, Clinical Practice Guidelines, Definitions of Recommendation Levels, 1996.

CHANGING THE WAY PHYSICIANS USE LABORATORY TESTS

It is difficult to change physicians' behavior. Efforts to combat laboratory overuse have included education in appropriate laboratory use, feedback of utilization and charge data to the clinician, administrative changes including display of guidelines and redesign of request forms, physician participation in limiting strategies, and penalties and rewards. Although each method has shown some success on its own, interventions that rely on more than one method appear to be the most successful.

Decision-Oriented Laboratory Testing

The use of decision-oriented laboratory testing represents an effective way to encourage physicians to use the right tests and eliminate unnecessary ones. Historically, efforts to modify physicians' behavior using various techniques, including education, have not been very successful. Interestingly, when house officers were reminded about the charges for tests, they ordered 14% fewer tests—apparently without adverse effects on patient outcomes.

In one study it was possible to decrease inappropriate serum triiodothyronine testing by 38% and thyrotropin testing by 61% through an educational program plus implementation of a medical decision-oriented test request form for hyperthyroidism and hypothyroidism in place of a menu of individual thyroid tests, as follows:

	T_3 uptake
	T_4 (RIA)
	T_3 (RIA)
A	TSH

	☐	Thyroid function screen (T_4 [RIA], T_3 uptake, plus index)
	☐	Hyperthyroid panel (T_4 [RIA], T_3 uptake, plus index)
	☐	Hypothyroid panel (T_4 [RIA], T_3 uptake, TSH, plus index)
B	☐	Other thyroid tests Specify:

A, Thyroid function tests as listed on the previous comprehensive laboratory test request form. *B,* Problem-oriented format for thyroid function tests on the new request form. T_3 = triiodothyronine; RIA = radioimmunoassay; TSH = thyrotropin (thyroid-stimulating hormone).

Source: Wong ET, McCarron MM, Shaw ST Jr: Ordering of laboratory tests in a teaching hospital: Can it be improved? JAMA 249:3076–3080, 1983. Copyright 1983, American Medical Association.

The new form accomplished the reduction by eliminating inappropriate testing. Moreover, the physicians were assured of obtaining the correct tests for the diagnosis they had in mind. A similar effort to improve the use of serum creatine kinase and lactate dehydrogenase isoenzyme tests for the diagnosis of AMI failed when the educational program was conducted but the medical decision-oriented test request form was omitted. New test request forms were also useful in reducing unnecessary ordering of tumor marker tests.

In another study, clerical and laboratory staff improved the appropriateness of physicians' requests for thyroid function tests, apparently because the clerical staff had access to computer-based help screens and laboratory technologists had some knowledge of appropriate testing strategies.

The development of a medical decision-oriented testing program not only benefits discrete medical choices but also enhances serially linked, test-dependent medical decisions. Some test-dependent medical decisions are not performed independently of one another but are linked in the context of an algorithm (for instance, maternal serum alpha-fetoprotein [MsAFP] testing), wherein one decision is linked to the results of a previous decision.

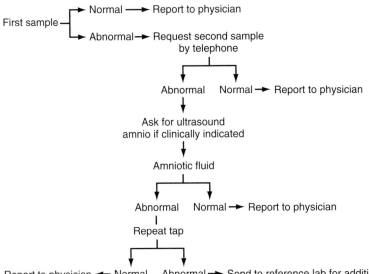

Algorithm for maternal serum α-fetoprotein testing.
Source: Speicher CE: Decision-oriented test request forms: A system for implementing practice parameters in laboratory medicine. Clin Lab Med 11:255–265, 1991.

In 1985, laboratory and clinical specialists at OSUMC collaborated to develop a decision-oriented MsAFP program. Following a community-wide educational effort conducted by the Departments of Obstetrics and Pathology of OSUMC, physicians became aware of the OSUMC MsAFP testing program and began using it. Physicians appreciate the program because OSUMC maintains a readily accessible data base that can be used for outcome studies. Test results are communicated in the context of a medical decision-oriented test request/report system. Every report includes not only the test result but also an interpretation of the meaning of the test result, as well as a prompt to direct the physician about what to do next.

By analogy, other serially linked, test-dependent medical decisions can benefit from the development of similar testing programs. For example, implementation of the National Cholesterol Education Program Expert Panel's recommendations could be expedited by a cholesterol testing program that would educate the physician, implement a medical decision-oriented request/report system, maintain the data base, ensure quality, and prompt the physician about what to do next.

Care Plans, Clinical Pathways, and Patient Care Management

A new vocabulary has emerged to describe management of the patient's episode of care. *Care plans* represent a way to map each step in the process, ensuring that it occurs at the right time and in the right way. *Care plan managers* are individuals charged with seeing that the care plan is carried out. At OSUMC care plan managers are called *patient care resource managers.*

Care plans are composed of pathways that are called clinical pathways or critical pathways. Clinical pathways exist for laboratory tests, the use of blood products, the length of hospital stay, and the use of drugs and other therapies. Moreover, these clinical pathways interact with one another, as follows:

Care Plan

Source: Speicher CE: Laboratory utilization: A discussion of the appropriate use of clinical laboratory tests by physicians. *In* Weinstein RS, Graham AR (eds): Advances in Pathology and Laboratory Medicine. St. Louis, Mosby-Year Book, 1995, Vol 8, pp 3–37.

One can analyze a care plan and isolate the component test-dependent clinical pathways. Practice guidelines can be used to benchmark these pathways and conduct outcome studies. Pathologists should actively participate in the development and improvement of care plans and test-dependent clinical pathways as one way of ensuring appropriate laboratory utilization. This activity will enhance physicians' laboratory-ordering practices in the context of total quality improvement.

Clinical Protocol Software

In the future, physicians will use computer workstations to validate their diagnostic testing, verify optimal treatments, and reduce the use of expensive and ineffective procedures. One cannot possibly remember all the guidelines—computer-based prompts are essential.

At OSUMC we have chosen the Kurzweil workstation to accomplish surgical pathology reports and intend to explore the use of this device for autopsy reports and clinical pathology consultations. These physician workstations will contain guidelines to help pathologists execute appropriate laboratory medicine testing strategies. For clinicians, we have chosen the Shared Medical System (SMS) workstation for hospital patients and the Clinical Micro-Systems (ClinScan) workstation for ambulatory-care patients.

Clinical protocol software is currently under development to assist physicians in their diagnostic, monitoring, and cost-saving efforts. Several software packages are now available. Strong evidence suggests that computer-based medical decision support systems can improve physician performance. Additional well-designed studies are needed to assess their effects, especially on patient outcomes and costs.

Decision-Oriented Panels and Profiles

A growing sense exists that physicians should request tests one by one for a particular medical decision. Nevertheless, as a point of departure, it is useful to group certain panels and profiles of tests that may be appropriate for common test-dependent medical decisions. These panels and profiles serve as reminders of tests to consider; that is, they may be useful as prompts for physicians on their workstations.

FORMAT FOR DISCUSSING MEDICAL PROBLEMS IN THIS BOOK

Problem Organization

In this book each medical problem is discussed in terms of individual clinical decisions: when to choose certain tests and which tests to choose, how to evaluate the tests and the results, what to do if test results are positive, what to do if test results are negative, and how to use tests to monitor the patient if the diagnosis is confirmed. The format is to state the decision recommendation in bold type, followed by a justification of the recommendation in regular type.

Which Tests to Choose

In this section, clues are presented that affect the pretest probability of the clinical condition under consideration. Information is provided about appropriate tests to request in a given screening or diagnostic decision-making situation. For diagnosis, sensitive clinical findings for the condition are given. Sometimes tests that should not be obtained are also mentioned. Unfortunately, in practice the use of a new test does not usually replace the other tests for which it provides an alternative. Rather, the new test often is done in addition to the old tests. This poor practice needs to be corrected.

If patient preparation or specimen collection and handling issues are important, instructions are provided on how to perform these tasks properly. For example, accurate measurement of the plasma activated partial thromboplastin time depends on filling the citrated collection tube completely with blood, thoroughly mixing it, and promptly delivering it to the laboratory.

How to Evaluate the Tests and the Results

Physicians should learn more about laboratory tests. The clinical laboratory is not simply a "black box" from which tests are requested and equivalent results are always received. There are pitfalls related to specimen collection and handling, methodologies, and the skills of the individuals performing the tests. All laboratory tests are not created equal, and test differences can affect results, which in turn can affect clinical decisions. Greater knowledge about laboratory tests not only will enable physicians to use tests more effectively but also will help them to understand better the nuances of office laboratory testing and home (self) testing. In some situations it is occasionally helpful for physicians actually to know how to interpret the tests themselves: (1) examination of a Gram-stained smear of sputum for pneumonia, of urine for urinary tract infection, and of wound drainage for an infected wound; (2) performance of a macroscopic reagent strip (dipstick) urinalysis and microscopic examination of the urinary sediment for urinary tract disorders; (3) examination of a Wright-stained peripheral blood smear for red cell, white cell, and platelet disorders; and (4) examination of a fecal sample for occult blood. For certain clinical decisions it is imperative to know not only which test or tests to request but also which method or methods to use and how the methods should be standardized and controlled. For example, the National Cholesterol Education Program recommendations for desirable, borderline-high, and high levels of serum cholesterol cannot be used unless a method for measuring cholesterol is used that is equivalent to the Program method. It is also important to know the diagnostic utility of tests (i.e., how effective they are in confirming or excluding a diagnosis).

Physicians should use the reference ranges of the laboratory that performs their tests because reference ranges vary with the methodology. Common reference ranges are provided inside the front and back covers of this book, and special reference ranges are included in the test evaluation section of each problem. Reference ranges and other laboratory values are given in conventional units followed by international units in parentheses. Reference ranges should address important variables (analytic; biologic, genetic, and ethnic; environmental; and life-style).

Clinical decision levels are also included in this section. The term *decision level* refers to a threshold value above which or below which a particular management action is recommended. The use of decision levels recognizes the importance of additional information in knowing not only whether a test result is high or low, but also how high or low. For example, the reference range for serum calcium is 8.4 to 10.2 mg/dL (2.10 to 2.55 mmol/L). The decision level above which hypercalcemic coma can occur is 13.5 mg/dL (3.37 mmol/L), and the decision level below which tetany can occur is 7 mg/dL (1.75 mmol/L). It would be inappropriate to assign the cause of a patient's coma to hypercalcemia if the level were 11.5 mg/dL (2.87 mmol/L); even though 11.5 mg/dL (2.87 mmol/L) is above the upper limit of the reference range for serum calcium, it is below the decision level for hypercalcemic coma. Moreover, decision levels can help in determining whether an unexpected or unexplained abnormal test result is a true positive or false positive—with markedly abnormal test results more likely to be true positive than slightly abnormal test results.

How to Interpret Positive and Negative Test Results

If a test result does not make sense or is indeterminate, a useful tactic is to repeat it. For example, when testing for HIV infection, if the enzyme-linked immunosorbent assay is positive and the Western blot analysis is indeterminate, repeat the Western blot test monthly. Another useful technique is to use a second test to confirm the significance of the indeterminate test (e.g., using a serum gamma-glutamyl transferase test to confirm the significance of an isolated high serum alkaline phosphatase value for diagnosing liver disease).

How to Monitor the Patient's Disorder

If a diagnosis is confirmed and the patient is treated, this section gives information on which tests are useful to monitor the patient's condition and how often these tests should be ordered. For example, in patients with acute hepatitis B who are e antigen positive, it is appropriate to test for anti-hepatitis B e antibody monthly because development of the antibody indicates when the patient is less infectious to others.

Additional Abnormal Test Results

Sometimes test results are available that are not really necessary for the diagnostic strategy, but they have been ordered as part of a profile or for some other reason. These test results are included and are organized according to whether they are increased or decreased. It is important to know whether or not these test results can occur in the condition under consideration and whether or not another disease process must be hypothesized to explain them. According to the scientific and philosophic rule of Occam's razor, the simplest explanation is often the best. If available, information on the pathophysiologic derangements responsible for these abnormal test results is included.

ADDITIONAL CONSIDERATIONS

Data in the medical literature support the approach used in this book, that is, a series of recommendations followed by an explanation of the underlying reasons. Individuals often have difficulty with rote memorization of recommendations unless they understand the underlying reasons. Further, physicians do not use recommendations for clinical decision-making unless they have confidence that the recommendations are correct. This confidence comes from an understanding of the underlying reasons and the credibility of the source of the recommendations.

Material for this book comes from several sources: the author's experience, general references at the end of the book, annotated references at the end of each problem, and occasional references included within the problem discussion. The annotated references and occasional references were chosen mainly, but not entirely, to highlight important information that has surfaced between the publication of the general references and the present time. Sometimes an older reference is included to emphasize information that has not found its way into standard texts.

Finally, it is hoped that a more scientific approach to medical decision-making using laboratory tests will help ensure quality patient care. This quality assurance through appropriate laboratory testing not only is good for patients but also is economical; that is, good medicine is cost-effective. Moreover, physicians' anxiety about medicolegal risk should be lessened because, to the extent possible, the recommendations in this book are based on the best information currently available. By following these recommendations, physicians are practicing the best clinical medicine they can.

BIBLIOGRAPHY

Anders G: Required surgery: Health plans force even elite hospitals to cut costs sharply. The Wall Street Journal, March 8, 1994, p A1.
    Expresses concern about excessive cost cutting.
Aronowitz R: To screen or not to screen: What is the question? J Gen Intern Med 10:295, 1995.
    Brett AS: The mammography and prostate-specific antigen controversies: Implications for patient-physician encounters and public policy. J Gen Intern Med 10:266, 1995.
    We need a single set of national screening recommendations.

Berger JT, Rosner F: The ethics of practice guidelines. Arch Intern Med 156:2051, 1996.
  Discusses the ethical implications of practice guidelines.
Blumenthal D: Total quality management and physicians' clinical decisions. JAMA 269:2775, 1993.
  Reviews care plans and clinical pathways in the context of total quality improvement.
Brecher G: Laboratory medicine 1953–1978 and the next ten years. Hum Pathol 9:615, 1978.
  Emphasizes the use of tests to monitor patients' progress.
Brook RH: Quality of care: Do we care? Ann Intern Med 115:486, 1991.
  Believes that physicians should develop practice guidelines and study outcomes.
Brook RH: Implementing medical guidelines. Lancet 346:132, 1995.
  We need to develop clinically sound and valid guidelines that can be implemented.
Burke MD: Clinical decision making and laboratory use. *In* Fenoglio-Preiser C, Weinstein RS (eds): Advances in Pathology, vol 3. St. Louis, Mosby–Year Book, 1990, p 207.
  Good review of medical decision-making by laboratory tests.
Burke MD: Clinical decision-making: The role of the laboratory. *In* Benson ES, Rubin M (eds): Logic and Economics of Clinical Laboratory Use. New York, Elsevier–North Holland, 1978, p 59.
  Test strategies for monitoring are generally lacking.
Capitation I: The New American Medicine. Washington, DC, The Advisory Board Company, The Governance Committee, 1994.
  Projects up to a 50% drop in laboratory tests under capitation.
Conn RB: Practice parameter—the lupus erythematosus cell test. Am J Clin Pathol 101:65, 1994.
  A practice parameter that recommends discontinuing performance of an obsolete test.
Directory of Clinical Practice Guidelines, 1997 ed. Chicago, American Medical Association.
  Compendium of practice guidelines.
Durand-Zaleski I, Rymer JC, Roudot-Thoraval F, et al: Reducing unnecessary laboratory use with new test request form: Example of tumor markers. Lancet 342:150, 1993.
  The test request form is important in the appropriate use of tumor markers.
Eddy DM (ed): Common Screening Tests. Philadelphia, American College of Physicians, 1991.
  Reviews the use of laboratory tests for screening.
Finn AF Jr, Valenstein PN, Burke MD: Alteration of physicians' orders by non-physicians. JAMA 259:2549, 1988.
  Clerical and laboratory staff can help to implement guidelines.
Galen PS, Gambino SR: Beyond Normality: The Predictive Value and Efficiency of Medical Diagnoses. Philadelphia, Churchill Livingstone, 1975.
  Reviews Bayes' theorem as it relates to medical decision-making.
Greco PJ, Eisenberg JM: Changing physicians' practices. N Engl J Med 329:1271, 1993.
  Discusses strategies to change physicians' behavior.
Grimshaw JM, Russell IT: Effect of clinical guidelines on medical practice: A systematic review of rigorous evaluations. Lancet 342:1317, 1993.
  Guidelines development must be careful and rigorous.
Hart R, Musfeldt C: MD-directed critical pathways: It's time. Hospitals 66:56, 1992.
  Discusses clinical (critical) pathways.
Hayward RSA, Steinberg EP, Ford DE, et al: Preventive care guidelines: 1991. Ann Intern Med 114:758, 1991.
  Compares practice guidelines for wellness screening.
Hilborne L, Lee H, Cathcart P: STAT testing? A guideline for meeting clinician turnaround time requirements. Am J Clin Pathol 105:671, 1996.
  The benefits and costs of stat testing must be carefully considered.
Johnston ME, Langton KB, Haynes B, et al: Effects of computer-based clinical decision support systems on clinician performance and patient outcome. Ann Intern Med 120:135, 1994.
  Computer-based medical decision support systems can improve physicians' performance.

Lee TH, Goldman L: Serum enzyme assays in the diagnosis of acute myocardial infarction: Recommendations based on a quantitative analysis. *In* Sox HC Jr (ed): Common Diagnostic Tests: Use and Interpretation, 2nd ed. Philadelphia, American College of Physicians, 1990, p 35.
Discusses the sensitivity of CK-MB testing for acute myocardial infarction.

Lundberg GD: Laboratory request forms (menus) that guide and teach. JAMA 249:3075, 1983.
Emphasizes the importance of the request form in choosing the right test.

Lundberg GD (ed): Using the Clinical Laboratory in Medical Decision-Making. Chicago, American Society of Clinical Pathologists Press, 1983.
Lists the reasons why doctors order laboratory tests.

McDonald CJ: Medical heuristics: The silent adjudicators of clinical practice. Ann Intern Med 124:56, 1996.
Scientific data cannot be expected to guide most medical decisions.

McDonald CJ, Overhage JM: Guidelines you can follow and can trust: An ideal and an example. JAMA 271:872, 1994.
Evidence-based guidelines are needed.

Moser R: No more "battered" patients: Blue Cross urges curb on hospital tests. Time, February 19, 1979, p 80.
Use a rifle, not a shotgun, approach.

Murphy J, Henry JB: Effective utilization of clinical laboratories. Hum Pathol 9:625, 1978.
In hospitals, monitoring is a major reason for testing.

Nardella A, Farrell M, Pechet L, et al: Continuous improvement, quality control, and cost containment in clinical laboratory testing. Arch Pathol Lab Med 118:965, 1994.
Reviews care plans and clinical pathways in the context of total quality improvement.

National Cholesterol Education Program: Detection, evaluation, and treatment of high blood cholesterol in adults (adult treatment panel II). Circulation 89:1329, 1994.
Update of 1988 guidelines emphasizing LDL-cholesterol.

Ohio State Faculty: Wellness screening and case finding. Columbus, The Ohio State University Health Plan Clinical Notes, vol 2, no 1, December 1992.
Ohio State University Medical Center has local wellness screening guidelines.

Panzer RJ, Black ER, Griner PF (eds): Diagnostic Strategies for Common Medical Problems. Philadelphia, American College of Physicians, 1991.
Reviews testing strategies for common medical problems.

Pear R: Cost is obscured in health debate. New York Times, August 7, 1994, p 1.
Projects the rising cost of health care.

Pearson SD, Goulart-Fisher D, Lee TH: Critical pathways as a strategy for improving care: Problems and potential. Ann Intern Med 123:941, 1995.
Physicians should understand the potential benefits and problems associated with critical pathways.

Portugal B: Benchmarking Hospital Laboratory Financial and Operational Performance. Chicago, American Hospital Association, 1993, p 1.
Laboratories' performance will be compared with that of their peers.

Puleo PR, Meyer D, Wathen C, et al: Use of a rapid assay of subforms of creatine kinase MB to diagnose or rule out acute myocardial infarction. N Engl J Med 331:561, 1994.
Better tests for acute myocardial infarction are needed.

Roberts RG, Rosof BM, Thompson RS: Practice guidelines: Coping with information overload. Patient Care 30:39, 1996.
Guidelines are coming at a relentless pace.

Robinson A: Rationale for cost-effective laboratory medicine. Clin Microbiol Rev 7:185, 1994.
Discusses cost-effective laboratory testing.

Sackett DL, Rosenberg WMC: The need for evidence-based medicine. J R Soc Med 88:620, 1995.
Recommends that physicians practice evidence-based medicine.

Shaw ST Jr, Miller JM: Cost containment and the use of reference laboratories. Clin Lab Med 5:725, 1985.
Estimates cost of laboratory tests.

Smith JW Jr, Speicher CE: Workstations for pathologists. Medical Electronics, June, 1985, p 90.
Pathologists' workstations are essential.

Sox HC Jr (ed): Common Diagnostic Tests: Use and Interpretation, 2nd ed. Philadelphia, American College of Physicians, 1990.
Reviews testing strategies for common medical problems.

Sox HC Jr, Blatt MA, Higgins MC, et al (eds): Medical Decision Making. Boston, Butterworth Publishers, 1988.
Good reference on medical decision-making.

Speicher CE: So duplicate chemistry profiles correlate with multiple physicians: Let's not blame the doctors! Arch Pathol Lab Med 112:235, 1988.
Discusses operational factors that cause excessive testing.

Speicher CE: Practice parameters: An opportunity for pathologists to take a leadership role in patient care. Arch Pathol Lab Med 114:823, 1990.
Discusses the impact of practice guidelines.

Speicher CE: Decision-oriented test request forms: A system for implementing practice parameters in laboratory medicine. Clin Lab Med 11:255, 1991.
The test request form is an important tool to facilitate ordering the right tests.

Speicher CE: The Right Test: A Physician's Guide to Laboratory Medicine, 2nd ed. Philadelphia, WB Saunders Company, 1993.
Recommends appropriate testing strategies.

Speicher CE: Laboratory utilization: A discussion of the appropriate use of clinical laboratory tests by physicians. *In* Weinstein RS, Graham AR (eds): Advances in Pathology and Laboratory Medicine. St Louis, Mosby–Year Book, 1995, vol 8, pp 3–37.
Reviews appropriate testing by physicians.

Speicher CE, Smith JW Jr: Interpretive reporting in clinical pathology. JAMA 243:1556, 1980.
Studies the use of interpretive reports.

Speicher CE, Smith JW Jr: Choosing Effective Laboratory Tests. Philadelphia, WB Saunders Company, 1983.
Explores the theoretical aspects of medical decision-making.

Speicher CE, Smith JW Jr: Interpretive reporting. Clin Lab Med 4:41, 1984.
Reviews interpretive reporting.

Speicher CE, Smith JW Jr: Helping physicians use laboratory tests. Clin Lab Med 5:653, 1985.
Discusses ways to improve physicians' choice of tests.

Statland BE: Clinical Decision Levels for Laboratory Tests. Oradell, NJ, Medical Economics Books, 1983.
Discusses and reviews clinical decision levels for common tests.

Tenery RM Jr: Should doctors treat patients like we make cars? American Medical News, October 10, 1994, p 20.
Discusses the industrialization of American medicine.

Tierney WM, Miller ME, Overhage M, et al: Physician inpatient order writing on microcomputer workstations. JAMA 269:379, 1993.
Feedback on test charges was effective in decreasing test requests.

Walker RD, Howard MO, Lambert MD, et al: Medical practice guidelines. West J Med 161:39, 1994.
Efforts to develop guidelines are likely to continue unabated for the foreseeable future. Additional research comparing different methods of developing and disseminating guidelines is needed.

Weinstein MC, Fineberg HV (eds): Clinical Decision Analysis. Philadelphia, WB Saunders Company, 1980.
Good reference on decision analysis.

Wertman BG, Sostrin SV, Pavlova Z, et al: Why do physicians order laboratory tests? A study of laboratory test request and use patterns. JAMA 243:2080, 1980.
Screening, diagnosis, and monitoring are the main reasons.

Wilkinson DS: Clinical pathology: Practice, consultation, and management issues. *In* Weinstein RS, Graham AR (eds): Advances in Pathology and Laboratory Medicine, vol 6. St. Louis, Mosby–Year Book, 1993, p 3.
Discusses care plans and care plan managers.

Winkelman JW, Hill RB: Clinical laboratory responses to reduced funding. JAMA 252:2435, 1984.
Creative responses to cost cutting are necessary.

Wong ET, McCarron MM, Shaw ST Jr: Ordering of laboratory tests in a teaching hospital: Can it be improved? JAMA 249:3076, 1983.
   Improved thyroid function testing using a medical decision-oriented test request form.
Woolf SH: Practice guidelines: A new reality in medicine. Arch Intern Med 153:2646, 1993.
   Expert opinion is the basis for many guidelines.

1

Screening

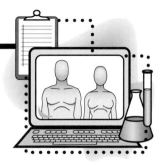

- Wellness Screening and Case Finding
- Unexplained Abnormal Test Result
- Pregnancy Testing
- Pap Test and Cervical Cancer
- Serum Cholesterol and Coronary Heart Disease
- Occult Fecal Blood Testing and Colorectal Cancer
- Digital Rectal Examination, Prostate-Specific Antigen, and Prostate Cancer
- Alcohol Abuse
- Drug Abuse
- Hemochromatosis
- Cancer Screening

WELLNESS SCREENING AND CASE FINDING

Recommendations for wellness screening and case finding are from the American Cancer Society, the American College of Obstetricians and Gynecologists, the American Diabetes Association, the American College of Physicians, the American Heart Association, the American Urological Association, the College of American Pathologists, the National Cholesterol Education Program, the University Hospital Consortium, the U.S. Preventive Services Task Force, and other medical groups—there is no consensus. The following recommendations represent the more aggressive screening advice.

1. In wellness screening, perform the following tests: serum cholesterol measurements every 5 years starting at age 20; fasting serum glucose every 3 years starting at age 45; fecal occult blood testing yearly starting at age 50; an annual Pap test on women starting at age 18; an annual digital rectal examination of the prostate in men after age 50; and an annual serum prostate-specific antigen measurement in men beginning at age 50. Consider testing older persons for thyroid dysfunction and all adults for hemochromatosis. See the College of American Pathologists (CAP) summary of recommendations for screening and case finding in asymptomatic adults and The Ohio State University Health Plan (OSUHP) guidelines for screening asymptomatic adults at low medical risk at the end of this discussion, as well as the rest of this chapter for additional discussion of these and other screening issues, including sigmoidoscopy for colorectal cancer and mammography for breast cancer.

27

Wellness screening is the testing of asymptomatic individuals who are basically healthy. The screening should be tailored to an individual's risk profile. For example, for persons who are at increased risk for a target condition, such as individuals with a family history of colon cancer, additional studies are indicated. One should screen for diseases that are prevalent, that can be detected before clinical findings develop, that are treatable, and that have harmful consequences if left untreated.

Baseline testing is a term applied to wellness screening that occurs at the time of the initial visit, and it requires a different rationale. Although all tests have a reference range for all subjects, each individual has his or her own particular reference range. For example, the reference range for hemoglobin in women is 12.0 to 16.0 g/dL (120 to 160 g/L). A woman could have an initial hemoglobin value of 16.0 g/dL (160 g/L) and a year later 12.0 g/dL (120 g/L), a highly significant change, yet still be in the general reference range for both determinations. Thus, it is important to know the hemoglobin level at the time of the initial visit—that is, the baseline testing value—so that the downward trend can be detected. Another example of baseline testing is the baseline electrocardiogram. Guidelines for baseline testing are generally lacking, and physicians vary in their practice of baseline testing depending on their education, experience, and opinion of its usefulness.

Under the influence of managed care, some physicians are doing less wellness screening and little baseline testing. Other physicians continue to do traditional wellness and baseline testing because they believe it provides important information. These are controversial issues without enough evidence to support conclusive recommendations. The CAP wellness screening and case finding guidelines and the OSUHP guidelines for asymptomatic adults are included at the end of this discussion. These may be used as templates for additions or deletions according to one's individual practice preferences. Computerized reminders may be useful to increase the use of wellness screening tests.

Hematology

Examples of individuals who are at risk for anemia and who may benefit from testing include infants—especially infants fed cow's milk; persons of low socioeconomic status; institutionalized and elderly persons; pregnant women; and recent immigrants from Third World countries. The complete blood count (CBC) is insensitive for detecting colorectal cancer. A recent study found that iron deficiency and iron deficiency anemia are still relatively common in toddlers, adolescent girls, and women of childbearing age.

If only the detection of anemia is of interest and a discrete hemoglobin or hematocrit measurement is available, one or both of these tests may be requested. A CBC is usually performed on an automated instrument that gives values for hemoglobin, hematocrit, red blood cell indices, and white blood cells—and often platelets and an electronic white cell differential count as well. Thus, a CBC may be available and cost little more than a hemoglobin or hematocrit determination. See Chapter 9 for additional discussion of anemia.

Chemistry

Screening for diabetes is beneficial, and screening for diabetes can be particularly helpful for all persons at high risk. See Chapter 8 for additional discussion of diabetes. Measurements of serum cholesterol in adults 20 years of age and over is worthwhile because of the prevalence of high serum cholesterol as a risk factor for coronary heart disease (CHD). Many authorities recommend high-density lipoprotein (HDL) cholesterol as well so that the total cholesterol:HDL cholesterol ratio can be calculated. See the discussion of serum cholesterol and CHD later in this chapter. Although some experts believe that screening serum calcium or uric acid determinations are valuable, others argue that because treating asymptomatic hyperparathyroidism or hyperuricemia has no advantage, screening for abnormal calcium and uric acid values should be omitted. In the elderly, low serum albumin is a risk factor for increased mortality. Screening for hemochromatosis using serum iron, transferrin saturation, and ferritin determinations may be productive. Thyroid function testing in older persons is appropriate, and testing in all adults aged 35 years and older has been recently suggested.

Urinalysis

Examples of individuals with a high prevalence of urinary tract disorders who may benefit from a urinalysis include pregnant women; older men with prostatic hypertrophy, obstruction, and possible infection; and anyone known to have a history of recurrent urinary tract disease. See Chapter 7 for additional discussion of urinalysis.

Miscellaneous

Because the prevalence of sexually transmitted diseases is increasing, consider testing for *Chlamydia* and gonorrhea in sexually active patients with multiple partners. *Chlamydia* screening in women can help prevent pelvic inflammatory disease. Screening for drug abuse, alcohol abuse, syphilis, and the human immunodeficiency virus (HIV) may be appropriate for groups at high risk. See the discussions of screening for alcohol and drug abuse later in this chapter, and see Chapter 2 for discussions of HIV and sexually transmitted diseases. For the early detection of cancer in asymptomatic people see the American Cancer

Society recommendations at the end of this chapter. A chest x-ray is not recommended for wellness screening.

2. In case finding, request tests that are appropriate for the clinical situation.

Case finding is the testing of patients seen for unrelated findings or diseases. In contrast to wellness screening, in which the individuals are asymptomatic, these persons have a medical problem—that is, they are patients. In case finding, appropriate testing depends on the good judgment of the attending physician. Testing may range from a few tests to a variety of routine and special laboratory studies. If an otherwise healthy patient is seen with a minor injury or for an elective minor surgical procedure, little testing may be necessary. Better systems are required to optimize physician use of preoperative laboratory tests because financial controls to reduce unneeded tests can potentially decrease needed tests as well.

The following preoperative testing recommendations originate with the University Hospital Consortium.

PREOPERATIVE TESTING

Test	Recommendation
Chest x-ray[1]	All patients over age 60 and all other patients with a specific clinical indication noted on the medical record should have a preoperative chest x-ray.
ECG	All men age 40 and older, women age 50 and older, and all other patients with a specific clinical indication noted on the medical record should have a preoperative ECG.
CBC[2]	Specific clinical indications should determine the need for these tests.
Serum chemistries[2]	Specific clinical indications should determine the need for these tests.
Urinalysis	Specific clinical indications should determine the need for these tests.
PT/PTT	Clinical history or specific clinical indications should determine the need for these tests.
Platelet count	Clinical history or specific clinical indications should determine the need for this test.

PREOPERATIVE TESTING *Continued*

Use of Prior Test Results

Chest x-ray	A chest x-ray showing normal results that was performed within 1 year of surgery can be used if there has been no intervening clinical event.
ECG	An ECG showing normal results that was performed within 6 months of surgery can be used if there has been no intervening clinical event.
Blood tests	Tests performed within 6 weeks of surgery that show normal results can be used if there has been no intervening clinical event.

PT = prothrombin time; PTT = partial thromboplastin time.

[1]The Mayo Clinic recommends spirometry (forced vital capacity) in patients ≥ 40 with a history of smoking who are scheduled for an upper abdominal or thoracic surgical procedure.

[2]The Mayo Clinic recommends serum glucose and creatinine measurements on otherwise healthy patients age 40 to 59; CBC, glucose, and creatinine measurements on patients ≥ age 60; a CBC on all patients who undergo blood typing and who are screened or cross-matched; and a serum potassium in patients taking diuretics or undergoing bowel preparation (Narr, 1991).

Source: Technology Assessment: Routine Preoperative Diagnostic Evaluations. University Hospital Consortium Technology Advancement Center, Oak Brook, IL, June, 1994.

3. Interpret test results in the context of the complete health examination.

Clinical laboratory test results are valuable, but they are only one part of the assessment of patients and are best used in the context of information from other sources such as (1) the general history and physical examination, (2) blood pressure, (3) weight, (4) hearing and vision, (5) oral examination, (6) breast examination, (7) electrocardiography, (8) mammography, (9) sigmoidoscopy, and (10) radiography.

Follow significantly abnormal test results with additional testing. Sometimes an abnormal test result (just outside the reference range) makes no sense in the context of the clinical findings, and it is questioned. This constitutes the problem of the unexplained abnormal test result, which should be approached as outlined in the next section.

CAP SUMMARY OF RECOMMENDATIONS FOR SCREENING AND CASE FINDING IN ASYMPTOMATIC ADULTS

Test	Recommendation
Atherosclerotic diseases and cholesterol[1]	Measure total serum cholesterol and high-density lipoprotein cholesterol using the original blood specimen on all adults 20 years of age and older at least once every 5 years. The blood specimen can be obtained at random. If the results are abnormal, test for secondary dyslipidemia due to hypothyroidism, diabetes mellitus, and renal disease using the original blood sample. If secondary dyslipidemia is not present, a definitive lipoprotein analysis is recommended.
Secondary dyslipidemia	To test for secondary dyslipidemia using the initial specimen, the laboratorian can measure creatinine, urea nitrogen, glucose, and a sensitive thyrotropin (S-TSH). Because neither creatinine nor urea nitrogen is highly sensitive, a creatinine clearance test along with a complete urinalysis with a microscopic study of sediments may be needed. Consider a 2-hour postprandial serum, plasma, or whole blood glucose measurement if diabetes mellitus is suspected. A S-TSH detects hypothyroidism.
Thyroid testing[2]	Test females age 50 years or older if they seek medical care. Test all geriatric unit patients on admission and at least every 5 years thereafter. Test any adult age 50 years or older who visits a medical facility complaining of other than minor transitory ailments. Test all adults with newly discovered dyslipidemia. Test for thyroid dysfunction using a third- or fourth-generation S-TSH as the initial, frontline analytic procedure, provided that the method meets American Thyroid Association guidelines. 1. If the S-TSH measurement is normal, the patient is euthyroid and further thyroid testing is unnecessary. 2. If the S-TSH measurement is undetectable (<0.1 IU/L), suspect primary hyperthyroidism. Confirm the diagnosis by detecting an elevation of free thyroxine (FT_4), free triiodothyronine (FT_3), or perhaps a total T_4 (TT_4), total T_3 (TT_3), or the FT_4 index, although these latter three tests are less optimal. 3. If the S-TSH measurement is subnormal but detectable, suspect borderline or fluctuating hyperthyroidism, which may be confirmed as in situation 2 (above). If these measurements fail to confirm hyperthyroidism, recommend repeat testing at a later date and/or consider recommending an endocrinologic work-up, which could include a radionuclide scan of the thyroid and a thyrotropin-releasing hormone stimulation test. 4. If the S-TSH and FT_4 (or TT_4) measurements are low, suspect secondary hypothyroidism. Refer for endocrinologic work-up. 5. If the S-TSH measurement is slightly elevated, suspect subclinical or fluctuating hypothyroidism. The diagnosis is confirmed if the FT_4 or TT_4 measurement is low. 6. If a patient has a significant non-thyroidal illness and the S-TSH measurement is undetectable, hyperthyroidism is probable, but an elevated FT_4 is a more reliable test in this situation. 7. If a patient has a significant non-thyroidal illness and the S-TSH measurement is elevated and the FT_4 is low, primary hypothyroidism is indicated. In seriously ill patients, thyroid function test results may be altered by the major disease or pituitary function that is suppressed by glucocorticoids, dopamine, or other medications. In general, these patients are not candidates for application of this parameter, which addresses asymptomatic disease.

Hemochromatosis and serum iron measurements[1]	Measure percent transferrin saturation (TS) in all adults using a random sample of serum. If TS exceeds 60%, retest using a serum sample following an overnight fast. If the repeat TS exceeds 60%, a serum ferritin measurement is indicated. If serum ferritin exceeds 400 ng/mL (400 µg/L) in men or postmenopausal women, or 200 ng/mL (200 µg/L) in premenopausal women, further evaluation is indicated. If serum TS and ferritin are both below these decision levels on two occasions, the likelihood of hereditary hemochromatosis is very low.
Gestational diabetes mellitus, diabetes mellitus, and glucose testing[2]	Case finding for diabetes mellitus is advised every 3 years, or more often in adults age 40 years or older if there is a history of the disease in a first-degree relative; in patients with obesity greater than 20% over ideal body weight; in Native Americans, Hispanics, or African-Americans with any of the cited risk factors; in patients with previously diagnosed glucose intolerance, unless related to prescription drug use; in patients with hypertension; in women with a history of newborn macrosomia or proven dyslipidemia; and if significant hypercholesterolemia or hypertriglyceridemia is present. If abnormal results are found, consider a glucose tolerance test and a glycohemoglobin test. Test all pregnant females for gestational diabetes, preferably between 24 and 28 weeks' gestation, using a 50-g oral glucose load and measuring whole blood, plasma, or serum glucose 1 hour later. Testing requires no preparation and is given without regard to time of last meal. If the 1-hour glucose measurement exceeds 140 mg/dL (7.77 mmol/L), consider retesting the patient using the traditional 100-g oral glucose tolerance test and measure whole blood, plasma, and serum glucose at 1, 2, and 3 hours.
Cervical carcinoma and cervical cytology[1]	All sexually active women and any woman 18 years of age or older should have an annual, adequate cervical smear. Postmenopausal women should be examined according to the same program. Follow-up studies are recommended for any degree of abnormality in squamous or glandular cells of undetermined significance.
Colorectal cancer and stool examination for occult blood[1]	Perform an annual fecal occult blood test on subjects 50 years of age or older, making two smears from separate locations on each of three consecutive stools. Use a guaiac method and hydrate each fecal smear with one drop of deionized water.* Patients must abstain from ingestion of red meat, fish, aspirin, vitamin C, and selected fruits and vegetables as suggested by the manufacturer of the test before and during specimen collection. Selective annual testing is advised for individuals 40 years of age and older who have a personal history of ulcerative colitis, Gardner's syndrome, familial colonic polyposis or history of polyps, prior colon cancer, or a family history of rectocolonic cancer. *Recently, some medical experts have recommended testing without hydration because hydration increases the false-positive rate.
Prostatic cancer and prostate-specific antigen testing[2]	Measurements of serum prostate-specific antigen testing should be obtained only if digital rectal examination is performed for the purpose of detecting prostatic cancer. Prostate-specific antigen testing is not recommended as a screening or case finding test on a stand-alone basis.

[1]Screening; [2]Case finding.
Source: Glenn GC, and the Laboratory Testing Strategy Task Force of the College of American Pathologists: Practice parameter on laboratory panel testing for screening and case finding in asymptomatic adults. Arch Pathol Lab Med 120:932, 1996.

OSUHP HEALTH MAINTENANCE "PHYSICAL EXAM" RECOMMENDATIONS FOR THE ASYMPTOMATIC ADULT FEMALE AT LOW MEDICAL RISK*

Age

Elements of the Exam	20	21	22	23	24	25	26	27	28	29	30	31	32	33	34	35	36	37	38	39	40	41	42	43	44	45	46	47	48	49	50	51	52	53	54	55	56	57	58	59	60	61	62	63	64	65
History, physical, and counseling regarding risk factors: Every 5 yrs to age 40, then every yr	□					□					□					□					□	□	□	□	□	□	□	□	□	□	□	□	□	□	□	□	□	□	□	□	□	□	□	□	□	□
Gyn exam: Begin age 18, yearly thereafter; or every 2 yrs after three negative Pap smears, until age 40. After age 40 every yr or every other yr	□		+|	+|		+|	+|	+|	+|	+|	+|	+|	+|	+|	+|	+|	+|	+|	+|	+|	+|	+|	+|	+|	+|	+|	+|	+|	+|	+|	+|	+|	+|	+|	+|	+|	+|	+|	+|	+|	+|	+|	+|	+|	+|	+|
Clinical breast exam: Same frequency as Gyn exam. Teach monthly self-exam	□		+|	+|		□	+|	+|	+|	+|	+|	+|	+|	+|	+|	+|	+|	+|	+|	+|	+|	+|	+|	+|	+|	+|	+|	+|	+|	+|	+|	+|	+|	+|	+|	+|	+|	+|	+|	+|	+|	+|	+|	+|	+|	+|
Pap smear: Same frequency as Gyn exam	□		+|	+|		+|	+|	+|	+|	+|	+|	+|	+|	+|	+|	+|	+|	+|	+|	+|	+|	+|	+|	+|	+|	+|	+|	+|	+|	+|	+|	+|	+|	+|	+|	+|	+|	+|	+|	+|	+|	+|	+|	+|	+|	+|
Blood pressure check: Each visit	□		+|	+|		+|	+|	+|	+|	+|	+|	+|	+|	+|	+|	□	□	□	□	□	□	□	□	□	□	□	□	□	□	□	□	□	□	□	□	□	□	□	□	□	□	□	□	□	□	□
Vision, dilated eye exam: Age 20–39, every 3–5 yrs; age 40–64 every 2–4 yrs	□	+|			+|				+|	+|			+|			□			+|				+|		+|		+|		□		+|			+|		+|		+|			+|			□	
Hearing, pure tone audiometry (if exposed chronically to excessively loud noises): Every 1–3 yrs; begin age 40																					+|	+|	+|	+|	+|	+|	+|	+|	+|	+|	+|	+|	+|	+|	+|	+|	+|	+|	+|	+|	+|	+|	+|	+|	+|	+|

34

Diagnostic/Screening Tests

Mammogram: 35–39 baseline; 40–49, every 1–2 yrs. Age 50 yearly

Stool for occult blood: Yearly after age 40, three consecutive stools, using Hemoccult II cards. Follow recommended diet and sampling procedure.

Urinalysis, multi-combination dipstick: Same frequency as Gyn exam

Sigmoidoscopy, with 60-cm flexible scope: Age 50 or older, for individuals with first-degree relatives with colorectal cancer or other high-risk conditions. Repeat every 5 yrs after two negative exams.

Blood work: FBS, cholesterol, CBC, BUN, creatinine, electrolytes; every 5–10 yrs

ECG: Baseline before age 40; every 5 yrs thereafter or at the physician's discretion

(One exam)

One ECG

□ = recommended age to be performed; ± = can be performed at the discretion of patient or physician.

*These recommendations have been recently modified to reflect the recommendations of the American College of Physicians, the U.S. Preventive Task Force, and the Canadian Task Force on the Periodic Health Examination, which advocate less laboratory testing, e.g., no routine urinalysis or blood work except cholesterol screening periodically from age 35 to 65.

Source: OSU Health Plan Clinical Notes, vol 1, no 1, Summer 1990.

OSUHP HEALTH MAINTENANCE "PHYSICAL EXAM" RECOMMENDATIONS FOR THE ASYMPTOMATIC ADULT MALE AT LOW MEDICAL RISK*

Elements of the Exam

Element	Age 20	21	22	23	24	25	26	27	28	29	30	31	32	33	34	35	36	37	38	39	40	41	42	43	44	45	46	47	48	49	50	51	52	53	54	55	56	57	58	59	60	61	62	63	64	65
History, physical, and counseling regarding risk factors: Every 5 yrs to age 40, then every yr	□					□					□					□					□	□	□	□	□	□	□	□	□	□	□	□	□	□	□	□	□	□	□	□	□	□	□	□	□	□
Rectal/Prostate exam: Included with physical exam	□					□					□					□					□	□	□	□	□	□	□	□	□	□	□	□	□	□	□	□	□	□	□	□	□	□	□	□	□	□
Blood pressure check: Each visit	□					□					□					□					□	□	□	□	□	□	□	□	□	□	□	□	□	□	□	□	□	□	□	□	□	□	□	□	□	□
Vision, dilated eye exam: Age 20–39, every 3–5 yrs; age 40–64, every 2–4 yrs		+|						+|					+|				+|		□		□		□		□		□		□		□		□		□		□		□		□		□	
Hearing, pure tone audiometry (if exposed chronically to excessively loud noises): Every 1–3 yrs; begin at age 40.																					+		+		+		+		+		+		+		+		+		+		+		+	
Diagnostic/Screening Tests **Stool for occult blood:** Yearly after age 40, three consecutive stools, using Hemoccult II cards. Follow recommended diet and sampling procedure.																					□	□	□	□	□	□	□	□	□	□	□	□	□	□	□	□	□	□	□	□	□	□	□	□	□	□

Urinalysis, multi-combination dipstick: Every 5–10 yrs

Sigmoidoscopy; with 60-cm flexible scope. Age 50 or older, for individuals with first-degree relatives with colorectal cancer or other high risk conditions. Repeat every 5 yrs after 2 negative exams.

Blood work: FBS, cholesterol, CBC, BUN, creatinine, electrolytes; every 5–10 yrs. CBC, PSA every year after age 50

ECG: Baseline before age 40; every 5 yrs thereafter or at the physician's discretion

One ECG (ages 20–39)

□ = recommended age to be performed; ± = can be performed at the discretion of patient or physician.
*These recommendations have been recently modified to reflect the recommendations of the American College of Physicians, the U.S. Preventive Task Force, and the Canadian Task Force on the Periodic Health Examination, which advocate less laboratory testing, e.g., no routine urinalysis or blood work except cholesterol screening periodically from ages 45 to 65.
Source: OSU Health Plan Clinical Notes, vol 1, no 1, summer 1990.

BIBLIOGRAPHY

ACR Standard for Adult Chest Radiography. Written policy of the American College of Radiology, 1993. ACR Publications, Reston, VA 22091.
The American College of Radiology does not recommend chest radiography for wellness screening.

Adams JG Jr, Weigelt JA, Poulos E: Usefulness of preoperative laboratory assessment of patients undergoing elective herniorrhaphy. Arch Surg 127:801, 1992.
Routine laboratory testing for patients undergoing elective inguinal herniorrhaphy is unwarranted.

Aghajanian A, Grimes DA: Routine prothrombin time determination before elective gynecologic operations. Obstet Gynecol 78:837, 1991.
Routine preoperative prothrombin time testing is not worthwhile.

Anía BJ, Suman VJ, Fairbanks VF, et al: Prevalence of anemia in medical practice: Community versus referral patients. Mayo Clin Proc 69:730, 1994.
Anemia is common in a typical US community and often may go undiagnosed in the general population.

Boland BJ, Wollan PC, Silverstein MD: Yield of laboratory tests for case-finding in the ambulatory general medical examination. Am J Med 101:142, 1996.
The yield was highest for the lipids (16.5%).

Branch WT Jr, Jacobson TA: Routine preventive studies: What to include, and how often? Consultant 36:2401, 1996.
Discusses minimum preventive measures for asymptomatic adults based on the U.S. Preventive Service Task Force recommendations.

Burness R, Horne G, Purdie G: Albumin levels and mortality in patients with hip fractures. N Z Med J 109:56, 1996.
Corti M-C, Guralnik JM, Salive ME, et al: Serum albumin level and physical disability as predictors of mortality in older persons. JAMA 272:1036, 1994.
Herrmann FR, Safran C, Levkoff SE, et al: Serum albumin level on admission as predictor of death, length of stay, and readmission. Arch Intern Med 152:125, 1992.
Ferguson RP, O'Connor P, Crabtree B, et al: Serum albumin and prealbumin as predictors of clinical outcomes of hospitalized elderly nursing home residents. J Am Geriatr Soc 41:545, 1993.
Gillum RF, Makuc DM: Serum albumin, coronary heart disease, and death. Am Heart J 123:507, 1992.
McEllistrum MC, Collins JC, Powers JS: Admission serum albumin level as a predictor of outcome among geriatric patients. South Med J 86:1360, 1993.
A low serum albumin is predictive of poor outcomes and increased mortality.

Burton AA, Flynn JA, Neumann TM, et al: Routine serologic screening for syphilis in hospitalized patients: High prevalence of unsuspected infection in the elderly. Sex Transm Dis 21:133, 1994.
Consider routine serologic screening for syphilis in hospitalized patients with a high prevalence of syphilis.

Charache P, Cameron JL, Maters AW, et al: Prevalence of infection with human immunodeficiency virus in elective surgery patients. Ann Surg 214:562, 1991.
Routine determination of HIV status for all patients for elective surgery is not indicated.

Chase M: As physicals turn lean and mean, you must turn demanding. The Wall Street Journal, January 30, 1995, p B1.
Screening should be tailored to an individual's risk profile.

Danese MD, Powe NR, Sawin CT, et al: Screening for mild thyroid failure at the periodic health examination: A decision and cost-effectiveness analysis. JAMA 276:285, 1996.
Consider measuring thyroid-stimulating hormone in patients aged 35 years and older undergoing routine periodic health examinations.

Eddy DM (ed): Common Screening Tests. Philadelphia, American College of Physicians, 1991.
Collection of position papers on screening for hypertension, coronary artery disease, cardiac risk factors, diabetes mellitus, thyroid disease, osteoporosis, breast cancer, cervical cancer, colorectal cancer, and lung cancer.

Expert Committee on the Diagnosis and Classification of Diabetes Mellitus: Report of the Expert Committee on the diagnosis and classification of diabetes mellitus. Diabetes Care 20:1183, 1997.

Grady D: Newer guidelines redefine diabetes in broader terms. New York Times, June 24, 1997, p A1.

The American Diabetes Association recommends screening for diabetes, and the recommendations are endorsed by the Centers for Disease Control and Prevention, the National Institute of Diabetes and Digestive and Kidney Disease, and the World Health Organization.

Frame PS, Berg AO, Woolf S: U.S. Preventive Services Task Force: Highlights of the 1996 report. Am Fam Physician 55:567, 1997.

Summarizes the evidence-based clinical preventive services that might be offered by primary care physicians.

Frame PS, Zimmer JG, Werth PL, et al: Computer-based vs manual health maintenance tracking: A controlled trial. Arch Fam Med 3:581, 1994.

Computer reminders enhance preventive care.

Gambino SR: Better system required to optimize physician use of preoperative laboratory tests to avoid excess reduction of indicated tests. Lab Report Physicians 16:71, 1994.

Pressures to reduce unnecessary preoperative testing may cause a reduction in appropriate tests as well.

Genç M, Ruusuvaara L, Mardh P-A: An economic evaluation for *Chlamydia trachomatis* in adolescent males. JAMA 270:2057, 1993.

Shafer M-A, Schachter J, Moncada J, et al: Evaluation of urine-based screening strategies to detect *Chlamydia trachomatis* among sexually active young males. JAMA 270:2065, 1993.

Workowski KA, Lampe MF, Wong KG, et al: Long-term eradication of *Chlamydia trachomatis* genital infection after antimicrobial therapy. JAMA 270:2071, 1993.

The leukocyte esterase urine dipstick can detect asymptomatic chlamydial infection in males.

Gewirtz AS, Miller ML, Keys TF: The clinical usefulness of the preoperative bleeding time. Arch Pathol Lab Med 120:353, 1996.

Preoperative bleeding time does not predict excessive perioperative bleeding.

Gold BS, Young ML, Kinman JL, et al: The utility of preoperative electrocardiograms in the ambulatory surgical patient. Arch Intern Med 152:301, 1992.

Paraskos JA: Who needs a preoperative electrocardiogram? Arch Intern Med 152:261, 1992.

Few patients benefit from ECGs before ambulatory surgery.

Golub R, Cantu R, Sorrento JJ, et al: Efficacy of preadmission testing in ambulatory surgical patients. Am J Surg 163:565, 1992.

Order tests based on the history and physical examination. Obtain a hematocrit if large blood loss is anticipated and an electrocardiogram for patients over 50.

Gomez JA, Diehl AK: Admission stool guaiac test: Use and impact on patient management. Am J Med 92:603, 1992.

Routine admission fecal occult blood testing is seldom useful. It is best reserved for patients with clinical indications.

Gravlee GP, Arora S, Lavender SW, et al: Predictive value of blood clotting tests in cardiac surgical patients. Ann Thorac Surg 58:216, 1994.

Preoperative coagulation tests correlate poorly with bleeding after cardiopulmonary bypass.

Guidelines for electrocardiography: A report of the American College of Cardiology/ American Heart Association Task Force on Assessment of Diagnostic and Therapeutic Cardiovascular Procedures (Committee on Electrocardiography). J Am Coll Cardiol 19:473, 1992.

Guidelines for reducing the number of baseline and preoperative ECGs performed in persons less than age 40 and the number of routine follow-up ECGs.

Hillis SD, Wasserheit JN: Screening for chlamydia: A key to the prevention of pelvic inflammatory disease. N Engl J Med 334:1399, 1996.

Chlamydia screening can lower the rate of subsequent pelvic inflammatory disease.

Houry S, Georgeac C, Hay J-M, et al: A prospective multi-center evaluation of preoperative hemostatic screening tests. Am J Surg 170:19, 1995.

Routine preoperative coagulation screening tests are of no value for otherwise normal patients.

Kim DE, Berlowitz DR: The limited value of routine laboratory assessments in severely impaired nursing home residents. JAMA 272:1447, 1994.

Routine laboratory assessments are of limited value in impaired nursing home patients.

Knud-Hansen CR, Dallabetta GA, Reichart C, et al: Surrogate methods to diagnose gonococcal and chlamydial cervicitis: Comparison of leukocyte esterase dipstick, endocervical Gram stain, and culture. Sex Transm Dis 18:211, 1991.

The leukocyte esterase dipstick on an endocervical swab in saline can be used to screen for gonococcal and chlamydial cervicitis.

Kozak EA, Brath LK: Do "screening" coagulation tests predict bleeding in patients undergoing fiberoptic bronchoscopy with biopsy? Chest 106:703, 1994.

Preoperative coagulation tests are poor predictors of bleeding after fiberoptic bronchoscopy.

Kundrotas LW, Clement DJ: Serum alanine aminotransferase elevation in asymptomatic U.S. Air Force basic trainee blood donors. Digest Dis Sci 38:2145, 1993.

A slight alanine aminotransferase elevation in an otherwise healthy individual may lead to expensive additional testing that is of no clinical value.

Larocque BJ, Maykut RJ: Implementation of guidelines for preoperative laboratory investigations in patients scheduled to undergo elective surgery. Can J Surg 37:397, 1994.

Only a CBC and urinalysis are indicated for all patients. Other tests should be ordered selectively.

Little DR: Hemochromatosis: Diagnosis and management. Am Fam Physician 53:2623, 1996.

Screening for hemochromatosis is recommended in affected families, and screening programs for wider populations are being evaluated.

Litzelman DK, Dittus RS, Miller ME, et al: Requiring physicians to respond to computerized reminders improves their compliance with preventive care protocols. J Gen Intern Med 8:311, 1993.

Chart reminders can improve compliance with cancer screening guidelines.

London SJ, Connolly JL, Schnitt SJ, et al: A prospective study of benign breast disease and the risk of breast cancer. JAMA 267:941, 1992.

Few patients benefit from ECGs before ambulatory surgery.

Looker AC, Dallman PR, Carroll MD, et al: Prevalence of iron deficiency in the United States. JAMA 277:973, 1997.

Iron deficiency and iron deficiency anemia are still relatively common in toddlers, adolescent girls, and women of childbearing age.

Luckmann R, Melville SK: Periodic health evaluation of adults: A survey of family physicians. J Fam Pract 40:547, 1995.

The periodic health evaluation—including unrecommended tests—is still widely used.

Lurie P, Avins AL, Phillips KA, et al: The cost-effectiveness of voluntary counseling and testing of hospital inpatients for HIV infection. JAMA 272:1832, 1994.

Inpatient HIV screening is not cost-effective.

Lyon AW, Greenway DC, Hindmarsh JT: A strategy to promote rational clinical chemistry test utilization. Am J Clin Pathol 103:718, 1995.

Chemistry testing can be reduced by banning the use of test panels.

Macario A, Roizen MF, Thisted RA, et al: Reassessment of preoperative laboratory testing has changed the test-ordering patterns of physicians. Surg Gynecol Obstet 175:539, 1992.

A better system is needed for preoperative test selection to improve appropriate test selection.

Mangano DT, Goldman L: Preoperative assessment of patients with known or suspected coronary disease. N Engl J Med 333:1750, 1995.

Discusses preoperative testing in patients with coronary artery disease.

Mates M, Heyd J, Souroujon M, et al: The hematologist as watchdog of community health by full blood count. Q J Med 88:333, 1995.

In high-risk ambulatory patients, a complete blood count is a good screen for serious clinical problems.

Monane M, Gurwitz JH, Lipsitz LA, et al: Epidemiologic and diagnostic aspects of bacteriuria: A longitudinal study in older women. J Am Geriatr Soc 43:618, 1995.

Transient bacteriuria is a common event in elderly women and can be excluded by inexpensive routine analysis.

Mulkerrin EC, Arnold JD, Dewar R, et al: Glycosylated hemoglobin in the diagnosis of diabetes mellitus in elderly people. Age Ageing 21:175, 1992.
Glycosylated hemoglobin was only 36% sensitive for detecting diabetes in elderly subjects.

Narr BJ, Hansen TR, Warner MA: Preoperative laboratory screening in healthy Mayo patients: Cost-effective elimination of tests and unchanged outcomes. Mayo Clin Proc 66:155, 1991.
Outlines minimal preoperative test requirements at the Mayo Clinic.

Naughton BJ, Moran MB: Patterns of syphilis testing in the elderly. J Gen Intern Med 7:273, 1992.
Syphilis testing in the elderly should be done for a specific reason and not routinely.

Neithercut WD, Chattington P: Routine clinical biochemistry tests collected from patients dying in hospital. Br J Clin Pract 49:241, 1995.
Dying patients have unnecessary laboratory tests.

Niv Y, Sperber AD: Sensitivity, specificity, and predictive value of fecal occult blood testing (Hemoccult II) for colorectal neoplasia in symptomatic patients: A prospective study with colonoscopy. Am J Gastroenterol 90:1974, 1995.
Fecal occult blood tests have limited value in symptomatic patients.

Nunns D, Smith ARB, Hosker G: Reagent strip testing urine for significant bacteriuria in a urodynamic clinic. Br J Urol 76:87, 1995.
Urine dipstick testing can screen for urinary tract infection.

Rüttimann S, Clémençon D, Dubach UC: Usefulness of complete blood counts as a case-finding tool in medical outpatients. Ann Intern Med 116:44, 1992.
Concludes from a study of 595 middle-aged medical outpatients that CBCs have limited use.

Rüttimann S, Dreifuss M, Clémençon D, et al: Multiple biochemical blood testing as a case-finding tool in ambulatory medical patients. Am J Med 94:141, 1993.
Only three tests are useful: serum cholesterol, glucose, and alanine aminotransferase.

Selby JV, Friedman GD, Quesenberry CP Jr, et al: Effect of fecal occult blood testing on mortality from colorectal cancer: A case-control study. Ann Intern Med 118:1, 1993.
Annual or biennial fecal occult blood testing may reduce mortality from colorectal cancer by 25 to 30%.

Shea S, DuMouchel W, Bahamonde L: A meta-analysis of 16 randomized controlled trials to evaluate computer-based clinical reminder systems for preventive care in the ambulatory setting. J Am Med Inform Assoc 3:399, 1996.
Computerized reminders increase the rate of use of most preventive services.

Sox HC Jr (ed): Common Diagnostic Tests: Use and Interpretation, 2nd ed. Philadelphia, American College of Physicians, 1990.
Reviews the CBC, biochemical profiles, and other common laboratory tests with American College of Physicians' guidelines for their appropriate use.

Sox HC Jr (ed): The baseline electrocardiogram. Am J Med 91:573, 1991.
Suggests that baseline testing constitutes a different reason for testing than screening to detect and thus requires a different rationale.

Sox HC Jr: Preventive health services in adults. N Engl J Med 330:1589, 1994.
Compares wellness screening guidelines from the American College of Physicians, the Canadian Task Force on the Periodic Health Examination, and the U.S. Preventive Services Task Force.

Speights VO, Johnson MW, Stoltenberg PH, et al: Complete blood count indices in colorectal carcinoma. Arch Pathol Lab Med 116:258, 1992.
The complete blood count is insensitive for detecting colorectal carcinoma.

Spence RK, Costabile JP, Young GS, et al: Is hemoglobin level alone a reliable predictor of outcome in the severely anemic surgical patient? Am Surg 58:92, 1992.
Unless it is very low (<3 g/dL [<30 g/L]), the hemoglobin level alone is not a predictor of outcome in surgical patients.

Tortella BJ, Lavery RF, Rekant M: Utility of routine admission serum chemistry panels in adult trauma patients. Acad Emerg Med 2:190, 1995.
Routine admission chemistry profiles for trauma patients are not productive.

Trivalle C, Doucet J, Chassagne P, et al: Differences in the signs and symptoms of hyperthyroidism in older and younger patients. J Am Geriatr Soc 44:50, 1996.
   Clinicians should have a low threshold for thyroid function testing in the elderly because they often have hyperthyroidism without classic signs and symptoms.
Velanovich V: The value of routine preoperative laboratory testing in predicting postoperative complications: A multivariate analysis. Surgery 109:236, 1991.
   Only a few preoperative tests are useful for predicting preoperative complications.
U.S. Preventive Services Task Force: Guide to Clinical Preventive Services, 2nd ed. Baltimore, Williams & Wilkins, 1996.
   A standard reference for evidence-based screening recommendations.

UNEXPLAINED ABNORMAL TEST RESULT

Recommendations for an unexplained abnormal test result are from the medical literature.

1. If a slightly abnormal test result (just outside the reference range) does not fit with the patient's clinical and other laboratory findings, consider that it may represent a statistical outlier that may be ignored.

Minor test result abnormalities are common during wellness screening and case finding. These results are often statistical outliers that may be ignored if they lie just outside the reference range (>2 but <3 standard deviations) and the patient has no other abnormal clinical, radiographic, or laboratory findings. The probability of occurrence for these statistical outliers increases with the number of different tests performed as follows:

Number of Tests Performed	Probability (%) of Finding Results Outside Reference Range*
1	5
6	24
12	43

*Using the mean ± 2 standard deviations (95% confidence limits) for the reference range.

For wellness screening, consider asking your laboratory for the mean ± 3 standard deviations (99.7% confidence limits) to define normal. This would considerably decrease false-positive test results.

The condition of a healthy person with a false-positive test result has been called the *Ulysses syndrome* because, like Ulysses, the patient must pass through a long journey of investigative procedures before returning to the previous state of health.

2. If, however, an abnormal test result might be more than a minor statistical outlier and could have real clinical significance, e.g., increased serum calcium, verify the result rather than ignoring it. Pay attention to abnormal test results for critical analytes.

It is important to distinguish test results that are markedly abnormal from those that are minimally abnormal (possible statistical outliers). HIV testing illustrates this important point. In a low-risk group a weak HIV antibody titer is almost always a false-positive result because the probability of disease is very low. On the other hand, a strong HIV antibody titer is predictive of disease most of the time. Another way to clarify the significance of an unexplained abnormal test result is to follow it with a confirmatory test, e.g., clarifying the meaning of a positive Venereal Disease Research Laboratory (VDRL) test for syphilis by performing a fluorescent treponemal antibody absorption test. Still another way is to wait a while and repeat the test to determine whether it becomes normal, stays the same, or becomes more abnormal.

3. A general approach for verifying an unexplained test result abnormality follows: Repeat the measurement (repeat only tests that are abnormal; i.e., if a 12-test biochemical profile reveals an abnormal serum calcium result, repeat only the serum calcium measurement, not the entire 12-test biochemical profile).

- Prepare the patient properly.
- Ensure correct patient identification.
- Obtain a proper sample (e.g., even slight hemolysis causes a significant increase in serum lactate dehydrogenase, potassium, and acid phosphatase).
- Ensure appropriate specimen handling.
- Use the best laboratory method available (e.g., for serum calcium, use the atomic absorption method, if available).
- Use the proper reference range for the age and sex of the patient.
- Consult the following references for information about unexplained test results: Young DS: Effects of Preanalytical Variables on Clinical Laboratory tests, 2nd ed; Effects of Drugs on Clinical Laboratory Tests, 4th ed; and Friedman RB, Young DS: Effects of Disease on Clinical Laboratory Tests, 3rd ed (AACC Press, 2101 L Street, NW, Suite 202, Washington, DC 20037-1526). If these references are not available in your library, ask the medical director of your clinical laboratory to make them available.

4. If the abnormal test result has been verified, consider a drug effect or a life-style effect. If these do not explain the abnormality, consider the significance of the abnormal test result in the context of the individual's clinical and other laboratory findings.

A common example of an unexplained abnormal test result is increased serum alkaline phosphatase (ALP). Sometimes the increase can be explained by a specimen collection and handling problem, or a laboratory error, or the patient is a growing child or a pregnant woman, which explains the increased result. Occasionally the increase is due to a drug effect that can occur with agents such as chlorpromazine and methyltestosterone. The increase can also be caused by the formation of a macroenzyme complex of ALP with immunoglobulin, and the increase can persist for years and have no clinical significance. This macroenzyme phenomenon can occur with amylase, creatine kinase, lactate dehydrogenase, and aspartate aminotransferase (AST). Except for AST, patients with macroenzymes are generally older than 60 years of age. Benign increase of ALP may be familial.

Life-style effects can be due to drugs, exercise, alcohol intake, and smoking. These effects are catalogued in the references by Young and Friedman previously mentioned. For example, vigorous exercise in an unconditioned person can increase serum creatine kinase; excessive alcohol intake can cause anemia, increased lipids, and numerous other test abnormalities; and smoking can increase serum carcinoembryonic antigen. Vigorous exercise may cause hematuria and a positive test for fecal occult blood; if enough blood is lost, anemia can occur.

Only if an unexplained abnormal test result such as a high level of serum ALP cannot be accounted for by factors such as those previously discussed should one consider obtaining a differential diagnosis and follow-up studies. Unrecognized disease may be the cause for an unexplained abnormality, such as Paget's disease for an unexpected high ALP level. In the United States, osteoporosis is the only bone disease that is more prevalent than Paget's disease. Paget's disease affects an estimated 3 to 4% of people over the age of 45 and up to 8% of those over 80. The ALP of sons, daughters, and siblings of people with Paget's disease should be measured every 2 or 3 years after they reach age 40.

The significance of an unexplained test result may be clarified by considering it in the context of the patient's clinical and other laboratory findings. For example, an unexplained high ALP level in an elderly man with a history of prostate cancer takes on a special significance because the patient is at risk for metastatic bone disease, which may be manifested by an increased serum ALP. Similarly, if an unexplained high ALP level occurs in a middle-aged, overweight woman who has a slightly high serum bilirubin level, the possibility of cholelithiasis comes to mind, and additional studies are appropriate. When an initial test result such as an ALP is abnormal, the presence of another related abnormal test result such as increased gamma-glutamyl transferase (GGT) helps to confirm that the initial abnormal test result is significant.

5. In a patient with an unexplained high serum ALP level, perform a careful history and physical evaluation and obtain a CBC, chemistry profile, and GGT test. Repeat the ALP test in 1 to 3 months if no diagnosis is obvious.

This work-up is designed to detect the cause of the increased ALP, which includes the following disorders: malignancy, drug (e.g., phenytoin sodium [Dilantin]) therapy, congestive heart failure, bone disease, and hepatobiliary disease. Increased serum GGT is especially sensitive in detecting hepatobiliary disease. In the final analysis, none of these disorders may be present, and the isolated high ALP level may be due to a condition called *benign familial hyperphosphatasemia*.

6. See the discussion of jaundice and abnormal liver function tests in Chapter 6 for recommendations on evaluating a patient with unexplained high transaminase levels.

Besides liver disease, consider myositis in patients with an increased serum transaminase level—the lactate dehydrogenase level may also be increased. An increased serum creatine kinase level is consistent with myositis.

BIBLIOGRAPHY

Brody JE: A fairly common bone disease that many sufferers may not recognize. The New York Times, October 2, 1991, p B9.
Points out the significant prevalence of Paget's disease and the role of increased alkaline phosphatase in its diagnosis.

Dalal BI, Nyokong AM: Hyperthrombocytosis: A clinicohematological study. Lab Med 23:811, 1992.
Discusses the differential diagnosis of an increased blood platelet count.

Delmas PD, Meunier PJ: The management of Paget's disease of bone. N Engl J Med 336:558, 1997.
Reviews Paget's disease of bone and discusses biochemical markers, including alkaline phosphatase.

Galasso PJ, Litin SC, O'Brien JF: The macroenzymes: A clinical review. Mayo Clin Proc 68:349, 1993.
Suspect macroenzymes when an isolated persistent serum enzyme elevation occurs in the absence of symptoms or when the symptoms are atypical for that level of serum enzyme.

Gambino SR: The misuse of predictive value: Or why you must consider the odds. Lab Report Physicians 11:65, 1989.
Describes different techniques for clarifying an unexplained abnormal test result. The likelihood of disease varies with the degree of abnormality.

Gambrell RC, Blount BW: Exercise-induced hematuria. Am Fam Physician 53:905, 1996.
Patients with exercise-induced hematuria can be reassured that the condition is benign and that they can return to full activity.

Helfgott SM, Karlson E, Beckman E: Misinterpretation of serum transaminase elevation in "occult" myositis. Am J Med 95:447, 1993.
Consider myositis in patients with increased serum transaminase and lactate dehydrogenase levels. An increased creatine kinase level suggests myositis.

Hutchinson RG, Barksdale B, Watson RI: The effects of exercise on serum potassium levels. Chest 101:398, 1992.
A significant number of individuals show increases of 0.3 mEq/L (0.3 mmol/L) or more after exercise.

Katkov WN, Friedman LS, Cody H, et al: Elevated serum alanine aminotransferase levels in blood donors: The contribution of hepatitis C virus. Ann Intern Med 115:882, 1991.
Discusses differential diagnosis for an elevated serum alanine aminotransferase in healthy blood donors.

Kundrotas LW, Clement DJ: Serum alanine aminotransferase elevation in asymptomatic U.S. Air Force basic trainee blood donors. Digest Dis Sci 38:2145, 1993.
A slight isolated increase in serum alanine aminotransferase (ALT) in a healthy

individual is of limited significance. A thorough work-up is indicated only in individuals having two ALT elevations separated by a period of time.

Lieberman D, Phillips D: "Isolated" elevation of alkaline phosphatase: Significance in hospitalized patients. J Clin Gastroenterol 12:415, 1990.
Recommends a work-up for an isolated high serum alkaline phosphatase test result and discusses possible causes.

Miles MP, Schneider CM: Creatine kinase isoenzyme MB may be elevated in healthy young women after submaximal eccentric exercise. J Lab Clin Med 122:197, 1993.
Healthy women can show a substantial increase in serum creatine kinase-MB after stressful exercise.

Nosaka K, Clarkson PM, Apple FS: Time course of serum protein changes after strenuous exercise of the forearm flexors. J Lab Clin Med 119:183, 1992.
Heavy exercise can cause elevations of serum creatine kinase, lactate dehydrogenase, aspartate aminotransferase, alanine aminotransferase, and myoglobin.

Rang M: The Ulysses syndrome. Can Med Assoc J 106:122, 1972.
Coined the term Ulysses syndrome to describe the state of a healthy person with a false-positive test result.

Shulkin DJ, DeTore AW: When laboratory tests are abnormal and the patient feels fine. Hosp Pract 25:85, 1990.
Points out that slightly abnormal results on routine biochemical screens often indicate a problem with the test results, not with the patient.

Siraganian PA, Mulvihill JJ, Mulivor RA, et al: Benign familial hyperphosphatasemia. JAMA 261:1310, 1989.
Describes the increased serum alkaline phosphatase in benign familial hyperphosphatasemia.

Yücel D, Dalva K: Effect of in vitro hemolysis on 25 common biochemical tests. Clin Chem 38:575, 1992.
Even slight hemolysis results in substantial changes in serum lactate dehydrogenase, potassium, acid phosphatase, and prostatic acid phosphatase.

Zaman Z, Van Orshoven A, Mariën G, et al: Simultaneous macroamylasemia and macrolipasemia. Clin Chem 40:939, 1994.
Describes the first case of simultaneous serum macroamylasemia and macrolipasemia.

• •

PREGNANCY TESTING

Recommendations for pregnancy testing are from the medical literature.

1. Perform a urine or serum pregnancy test to screen for or to confirm the diagnosis of pregnancy. Perform a serum pregnancy test if the earliest possible detection of pregnancy is important, if an ectopic pregnancy is suspected, or if there is any question about the validity of a previous urine pregnancy test. Serial quantitative serum human chorionic gonadotropin (hCG) determinations are useful to diagnose ectopic pregnancy.

Selective screening for pregnancy is appropriate when a woman is contemplating the performance of a procedure that is potentially harmful to the fetus (e.g., having a radiographic study or ingesting a potentially teratogenic drug). Even if the pregnancy test is negative, many women may benefit from routine assessment of prenatal risk factors.

Modern pregnancy tests for serum or urinary hCG are very sensitive and specific. Keep several points in mind: (1) use serum or a concentrated first-morning urinary specimen collected in a clean, dry container; (2) carefully label the specimen; (3) choose a method that incorporates controls; (4) meticulously follow the directions; and (5) perform the test promptly.

2. Evaluate the tests.

Important differences exist between urine and serum tests for hCG. Obtaining accurate and precise serum hCG assays is necessary for the diagnosis of ectopic pregnancy.

Urine Pregnancy Test

Most current methods use monoclonal antibody to hCG. Urine pregnancy tests are qualitative—the results are either positive or negative. The most sensitive methods give positive results at or before the time of the first missed menstrual period (hCG level, 20 to 50 mIU/mL [20–50 IU/L]), and most methods give positive results within 2 to 3 weeks after the first missed period. Blood, protein, or detergents in the urine can interfere with the test.

Serum Pregnancy Test

Most current methods use monoclonal antibody to hCG. Serum pregnancy tests may be either qualitative or quantitative. Serum hCG becomes detectable within 24 hours after implantation and increases progressively. Higher-than-expected levels are found with multiple pregnancies, polyhydramnios, eclampsia, and erythroblastosis fetalis.

SERUM hCG LEVELS

Weeks of Gestation	Level
<1	5–50 mIU/mL (5–50 IU/L)
2	50–500 mIU/mL (50–500 IU/L)
3	100–10,000 mIU/mL (100–10,000 IU/L)
4	1,000–30,000 mIU/mL (1000–30,000 IU/L)
5	3,500–115,000 mIU/mL (3500–115,000 IU/L)
6–8	12,000–270,000 mIU/mL (12,000–270,000 IU/L)
12	15,000–220,000 mIU/mL (15,000–220,000 IU/L)

Source: Tietz NW (ed): Clinical Guide to Laboratory Tests, 3rd ed. Philadelphia, WB Saunders Company, 1995, p 134.

Serum hCG can be increased in the following conditions:

• Normal pregnancy
• Ectopic pregnancy
• Abortion

- Gestational trophoblastic tumors: hydatidiform mole and chorio-carcinoma
- Testicular tumors, germinal cell origin: choriocarcinoma, embryonal carcinoma with syncytiotrophoblastic giant cells, and seminoma with syncytiotrophoblastic giant cells
- Other tumors: breast, ovarian, pancreatic, cervical, gastric, and hepatic cancers

Ectopic Pregnancy

Between 1970 and 1980 the rate of diagnosis of ectopic pregnancies increased from 4.5 to 16.8 ectopic pregnancies per 1000 pregnancies. In 1989, an estimated 88,400 ectopic pregnancies were diagnosed in the United States. Three diagnostic techniques have helped: high-resolution ultrasonography, laparoscopy, and serum quantitative hCG assays. Currently available assays are more than 99% sensitive for detecting the presence of a pregnancy. Suspect ectopic pregnancy if serum hCG fails to increase to values seen in a normal pregnancy and if the rate of increase is less than that of a normal pregnancy. A normal intrauterine pregnancy should have at least a 66% increase of serum hCG over a 48-hour observation period. A lower rate of increase indicates an ectopic pregnancy or an intrauterine pregnancy destined to abort in approximately 85% of cases, whereas a significantly higher rate of increase may indicate a multiple pregnancy. Accurate and precise quantitative measurements of serum hCG are essential to assess the rate of increase. A high hCG peritoneal fluid:serum ratio may be helpful to diagnose ectopic pregnancy (mean ratio for ectopic pregnancy was 19.1, compared with 1.15 for patients with intrauterine pregnancy).

A single serum progesterone level can be used to diagnose early pregnancy failure and the short- and long-term prognosis of viability in threatened abortion. A progesterone level of 25 ng/mL ($\geq$79.5 nmol/L) or more excludes ectopic pregnancy (97.5% sensitivity), and a level of 5 ng/mL ($\leq$15.9 nmol/L) or less allows diagnostic uterine evacuation to be performed when ectopic pregnancy cannot be otherwise distinguished from a nonviable spontaneous intrauterine abortion. With values between 5 and 25 ng/mL (15.9 and 79.5 nmol/L), viability must be established by ultrasonography.

3. Remember that either false-positive or false-negative results can occur.

Modern pregnancy tests have pitfalls that may cause false-positive or false-negative results. They include mislabeled specimens, using dilute urine, dirty containers, deterioration of specimens kept at room temperature, outdated reagents, failure to follow directions, and subjective bias when a woman performs a test on her own urine. See the Introduction of this book for a table that gives the relationships for predictive value, sensitivity, specificity, and prevalence for pregnancy testing.

4. In pregnant women, the following blood test results may be increased:

- **Leukocytes** during late pregnancy and labor. Myelocytes may be found in the peripheral blood in pregnancy.
- **Platelets** with increased risk of first trimester abortion
- **Chloride** caused by decreased bicarbonate secondary to respiratory alkalosis, which is especially prominent during labor
- **Erythrocyte sedimentation rate** from the third month to 3 weeks postpartum because of increased fibrinogen
- **Glucose** from glucose intolerance caused by ovarian and placental hormones
- **Creatine kinase** during the last few weeks that remains high during parturition and becomes normal 5 days postpartum. Earlier, it may be a marker for tubal pregnancy.
- **Lactate dehydrogenase**
- **Alkaline phosphatase** from the placenta. First appears in second trimester, increases in third trimester, and disappears 4 weeks postpartum.
- **Cholesterol,** probably related to increased hepatic synthesis
- **Erythropoietin** in pregnant women with iron deficiency anemia

5. In pregnant women, the following blood test results may be decreased:

- **Hemoglobin and hematocrit** related to increased plasma volume that can be aggravated by iron deficiency anemia
- **Platelets** with good outcomes as long as counts are greater than $50 \times 10^3/\mu L$ ($>50 \times 10^9/L$)
- **Bicarbonate** caused by respiratory alkalosis
- **Calcium** related to insufficient ingestion of calcium, phosphorus, and vitamin D
- **Partial pressure of carbon dioxide** from respiratory alkalosis caused by increasing enlargement of the uterus and a stimulating effect on respiration by pregnancy hormones
- **Urea nitrogen** because of expanded intravascular space and increased glomerular filtration rate: a decreased urea nitrogen:creatinine ratio ($<10:1$)
- **Creatinine:** a creatinine level of 1.2 mg/dL (106 μmol/L) or greater in pregnancy represents an increased level
- **Sodium** caused by expanded intravascular space
- **Phosphorus,** slight, with no significant implications
- **Creatine kinase** during 8th to 20th week, with minimal value at 12th week
- **Aspartate aminotransferase** caused by decreased pyridoxine levels during pregnancy
- **Albumin** caused by expanded intravascular space

BIBLIOGRAPHY

Abramov Y, Abramov D, Abrahamov A, et al: Elevation of serum creatine phosphokinase and its MB isoenzyme during normal labor and early puerperium. Acta Obstet Gynecol Scand 75:255, 1996.
Recognizing the elevations of creatine kinase (CK) and CK-MB in normal vaginal delivery should prevent the erroneous diagnosis of myocardial ischemia without other evidence to support this diagnosis.

Al-Sebai MAH, Kingsland CR, Diver M, et al: The role of a single progesterone measurement in the diagnosis of early pregnancy failure and the prognosis of fetal viability. Br J Obstet Gynaecol 102:364, 1995.
A single serum progesterone level provides an immediate diagnosis of early pregnancy failure and the short- and long-term prognosis of viability in threatened abortion.

Anteby E, Shalev O: Clinical relevance of gestational thrombocytopenia of <100,000/μL. Am J Hematol 47:118, 1994.
Gestational thrombocytopenia can be conservatively managed as long as the platelet counts are greater than $50 \times 10^3/μL$ ($>50 \times 10^9/L$).

Bakerman S: ABC's of Interpretive Laboratory Data, 2nd ed. Greenville, NC, Interpretive Laboratory Data, 1984, p 239.
Summarizes conditions in which hCG is increased.

Barnhart K, Mennuti MT, Benjamin I, et al: Prompt diagnosis of ectopic pregnancy in an emergency department setting. Obstet Gynecol 84:1010, 1994.
Quantitative hCG measurements are useful for diagnosing ectopic pregnancy with transvaginal ultrasonography for all patients with hCG levels greater than 1500 mIU/mL (>1500 IU/L).

Beressi AH, Tefferi A, Silverstein MN, et al: Outcome analysis of 34 pregnancies in women with essential thrombocythemia. Arch Intern Med 155:1217, 1995.
Women with essential thrombocythemia have an increased risk of first-trimester abortion.

Berkowitz RS, Goldstein DP: Chorionic tumors. N Engl J Med 335:1740, 1996.
Reviews gestational trophoblastic tumors.

Bluestein D: Monoclonal antibody pregnancy tests. Am Fam Physician 38:197, 1988.
Discusses the advantages of using a monoclonal antibody to hCG.

Carson SA, Buster JE: Ectopic pregnancy. N Engl J Med 329:1174, 1993.
Reviews the use of serum progesterone and β-hCG measurements in the diagnosis of ectopic pregnancy. Discusses decision levels for a single progesterone level.

Chandra L, Jain A: Maternal serum creatine kinase as a biochemical marker of tubal pregnancy. Int J Gynaecol Obstet 49:21, 1995.
An elevated creatine kinase level may be an important test for diagnosing tubal pregnancy.

Copplestone JA: Asymptomatic thrombocytopenia developing during pregnancy (gestational thrombocytopenia)—a clinical study. Q J Med 84:593, 1992.
The lower limit of normal of the platelet count in pregnancy should be $120 \times 10^3/μL$ ($120 \times 10^9/L$).

Daily CA, Laurent SL, Nunley WC: The prognostic value of serum progesterone and quantitative β-human chorionic gonadotropin in early human pregnancy. Am J Obstet Gynecol 171:380, 1994.
Serum progesterone in early pregnancy predicts outcome.

Fields SA, Toffler WL: Pregnancy testing: Home and office. West J Med 154:327, 1991.
Highlights the advantages and pitfalls of modern pregnancy tests.

Gronlund B, Marushak A: Serial human chorionic gonadotropin determination in the diagnosis of ectopic pregnancy. Aust NZ Obstet Gynaecol 33:312, 1993.
A discrimination limit of hCG increasing 980 mIU/mL (980 IU/L) in 2 days provided a predictive value for ectopic pregnancy of 90% when below this value.

Hellemans P, Gerris J, Joostens M, et al: Serum hCG decline following salpingotomy or salpingectomy for extrauterine pregnancy. Eur J Obstet Gynecol Reprod Biol 53:59, 1994.
Monitoring the decline in serum hCG values is useful in following women treated for ectopic pregnancy.

Jack BW, Campanile C, McQuade W, et al: The negative pregnancy test: An opportunity for preconception care. Arch Fam Med 4:340, 1995.
Negative pregnancy tests: A time to evaluate prenatal risk.

Lavie O, Beller U, Neuman M, et al: Maternal serum creatine kinase: A possible predictor of tubal pregnancy. Am J Obstet Gynecol 169:1149, 1993.
A high serum creatine kinase level may occur in tubal pregnancy.

Leiserowitz GS, Evans AT, Samuels SJ, et al: Creatine kinase and its MB isoenzyme in the third trimester and the peripartum period. J Reprod Med 37:910, 1992.
Be careful about the use of elevated serum creatine kinase and its MB isoenzyme to evaluate myocardial ischemia during the peripartum period.

Maccato M, Estrada R, Faro S: Ectopic pregnancy with undetectable serum and urine β-hCG and the detection of β-hCG in the ectopic trophoblast by immunocytochemical evaluation. Obstet Gynecol 81:878, 1993.
Ectopic pregnancy may occur with undetectable β-hCG levels.

Oettinger M, Odeh M, Tarazova L, et al: β-HCG concentration in peritoneal fluid and serum in ectopic and intrauterine pregnancy. Acta Obstet Gynecol Scand 74:212, 1995.
The mean peritoneal fluid:serum ratio for patients with ectopic pregnancy was 19.1, compared with 1.15 for patients with intrauterine pregnancy.

Ory SJ: New options for diagnosis and treatment of ectopic pregnancy. JAMA 267:534, 1992.
Mayo Clinic recommendations for the diagnosis of ectopic pregnancy using serum hCG concentrations and other techniques.

Riikonen S, Saijonmaa O, Järvenpää AL, et al: Serum concentrations of erythropoietin in healthy and anemic pregnant women. Scand J Clin Lab Invest 54:653, 1994.
Discusses elevated serum concentrations of erythropoietin in pregnancy.

Rodriguez GC, Hughes CL, Soper JT, et al: Serum progesterone for the exclusion of early pregnancy in women at risk for recurrent gestational trophoblastic neoplasia. Obstet Gynecol 84:794, 1994.
Serum progesterone differentiates early pregnancy from recurrent trophoblastic disease.

Satin AJ, Hankins GDV, Patterson WR, et al: Creatine kinase and creatine kinase isoenzymes as a marker of uterine activity. Am J Perinatol 9:456, 1992.
Serum creatine kinase cannot be used to assess myocardial damage during labor. An early rise in creatine kinase may signal the onset of spontaneous labor that does not require oxytocin augmentation.

Stewart BK, Nazar-Stewart V, Toivola B: Biochemical discrimination of pathologic pregnancy from early, normal intrauterine gestation in symptomatic patients. Am J Clin Pathol 103:386, 1995.
A low rate of change of the β-hCG level and a progesterone level less than 8 ng/mL (<25.4 mmol/L) are suggestive of ectopic pregnancy.

PAP TEST AND CERVICAL CANCER

Recommendations for the Papanicolaou (Pap) test to detect cervical cancer are from the American Cancer Society and are similar to those of other groups such as the College of American Pathologists, the American College of Obstetricians and Gynecologists (ACOG), the American Medical Association, the National Cancer Institute, the U.S. Preventive Services Task Force, and the Canadian Task Force on the Periodic Health Examination.

1. Use an annual Pap test and pelvic examination to screen for cervical cancer in all women 18 years of age and older. After three or more consecutive satisfactory examinations with normal findings, the Pap test may be performed less frequently. The patient should discuss the matter with her physician. According to ACOG, more

frequent Pap tests may be required when one or more of the following high-risk factors is present.

- Women who have had multiple sexual partners or whose male sexual partners have had multiple partners
- Women who began sexual intercourse at an early age
- Women whose male sexual partners have had other sexual partners with cervical cancer
- Women with current or prior human papillomavirus infection or condylomata or both
- Women with current or prior herpes simplex virus infections
- Women who are infected with HIV
- Women with a history of other sexually transmitted diseases
- Women who are immunosuppressed (such as those who have received renal transplants)
- Smokers and abusers of other substances, including alcohol
- Women who have a history of cervical dysplasia or cervical cancer or endometrial, vaginal, or vulvar cancer
- Women of lower socioeconomic status (a surrogate for other closely related risk factors)

In 1995, 15,800 women developed cervical cancer in the United States, and approximately 4800 died of the disease. Worldwide, cervical cancer kills more than half a million women each year. Cervical cancer screening can reduce the incidence and mortality rate by up to 90%.

Poor technique is a significant cause of false-negative Pap tests. Common causes of poor tests are (1) using a thick smear from an abundance of red blood cells or inflammatory cells; (2) poor fixation, often caused by air drying the smear before fixation; (3) a scarcity of cells, caused by wiping the cervix before obtaining the smear; (4) an absence of endocervical cells, which results from failure to obtain an endocervical sample. The recently approved ThinPrep Pap Test (Cytyc Corporation) may decrease the number of errors currently associated with the Pap smear.

The reported sensitivity of the Pap test for cervical cancer and precancerous lesions is as low as 70% and may not be much above 95% even under the most ideal conditions.

2. Consider testing for human papillomavirus (HPV) in cervical smear and biopsy specimens as tests become available. On the basis of currently available information, women with cervical abnormalities should receive evaluation, treatment, and follow-up using current Pap test and biopsy technology for these abnormalities. HPV typing may be useful in patient management when Pap test results indicate atypical squamous cells of undetermined significance (ASCUS) or low-grade squamous intraepithelial lesions (LSIL).

HPV is the fastest growing sexually transmitted disease in the United States—up to one in three Americans is affected. The Hybrid

Capture System (Digene Corporation) is a method to identify HPV DNA in Pap test samples. A suggested approach is to use PreservCyt of the ThinPrep Pap Test (Cytyc Corporation) to collect the sample. The Pap test is then interpreted in the traditional manner. If the result is ASCUS or LSIL, the laboratory performs a reflexive HPV test from the sediment of the remaining original PreservCyt solution.

3. Request cervical cytologic reports that evaluate the Pap test in terms of diagnostic implications rather than arcane numerical systems.

The "Bethesda system," developed in 1988 at a National Cancer Institute–sponsored workshop in Bethesda, Maryland, is the recommended format for reporting cervical and vaginal cytologic diagnoses. The report includes three elements: (1) a statement of the adequacy of the specimen; (2) a general categorization of whether the findings are normal or not; and (3) a descriptive diagnosis of the infection and/or neoplastic process.

THE 1991 BETHESDA SYSTEM

Adequacy of the specimen	• Satisfactory for evaluation • Satisfactory for evaluation but limited by . . . (specify reason) • Unsatisfactory for evaluation . . . (specify reason)
General categorization (optional)	• Within normal limits • Benign cellular changes: See descriptive diagnoses • Epithelial cell abnormalities: See descriptive diagnoses

Descriptive diagnoses	• Benign cellular changes
	• Infection:
	  (1) *Trichomonas vaginalis*
	  (2) Fungal organisms morphologically consistent with *Candida* species
	  (3) Predominance of coccobacilli consistent with shift in vaginal flora
	  (4) Bacteria morphologically consistent with *Actinomyces* species
	  (5) Cellular changes associated with herpes simplex virus
	  (6) Other

Reactive changes	• Reactive cellular changes associated with:
	  (1) Inflammation (includes typical repair)
	  (2) Atrophy with inflammation ("atrophic vaginitis")
	  (3) Radiation
	  (4) Intrauterine contraceptive device
	  (5) Other

Table continued on following page

THE 1991 BETHESDA SYSTEM *Continued*

Epithelial cell abnormalities	• Squamous cell:
	  (1) Atypical squamous cells of undetermined significance: Qualify[2]
	  (2) Low-grade squamous intraepithelial lesion encompassing HPV,[1] mild dysplasia/CIN 1
	  (3) High-grade squamous intraepithelial lesion encompassing moderate and severe dysplasia, CIS/CIN 2 and CIN 3
	  (4) Squamous cell carcinoma
	• Glandular cell:
	  (1) Endometrial cells, cytologically benign, in a postmenopausal woman
	  (2) Atypical glandular cells of undetermined significance: Qualify[2]
	  (3) Endocervical adenocarcinoma
	  (4) Endometrial adenocarcinoma
	  (5) Extrauterine adenocarcinoma
	  (6) Adenocarcinoma, NOS

Other malignant neoplasms	• Specify
Hormonal evaluation (applies to vaginal smears only)	(1) Hormonal pattern compatible with age and history (2) Hormonal pattern incompatible with age and history: Specify (3) Hormonal evaluation not possible due to: Specify

HPV = human papillomavirus; CIN = cervical intraepithelial neoplasia; CIS = carcinoma in situ; and NOS = non–organ specific.

[1]Cellular changes of HPV previously termed koilocytosis, koilocytotic atypia, or condylomatous atypia are included in the category of low-grade squamous intraepithelial lesion.

[2]Atypical squamous or glandular cells of undetermined significance should be further qualified, if possible, as to whether a reactive or a premalignant/ malignant process is favored.

Source: Kurman RJ, Henson DE, Herbst AL, et al: Interim guidelines for management of abnormal cervical cytology. JAMA 271:1866–1869, 1994. Copyright 1994, American Medical Association.

4. Evaluate every significantly abnormal result. A single negative report on a repeat test does not eliminate the need for a thorough diagnostic evaluation.

A significantly abnormal result means atypia or worse, including inflammatory atypia. The diagnostic evaluation may include treatment of an inflammatory condition, visual inspection, colposcopically directed biopsy, endocervical curettage, and, when indicated, cervical conization. Inflammatory change may be a clue to important disorders, including sexually transmitted diseases, especially in women less than 25 years of age.

5. If the cervical cytologic report is normal, repeat cervical cytologic screening annually. After therapy for preinvasive and invasive cancer, repeat screening every 3 months for 2 years and then every 6 months.

Women who have had cervical cancer require more frequent testing. The recently approved PAPNET (Neuromedical Systems, Inc.) test is an automated examination that may be performed after conventional screening as a quality assurance measure to make certain that no abnormal cells have been missed.

6. In patients who have had a hysterectomy for benign conditions, screen every 10 years. For women with abnormal cytology, screen within 3 years of hysterectomy and every 5 years thereafter.

7. In patients with cervical cancer, the following blood test results may be increased:

- **Platelets** related to the cancer
- **Lactate dehydrogenase** related to the cancer
- **Carcinoembryonic antigen** related to the cancer
- **Alkaline phosphatase.** As a group, cancers of the ovary, endometrium, cervix, and breast exhibit the highest frequency of the Regan alkaline phosphatase isoenzyme.

BIBLIOGRAPHY

American College of Obstetricians and Gynecologists: Recommendations on frequency of Pap test screening. Washington, DC, ACOG Committee Opinion, No 152, March 1995.
  ACOG guidelines for the Pap test.
Anderson GH, Benedet JL, Le Riche JC, et al: Invasive cancer of the cervix in British Columbia: A review of the demography and screening histories of 437 cases seen from 1985–1988. Obstet Gynecol 80:1, 1992.
  Reminds us that some women—especially members of indigent and minority populations—are not being screened and that false-negative test results still occur.
Austin RM, McLendon WW: The Papanicolaou smear: Medicine's most successful cancer screening procedure is threatened. JAMA 277:754, 1997.
  Litigation, low reimbursement, and automation are threatening the availability of the traditional Pap test.
Bauer HM, Ting Y, Greer CE, et al: Genital human papillomavirus infection in female university students as determined by a PCR-based method. JAMA 265:472, 1991.
  HPV infection is very common in university students, as determined by PCR-based assays.
Bertolino JG, Rangel JE, Blake RL Jr, et al: Inflammation on the cervical Papanicolaou smear: The predictive value for infection in asymptomatic women. Fam Med 24:447, 1992.
  Inflammation on a Pap test is not a reliable predictor of significant vaginal pathogens in asymptomatic women.
Brody JE: New guidelines and techniques help to increase the reliability of the Pap smear. The New York Times, November 6, 1996, p B9.
  PAPNET is a computer-based Pap test system that has been approved by the Food and Drug Administration to screen smears deemed "normal" by cytology technicians.
Brotzman GL, Julian TM: The minimally abnormal Papanicolaou smear. Am Fam Physician 53:1154, 1996.

New guidelines suggest a conservative and expectant approach for these mild abnormalities.

Campion MJ, Greenberg MD, Turner F: New horizons in cervical cancer screening. Symposium excerpts of the 1996 Annual Clinical Meeting of the American College of Obstetrics and Gynecology, May 1, 1996, Denver, CO.
Suggests a strategy for reflex HPV testing in patients with ASCUS and LSIL.

Cannistra SA, Niloff JM: Cancer of the uterine cervix. N Engl J Med 334:1030, 1995.
Reviews the pathophysiology, detection, and management of cervical cancer.

Carter PM, Coburn TC, Luszczak M: Cost-effectiveness of cervical cytologic examination during pregnancy. J Am Board Fam Pract 6:537, 1993.
Recommends eliminating routine prenatal Pap testing in women who have had a normal smear within the past 2 to 3 years.

Cates W Jr, Hinman AR: Sexually transmitted disease in the 1990's. N Engl J Med 325:1368, 1991.
Centers for Disease Control experts estimate that up to one in three Americans have HPV.

Crum CP, Newkirk GR: Abnormal Pap smears, cancer risk, and HPV. Patient Care 29:35, 1995.
Discusses the relevance of HPV to abnormal Pap tests and cervical cancer.

Cuzick J, Terry G, Ho L, et al: Human papillomavirus type 16 DNA in cervical smears as predictor of high-grade cervical cancer. Lancet 339:959, 1992.
Suggests clinical indications for use of HPV testing.

Eddy DM: Screening for cervical cancer. Ann Intern Med 113:214, 1990.
Excellent review of the data that support the use of Pap tests to diagnose cervical cancer.

Fetters MD, Fischer G, Reed BD: Effectiveness of vaginal Papanicolaou smear screening after total hysterectomy for benign disease. JAMA 275:940, 1996.
Routine screening is not indicated.

Fontaine PL: Pap smears: Controversies and challenges in interpreting abnormal results. Consultant 36:1976, 1996.
Cost-effective management of low-grade abnormalities is particularly challenging.

Gambino SR, Krieger P: False-negative fractions in cytology screening. Lab Report Physicians 10:61, 1988.

Gambino SR: The imperfect Pap test. Lab Report Physicians 17:16, 1995.
Estimates the sensitivity of a Pap test at 70 to 95%. No one has yet been able to reduce the false-negative fraction below 5%.

Hayward RSA, Steinberg EP, Ford DE, et al: Preventive care guidelines: 1991. Ann Intern Med 114:758, 1991.
Authoritative recommendations for the use of the Pap test to screen for cervical cancer.

Hernandez E, Lavine M, Dunton CJ, et al: Poor prognosis associated with thrombocytosis in patients with cervical cancer. Cancer 69:2975, 1992.
Thrombocytosis indicates poor prognosis in cervical cancer.

King A, Clay K, Felmar E, et al: The Papanicolaou smear. West J Med 156:202, 1992.
Good summary of recommendations by the American Cancer Society California Division's Ad Hoc Committee on Cervical Cancer.

Lopes A, Daras V, Cross PA, et al: Thrombocytosis as a prognostic factor in women with cervical cancer. Cancer 74:90, 1994.
In patients with cervical cancer, thrombocytosis is associated with a poorer survival rate.

Mandelblatt J: Papanicolaou testing following hysterectomy. JAMA 266:1289, 1991.
Recommendations for the Pap test in a not uncommon situation.

Mayeaux EJ Jr, Harper MB, Abreo F, et al: A comparison of the reliability of repeat cervical smears and colposcopy in patients with abnormal cervical cytology. J Fam Pract 40:57, 1995.
Repeat Pap tests are inadequate for following women with previously abnormal smears.

Miller KE, Losh DP, Folley A: Evaluation and follow-up of abnormal Pap smears. Am Fam Physician 45:143, 1992.
Practical discussion of the management of patients with abnormal Pap tests.

Piscitelli JT, Bastian LA, Wilkes A, et al: Cytologic screening after hysterectomy for benign disease. Am J Obstet Gynecol 173:424, 1995.

After hysterectomy, screening every 10 years is recommended for women with no previous abnormal cytology and within 3 years and then every 5 years for women with prior abnormalities.

Prasad CJ: Pathobiology of human papillomavirus. Clin Lab Med 15:685, 1995.
Reviews the role of human papillomavirus in the development of cervical cancer.

Shingleton HM, Patrick RL, Johnston WW, et al: The current status of the Papanicolaou smear. CA Cancer J Clin 45:305, 1995.
A scholarly review of the role of the Pap smear in patient care.

Slawson DC, Bennett JH, Herman JM: Follow-up Papanicolaou smear for cervical atypia: Are we missing significant disease? J Fam Pract 36:289, 1993.
Noel ML, Kazal LA Jr, Glenday MC: Papanicolaou smear adequacy: The effect of the sampling sequence. J Am Board Fam Pract 2:103, 1993.
In women with cervical atypia, a negative follow-up Pap test is not enough to rule out disease.

Slawson DC, Bennett JH, Simon LJ, et al: Should all women with cervical atypia be referred for colposcopy: A HARNET study. J Fam Pract 38:387, 1994.
The Pap test is not enough to follow cervical atypia.

Solomon D: The Bethesda System and Its Consequences. New Orleans, LA, American Society of Clinical Pathologists/College of American Pathologists Symposium, September 24, 1991.
Koss LG: The new Bethesda system for reporting results of smears of the uterine cervix. J Natl Cancer Inst 82:988, 1990.
National Cancer Institute Workshop: The 1988 Bethesda system for reporting cervical/vaginal cytologic diagnoses. JAMA 262:931, 1989.
Key articles on the Bethesda system. As late as 1987, 72% of laboratories in one metropolitan area were using an outmoded numerical system for cytology reports.

Stack PS: Pap smears. Postgrad Med 101:297, 1997.
Summarizes the current guidelines for the Pap test and discusses classification systems and interpretation.

Unger ER, Vernon SD, Thoms WW, et al: Human papillomavirus and disease-free survival in FIGO stage Ib cervical cancer. J Infect Dis 172:1184, 1995.
Absence of HPV by in situ hybridization is predictive of disease-free survival.

Wilson JD, Robinson AJ, Kinghorn SA, et al: Implications of inflammatory changes on cervical cytology. BMJ 300:638, 1990.
Inflammatory changes are an important clue to sexually transmitted diseases and other colposcopic abnormalities, especially in women under 25.

SERUM CHOLESTEROL AND CORONARY HEART DISEASE

Recommendations for cholesterol screening are from the National Cholesterol Education Program, the American Heart Association, the American Society of Clinical Pathologists, and the College of American Pathologists. The American College of Physicians and the U.S. Preventive Services Task Force disagree and recommend screening men age 35 to 65 and women age 45 to 65. Kaiser Permanente recommends screening once at age 20, at 45 and older for men, and at 55 and older for women.

1. In screening programs, consider measuring serum total cholesterol at least once every 5 years in all adults 20 years of age and over. If the individual visits a physician, measure serum total cholesterol and HDL cholesterol in the context of an assessment of other CHD risk factors. Consider measuring serum total cholesterol in children who have a strong family history of high cholesterol or CHD. Do not screen patients who are acutely ill or pregnant, and do

not use serum apolipoprotein studies or lipoprotein electrophoresis for general screening.

Most authorities recommend wellness screening for hypercholesterolemia using serum total cholesterol values. CHD causes more than 500,000 deaths in the United States each year, and because up to 80% of the population may have high serum total cholesterol levels, screening is worthwhile. Each 1% reduction in serum total cholesterol reduces the CHD rate by approximately 2%. Many authorities believe that the serum total cholesterol:HDL cholesterol ratio is better than total cholesterol to estimate risk of CHD. The risk of CHD decreases by 2 to 3% for each increase of 1 mg/dL (0.026 mmol/L) of HDL cholesterol.

Apolipoprotein A (Apo A) is associated with HDL cholesterol and apolipoprotein B (Apo B) with low-density lipoprotein (LDL) cholesterol. Thus, the ratio of Apo A1:Apo B has been proposed as a highly predictive measure of risk for CHD. However, at this time, good assays are not widely available, and these measurements are not recommended for general clinical use.

Use either serum or plasma; plasma values are about 3% lower. Draw blood in patients who have been sitting for at least 5 minutes, using a tourniquet for as brief a period as possible. Serum cholesterol is quite stable at room temperature, but if delays in testing are anticipated, the specimen should be refrigerated.

The serum total cholesterol concentration is not significantly increased after a meal; therefore, the screening specimen may be drawn any time the patient is seen. Because cholesterol values may be affected by an acute medical or surgical illness, do not screen acutely ill patients; evaluate only individuals who are ambulatory, in their usual state of health, on their normal diet, and not pregnant. In the first 24 hours after acute myocardial infarction the serum cholesterol concentration reflects preinfarction levels; after that time, the cholesterol levels may be lower than usual for as long as 12 weeks.

Childhood cholesterol screening is controversial. Some propose that all children be screened for high cholesterol values, whereas others suggest that the risk:benefit ratio of childhood cholesterol screening is unfavorable and that children should not be screened. At this time it seems prudent to screen selectively, based on a family history of high cholesterol or premature CHD.

2. Evaluate the test results.

RECOMMENDATIONS FOR CLASSIFICATION OF ADULTS

Serum Total Cholesterol

Desirable blood cholesterol	<200 mg/dL (<5.2 mmol/L)
Borderline-high blood cholesterol	200–239 mg/dL (5.2–6.18 mmol/L)
High blood cholesterol	≥240 mg/dL (≥6.21 mmol/L)

RECOMMENDATIONS FOR CLASSIFICATION OF ADULTS *Continued*

Serum HDL Cholesterol

Desirable HDL cholesterol	≥35 mg/dL (≥0.91 mmol/L)
Desirable total cholesterol/HDL cholesterol ratio	≤4.5:1*

*A ratio <3 = the lowest risk; a ratio ≥9 = the highest risk.

Source: Adapted from National Cholesterol Education Program: Detection, evaluation, and treatment of high blood cholesterol in adults (Adult Treatment Panel II). Circulation 89:1329–1445, 1994. Reproduced with permission of Circulation, American Heart Association, 1994.

RECOMMENDATIONS FOR CLASSIFICATION OF CHILDREN AND ADOLESCENTS

Serum Total Cholesterol

Desirable blood cholesterol	<170 mg/dL (<4.42 mmol/L)
Borderline-high blood cholesterol	170–199 mg/dL (4.42–5.17 mmol/L)
High blood cholesterol	≥200 mg/dL (≥5.2 mmol/L)

Source: Adapted from Benuck I, Gidding SS, Donovan M: Year-to-year variability of cholesterol levels in a pediatric practice. Arch Pediatr Adolesc Med 149:292–296, 1995. Copyright 1995, American Medical Association.

To use these reference ranges properly, your laboratory's results must be accurate, that is, appropriately standardized through one of the National Network Laboratories of the Centers for Disease Control and Prevention.

In public screening programs, all individuals with a serum cholesterol concentration of 200 mg/dL (5.2 mmol/L) or greater should be referred to their physician for remeasurement and evaluation. Remember that all serum cholesterol values should be confirmed by repeat measurements, with the average used to guide clinical decisions. Baseline lipid values are best determined by averaging two or three measurements, 1 to 8 weeks apart. If the initial serum cholesterol concentration is 200 mg/dL (5.2 mmol/L) or greater, the individual should return in 1 to 8 weeks for confirmation. If the confirmation value is within 30 mg/dL (0.8 mmol/L) of the first test result, use the average of the two results to guide subsequent decisions. If the second value differs from the first by more than 30 mg/dL (0.8 mmol/L), obtain a third test within 1 to 8 weeks and average the three values.

A low serum cholesterol concentration may be a sign of good health, proper diet, and appropriate exercise. On the other hand, it may signal disease because the following disorders can be associated with low cholesterol values: acquired immunodeficiency, severe liver damage, hyperthyroidism, malnutrition, chronic anemia, cerebral hemorrhage, and malignancy. Drugs are an additional cause of hypocholesterolemia. Nursing home residents and patients in acute care hospitals who have serum cholesterol concentrations less than 120 mg/dL (<3.10 mmol/L) are at increased risk of premature death. Moreover, the development of hypocholesterolemia after admission to the hospital may be a unique marker for poor prognosis in older hospitalized patients. A precipitous decline of more than 45 mg/dL (>1.16 mmol/L) per year or more than 20% per year is a marker for high mortality.

3. If the serum total cholesterol concentration is below 200 mg/dL (5.2 mmol/L), remeasure within 5 years or with subsequent physical examination. In patients with serum total cholesterol of 200 mg/dL (≥5.2 mmol/L) or above or HDL cholesterol of less than 35 mg/dL (<0.9 mmol/L), obtain a fasting (12 to 14 hours) lipoprotein analysis to include measurements of total cholesterol, HDL cholesterol, triglycerides, and an estimate of LDL cholesterol.

Although non-fasting total cholesterol and HDL cholesterol levels are adequate for screening, definitive measurements should be made on fasting samples. The serum cholesterol concentration can vary with age, diet, weight, physical activity, and medications, and it is prudent to remeasure the level periodically.

The cholesterol concentration should be evaluated in the context of the following additional risk factors:

- Male sex
- Family history of premature CHD (definite myocardial infarction or sudden death before 55 years of age in a parent or sibling)
- Cigarette smoking (currently smokes more than 10 cigarettes per day)
- Hypertension; ideally not greater than 130/85 mm Hg
- Low serum HDL cholesterol concentration (<35 mg/dL [<0.91 mmol/L])
- Diabetes mellitus
- History of definite cerebrovascular or occlusive peripheral vascular disease
- Severe obesity (≥30% overweight)

Other risk factors, which have been mentioned in the literature, include the following:

- High serum lipoprotein (a) [Lp(a)], greater than 30 mg/dL (>0.3 g/L)
- High plasma homocysteine, greater than 12 μmol/L. Dietary folate can decrease elevated plasma homocysteine levels.
- High serum C-reactive protein (recently implicated as a risk factor, probably related to the presence of inflammation)
- High serum C3
- High serum ferritin: greater than 200 ng/mL (>200 μg/L)
- High plasma fibrinogen
- High hematocrit

- High serum uric acid
- High blood leukocyte count
- Low serum bilirubin
- Low serum folate
- Low serum iron-binding capacity

It may be appropriate to revise current recommendations for the treatment of hypercholesterolemia to reflect the effects of alternative interventions that decrease overall risk for CHD but are not used specifically to alter blood lipids.

There are a number of causes for a low HDL cholesterol concentration, some of which are reversible: heavy cigarette smoking, obesity, lack of exercise, hypertriglyceridemia, anabolic steroids, progestational agents, antihypertensive agents, and genetic factors (e.g., primary hypoalphalipoproteinemia). If HDL cholesterol is low, try to increase it by managing the above variables.

Light to moderate drinking of alcohol appears to reduce the risk of CHD by increasing the concentrations of two types of HDL cholesterol and possibly by decreasing the concentration of LDL cholesterol. A reduction in the risk of CHD occurred in those who drank more than 5 g but less than 30 g of pure alcohol daily (one drink equals approximately 10 to 15 g of alcohol). All benefits vanish and alcohol can seriously injure the heart when the daily intake exceeds 50 g. Heavy drinking is associated with a higher incidence of cancer and overall mortality. Interestingly, an increased CHD mortality is seen in men with HDL cholesterol greater than 68 mg/dL ($>$1.75 mmol/L), with the greatest effect in heavy drinkers but some effect in light drinkers.

4. In patients with hyperlipidemia, the following blood test result may be increased:

- **Calcium** due to an increase in the calcium bound to lipoproteins

5. In patients with hyperlipidemia, the following blood test result may be decreased:

- **Sodium (artifactual).** Pseudohyponatremia caused by lipemia (when sodium is measured with a flame photometer but not with an ion-specific electrode). The serum osmotic pressure is normal.

6. Evaluate the serum LDL cholesterol and triglycerides. If the serum LDL cholesterol concentration is less than 130 mg/dL ($<$3.4 mmol/L), remeasure within 5 years. If it is 130 to 159 mg/dL (3.4 to 4.1 mmol/L) and fewer than two additional risk factors and no CHD are present, remeasure annually and prescribe a step-1 diet. Provide dietary and risk factor education.

The usual serum cholesterol measurement estimates total cholesterol. In estimating the risk of CHD, it is more informative to estimate the level of LDL cholesterol.

RECOMMENDATION FOR CLASSIFICATION OF ADULTS

Serum LDL Cholesterol*

Desirable LDL cholesterol	<130 mg/dL (<3.4 mmol/L)
Borderline-high LDL cholesterol	130–159 mg/dL (3.4–4.1 mmol/L)
High LDL cholesterol	≥160 mg/dL (≥4.1 mmol/L)

*Two measurements of LDL cholesterol after a 12- to 14-hour fast are made 1 to 8 weeks apart, and the average is used for clinical decisions unless the two values differ by more than 30 mg/dL (0.8 mmol/L), in which case a third test is carried out, and the average of all three is used. If the triglycerides are <400 mg/dL (<4.57 mmol/L), calculate LDL cholesterol as follows (all quantities are in milligrams per deciliter): LDL cholesterol = Total cholesterol − HDL cholesterol − 0.2 × Triglycerides.

Source: Adapted from National Cholesterol Education Program: Detection, evaluation, and treatment of high blood cholesterol in adults (Adult Treatment Panel II). Circulation 89:1329–1445, 1994. Reproduced with permission of Circulation, American Heart Association, 1994.

Remember to evaluate the patient for secondary (and possibly reversible) causes of high LDL cholesterol, which include the following conditions:

- Diabetes mellitus
- Hypothyroidism
- Nephrotic syndrome
- Obstructive liver disease
- Drugs that may raise LDL cholesterol levels or lower HDL cholesterol levels, particularly progestins, anabolic steroids, corticosteroids, and certain antihypertensive agents.

Hypertriglyceridemia is a risk factor for CHD, especially in the presence of other lipid risk factors. For example, individuals with relatively normal serum total cholesterol concentrations but with a low HDL cholesterol value and a high triglyceride value are at increased risk for CHD.

RECOMMENDATION FOR CLASSIFICATION OF ADULTS

Triglycerides

Desirable triglycerides	<200 mg/dL (<2.3 mmol/L)
Borderline-high triglycerides	200–400 mg/dL (2.3–4.5 mmol/L)
High triglycerides	400–1000 mg/dL (4.5–11.3 mmol/L)
Very high triglycerides	≥1000 mg/dL (≥11.3 mmol/L)

Source: National Cholesterol Education Program: Detection, evaluation, and treatment of high blood cholesterol in adults (Adult Treatment Panel II). Circulation 89:1329–1445, 1994. Reproduced with permission of Circulation, American Heart Association, 1994.

Hypertriglyceridemia frequently is associated with obesity, uncontrolled diabetes mellitus, liver disease, alcohol ingestion, uremia, and the use of estrogen-containing contraceptives, steroids, isotretinoin, and some antihypertensive agents. Very high triglyceride values (>1000 mg/dL [>11.3 mmol/L]) are associated with pancreatitis. A common problem with obtaining valid serum triglyceride studies is failure of the patient to observe the 12- to 14-hour fast.

7. If serum LDL cholesterol is 160 mg/dL ($\geq$4.1 mmol/L) or above or if it is 130 to 159 mg/dL (3.4 to 4.1 mmol/L) and the patient has CHD or two or more additional risk factors, the patient should undergo a clinical evaluation and enter a more intensive lipid intervention program.

The following treatment decisions are based on LDL cholesterol levels.

TREATMENT FOR ELEVATED LDL CHOLESTEROL

	Initiation Level	LDL Goal
Dietary therapy		
Without CHD and with fewer than two risk factors	$\geq$160 mg/dL	<160 mg/dL
Without CHD and with two or more risk factors	$\geq$130 mg/dL	<130 mg/dL
With CHD	>100 mg/dL	$\leq$100 mg/dL
	Consideration Level	**LDL Goal**
Drug treatment		
Without CHD and with fewer than two risk factors	$\geq$190 mg/dL[1]	<160 mg/dL
Without CHD and with two or more risk factors	$\geq$160 mg/dL	<130 mg/dL
With CHD	$\geq$130 mg/dL[2]	$\leq$100 mg/dL

[1]In men less than 35 years old and premenopausal women with LDL cholesterol levels of 190 mg/dL to 219 mg/dL, drug therapy should be delayed except in high-risk patients such as those with diabetes.

[2]In patients with CHD and LDL cholesterol levels of 100 mg/dL to 120 mg/dL, the physician should exercise clinical judgment in deciding whether to initiate drug treatment.

Source: National Cholesterol Education Program: Detection, evaluation, and treatment of high blood cholesterol in adults (Adult Treatment Panel II). Circulation 89:1329–1445, 1994. Reproduced with permission of Circulation, American Heart Association, 1994.

The triad of hypercholesterolemia, xanthomas, and a familial incidence is typical of familial hypercholesterolemia. Other familial dyslipidemias should be considered. Because an accurate diagnosis is important for proper therapy, you may wish to refer patients suspected of having familial dyslipidemia to a lipid specialist.

8. After treatment with dietary modification and/or drugs, monitor lipid levels at appropriate intervals.

The effects of selected drugs on lipid values follow:

EFFECTS OF DRUGS ON LIPID VALUES

Drug	Total Cholesterol	LDL Cholesterol	HDL Cholesterol	Triglycerides
Androgens	—	↑	↓	—
Antiepileptics	—	↑	↑	↑
Antihypertensives				
Thiazide diuretics	↑/—	↑	—	↑
Beta blockers	—	—	↓	↑
Alpha blockers	↓/—	↓/—	↑	↓
Corticosteroids	↑	↑	↑	↑
Cyclosporin A	↑	↑	—	—
Cyproterone acetate	↓	↓	—	—
C-19 Progestin	—	↑	↓	—
C-21 Progestin	—	—	↓	—
Oral estrogens	↓	↓	↑	↑
Phenothiazines	↑	—	↓	↑
Retinoids	↑	↑	↓	↑

Source: Adapted from Henkin Y, Como JA, Oberman A: Secondary dyslipidemia: Inadvertent effects of drugs in clinical practice. JAMA 267:961–968, 1992. Copyright 1992, American Medical Association.

It takes at least 4 to 6 weeks before lipid levels respond to dietary and/or drug therapy. If the LDL cholesterol goal is achieved, monitor total cholesterol every 4 months and remeasure LDL cholesterol annually. More frequent monitoring of lipid levels is unnecessary in the absence of changes in dietary and/or drug therapy.

BIBLIOGRAPHY

Avins AL, Browner WS: Lowering risk without lowering cholesterol: Implications for national cholesterol policy. Ann Intern Med 125:502, 1996.
   Alternative interventions not focused on altering blood lipids can decrease risk for CHD.
Benuck I, Gidding SS, Donovan M: Year-to-year variability of cholesterol levels in a pediatric practice. Arch Pediatr Adolesc Med 149:292, 1995.

One third of children with three separate measurements had at least one value of 200 mg/dL (5.2 mmol/L) or greater.

Bolibar I, Kienast J, Thompson SG, et al: Relation of fibrinogen to presence and severity of coronary artery disease is independent of other coexisting heart disease. Am Heart J 125:1601, 1993.
Elevated fibrinogen is risk factor for cardiovascular disease.

Bostom AG, Cupples LA, Jenner JL, et al: Elevated plasma lipoprotein(a) and coronary heart disease in men aged 55 years and younger. JAMA 276:544, 1996.
These findings suggest that lipoprotein(a) may soon make the leap from research test to clinical screening tool.

Castelli WP, Ockene JK, Roberts WC: Cardiovascular risk reduction: What really works? Patient Care 31:47, 1997.
A practical discussion of cardiovascular risk factors and their management.

Davidoff F: Evangelists and snails redux: The case of cholesterol screening. Ann Intern Med 124:513, 1996.
LaRosa JC: Cholesterol agonistics. Ann Intern Med 124:505, 1996.
American College of Physicians: Clinical Guideline, Part 1: Guidelines for using serum cholesterol, high-density lipoprotein cholesterol, and triglyceride levels as screening tests for preventing coronary heart disease in adults; and Garber AM, Browner WS, Hulley SB: Clinical Guideline, Part 2: Cholesterol screening in asymptomatic adults, revisited. Ann Intern Med 124:515, 1996.
Experts disagree on cholesterol screening recommendations.

Diekman T, Lansberg PJ, Kastelein JJP, et al: Prevalence and correction of hypothyroidism in a large cohort of patients referred for dyslipidemia. Arch Intern Med 155:1490, 1995.
Hypothyroidism is a well-known cause of dyslipidemia.

Doll R, Peto R, Hall E, et al: Mortality in relation to consumption of alcohol: 13 years' observations on male British doctors. BMJ 309:911, 1994.
Light to moderate drinkers have lower mortality, in part because of significantly reduced cardiovascular deaths.

Erikssen G, Thaulow E, Sandvik L, et al: Haematocrit: A predictor of cardiovascular mortality? J Intern Med 234:493, 1993.
Increased hematocrit is a risk factor for cardiovascular mortality.

Frohlich ED: Uric acid: A risk factor for coronary heart disease. JAMA 270:378, 1993.
Cappuccio FP, Strazzullo P, Farinaro E, et al: Uric acid metabolism and tubular sodium handling. JAMA 270:354, 1993.
Hyperuricemia is a well-documented risk factor for coronary artery disease.

Gambino SR, Rosen M: NIH Consensus Development Conference on triglycerides, high density lipoprotein, and coronary heart disease. Lab Report Physicians 14:17, 1992.
Panel recommends always measuring HDL cholesterol and total cholesterol together. Triglyceride measurement is recommended in patients with diabetes, obesity, peripheral vascular disease, high blood pressure, and kidney disease.

Gaziano JM, Buring JE, Breslow JL, et al: Moderate alcohol intake, increased levels of high density lipoprotein and its subfractions and decreased risk of myocardial infarction. N Engl J Med 329:1829, 1993.
Alcohol decreases risk of myocardial infarction by effect on HDL cholesterol.

Graham IM, Daly LE, Refsum HM, et al: Plasma homocysteine as a risk factor for vascular disease. JAMA 277:1775, 1997.
An increased plasma total homocysteine level confers an independent risk of vascular disease similar to that of smoking or hyperlipidemia.

Grant MD, Piotrowski ZH, Miles TP: Declining cholesterol and mortality in a sample of older nursing home residents. J Am Geriatr Soc 44:31, 1996.
Rapidly falling cholesterol is marker for high mortality in older nursing home residents.

Gronbaek M, Deis A, Sorensen TIA, et al: Influence of sex, age, body mass index, and smoking on alcohol intake and mortality. BMJ 308:302, 1994.
Goldberg RJ, Burchfiel CM, Reed DM, et al: A prospective study of the health effects of alcohol consumption in middle-aged and elderly men: The Honolulu Heart Program. Circulation 89:651, 1994.
In middle-aged and elderly men, coronary mortality fell with greater alcohol consumption, but cancer incidence and total mortality rose.

Grover SA, Coupal L, Hu X-P: Identifying adults at increased risk of coronary disease: How well do the current cholesterol guidelines work? JAMA 274:801, 1995.

Future guidelines should better incorporate HDL cholesterol levels and nonlipid risk factors to target high-risk individuals accurately.

Grundy SM: Cholesterol and coronary heart disease: The 21st century. Arch Intern Med 157:1177, 1997.

Aggressive lowering of LDL levels in high-risk patients promises to reduce morbidity and mortality from coronary heart disease significantly in the first third of the 21st century.

Guba SC, Fink LM, Fonseca V: Hyperhomocysteinemia: An emerging and important risk factor for thromboembolic and cardiovascular disease. Am J Clin Pathol 105:709, 1996.

Reviews this new and important risk factor.

Hostetter AL: Screening for dyslipidemia: Practice parameter. Am J Clin Pathol 103:380, 1995.

Recommendations by the author and the American Society of Clinical Pathologists.

Kasiske BL, Ma JZ, Kalil RSN, et al: Effects of antihypertensive therapy on serum lipids. Ann Intern Med 122:133, 1995.

With the exception of calcium antagonists, nearly all antihypertensive agents affect serum lipids. These effects differ among patient populations.

Kinosian B, Glick H, Garland G: Cholesterol and coronary heart disease: Predicting risks by levels and ratios. Ann Intern Med 121:641, 1994.

The total cholesterol:HDL cholesterol ratio is an excellent predictor of risk of CHD.

Klag MJ, Ford DE, Mead LA, et al: Serum cholesterol in young men and subsequent cardiovascular disease. N Engl J Med 328:313, 1993.

The serum cholesterol level in young men predicts cardiovascular disease 25 or more years later.

Klatsky AL: Can "a drink a day" keep a heart attack away? Patient Care 29:39, 1995.

Discusses safe levels of alcohol to prevent cardiovascular disease.

Levine GN, Keaney JF Jr, Vita JA: Cholesterol reduction in cardiovascular disease. N Engl J Med 332:512, 1995.

Reviews the relationship between an elevated cholesterol and coronary artery disease as well as the effects of the decreasing cholesterol levels.

Magnusson MK, Sigfusson N, Sigvaldason H, et al: Low iron-binding capacity as a risk factor for myocardial infarction. Circulation 89:102, 1994.

Low iron-binding capacity may increase risk of myocardial infarction.

Mänttäri M, Manninen V, Koskinen P, et al: Leukocytes as a coronary risk factor in a dyslipidemic male population. Am Heart J 123:873, 1992.

An elevated leukocyte count is a coronary risk factor, even in dyslipidemic subjects.

Morrison HI, Schaubel D, Desmeules M, et al: Serum folate and risk of fatal coronary heart disease. JAMA 275:1893, 1996.

Increased rate of fatal CHD is associated with low serum folate.

Muscari A, Bozzoli C, Puddu GM, et al: Association of serum C3 levels with risk of myocardial infarction. Am J Med 98:357, 1995.

An increased risk of myocardial infarction occurs in men with high serum C3 levels.

National Cholesterol Education Program: Detection, evaluation, and treatment of high blood cholesterol in adults (Adult Treatment Panel II). Circulation 89:1329, 1994.

The National Cholesterol Education Program has issued updated recommendations for cholesterol management.

Newman TB, Browner WS, Hulley SB: The case against childhood cholesterol screening. JAMA 264:3039, 1990.

Starc TJ, Belamarich PF, Shea S, et al: Family history fails to identify many children with severe hypercholesterolemia. Am J Dis Child 145:61, 1991.

Reviews the controversy about routine childhood cholesterol screening.

Noel MA, Smith TK, Ettinger WH: Characteristics and outcomes of hospitalized older patients who develop hypocholesterolemia. J Am Geriatr Soc 39:455, 1991.

Documents the poor prognosis in patients with hypocholesterolemia, especially in older patients recently admitted to the hospital.

Nygård O, Vollset SE, Refsum H, et al: Total plasma homocysteine and cardiovascular risk profile: The Hordaland Homocysteine Study. JAMA 274:1526, 1995.

Robinson K, Mayer EL, Miller DP, et al: Hyperhomocysteinemia and low pyridoxal phosphate: Common and independent reversible risk factors for coronary artery disease. Circulation 92:2825, 1995.
Homocysteine may be the next major risk factor for cardiovascular disease.

Paunio M, Virtamo J, Gref C-G, et al: Serum high-density lipoprotein cholesterol, alcohol, and coronary mortality in male smokers. BMJ 312:1200, 1996.
Increased mortality associated with high HDL cholesterol and drinking.

Ridker PM, Cushman M, Stampfer MJ, et al: Inflammation, aspirin, and the risk of cardiovascular disease in apparently healthy men. N Engl J Med 336:973, 1997.
The baseline plasma concentration of C-reactive protein predicts the risk of future myocardial infarction and stroke.

Rubins HB, Robins SJ, Collins D, et al: Distribution of lipids in 8,500 men with coronary artery disease. Am J Cardiol 75:1196, 1995.
The levels of HDL cholesterol, triglycerides, or both are better discriminators of CAD than are total and LDL cholesterol.

Salonen JT, Nyyssönen K, Korpela H, et al: High stored iron levels are associated with excess risk of myocardial infarction in Eastern Finnish men. Circulation 86:803, 1992.
High serum ferritin may be a risk factor for acute myocardial infarction.

Schwertner HA, Jackson WG, Tolan G: Association of low serum concentrations of bilirubin with increased risk of coronary artery disease. Clin Chem 40:18, 1994.
Low serum concentration of bilirubin increases risk of coronary artery disease.

Sempos CT, Looker AC, Gillum RF, et al: Body iron stores and the risk of coronary artery disease. N Engl J Med 330:1119, 1994.
Risk of coronary artery disease is unrelated to iron stores.

Stein JH, Rosenson RS: Lipoprotein Lp(a) excess and coronary heart disease. Arch Intern Med 157:1170, 1997.
Lipoprotein Lp(a) excess has been identified as a powerful predictor of premature atherosclerotic vascular disease in several large, prospective studies.

Tenkanen L, Pietilä K, Manninen V, et al: The triglyceride issue revisited: Findings from the Helsinki Heart Study. Arch Intern Med 154:2714, 1994.
High triglyceride level is a risk factor for coronary heart disease.

Tsai MY: Laboratory assessment of mild hyperhomocysteinemia as an independent risk factor for occlusive vascular diseases. Clin Chem 42:492, 1996.
Mild hyperhomocysteinemia is an independent risk factor for occlusive vascular disease, and laboratories should make a test available for this condition.

Wannamethee G, Shaper AG, Whincup PH, et al: Low serum cholesterol concentrations and mortality in middle-aged British men. BMJ 311:409, 1995.
Men with the lowest cholesterol levels had the highest mortality—mostly due to cancer and noncardiovascular deaths.

Wilder LB, Bachorik PS, Finney CA, et al: The effect of fasting status on the determination of low-density and high-density lipoprotein cholesterol. Am J Med 99:374, 1995.
A fasting sample is preferable for definitive measurement of lipids.

Wilson PWF: Cholesterol screening: Once is not enough. Arch Intern Med 155:2146, 1995.
Forrow L, Calkins DR, Allshouse K, et al: Evaluating cholesterol screening: The importance of controlling for regression to the mean. Arch Intern Med 155:2177, 1995.
Discusses the importance of measuring cholesterol twice, or even three or more times, before labeling the value abnormal.

Windler E, Ewers-Grabow U, Thiery J, et al: The prognostic value of hypocholesterolemia in hospitalized patients. Clin Invest 72:939, 1994.
Patients with cholesterol levels of 100 mg/dL (2.6 mmol/L) or less showed an increased mortality.

OCCULT FECAL BLOOD TESTING AND COLORECTAL CANCER

Recommendations for the early detection of colorectal cancer are from the American Cancer Society. The National Cancer Institute, the College of American Pathologists, the U.S. Preventive Services Task Force, and The World Health Organization support the use of occult fecal blood testing and flexible sigmoidoscopy. There is less support for annual digital rectal examination.

1. To screen for colorectal cancer in men and women age 50 or older, use one of the following examination schedules:

- A fecal occult blood test every year and a flexible sigmoidoscopy every 5 years.
- A colonoscopy every 10 years.
- A double-contrast barium enema every 5 to 10 years.
- A digital rectal exam should be done at the same time as sigmoidoscopy, colonoscopy, or double-contrast barium enema. People who are at moderate or high risk for colorectal cancer should talk with a doctor about a different testing schedule.

Risk factors for colorectal cancer include inflammatory bowel disease, hereditary polyposis and nonpolyposis syndromes, female genital or breast cancer; and first-degree relatives with colorectal cancer that occurred at 55 years or younger.

Approximately 160,000 new cases of and 60,000 deaths from colorectal cancer occur annually in the United States. Regular aspirin use appears to decrease the risk. Annual fecal occult blood testing can decrease mortality from colorectal cancer by 33%. The addition of flexible sigmoidoscopy reduces mortality by 40 to 50%. Colonoscopy has been advocated as the most sensitive screening procedure, and barium enema has been suggested as a cost-effective screening test. Most cases of colorectal cancer are diagnosed in patients with normal hemoglobin and normal erythrocyte mean corpuscular volume and red cell distribution width values. A low serum ferritin may indicate colorectal cancer.

2. To perform fecal occult blood testing, place the individual to be tested on a diet (see below) 2 days before the first stool collection, and continue this diet throughout the collection period. Instruct the individual about specimen collections. A positive test result on stool obtained via digital rectal examination should be regarded as a true positive.

The individual should be instructed as follows:
The diet should eliminate certain drugs (aspirin, nonsteroidal anti-inflammatory agents, vitamin C, iron, laxatives), rare red meat, raw fruits and vegetables high in peroxidase (broccoli, cantaloupe, cauliflower, horseradish, radishes, turnips), and excessive amounts of foods moderately high in peroxidase (artichokes, cabbage, carrots, cucumbers, grapefruit, mushrooms, potatoes). Consumption of ethanol (up to three bottles of beer per day or the equivalent) should not invalidate the test. Therapeutic doses of aspirin should be withheld at least 4 days before the collection of specimens, but one aspirin or less a day should not affect the results, provided that ethanol is excluded.

Beginning on the third day of the diet, using specimen cards, take two specimens from each of three consecutive stools. Because specimen collection is unpleasant and may adversely affect compliance, a suggested solution is to dab a small amount of stool from the toilet paper directly onto the card.

Promptly return these three completed cards (six samples) to the laboratory within 7 days—never over 14 days.

Test samples promptly. At the present time, the best test is Hemoccult II (SmithKline Diagnostics) without rehydration. Hemoccult II with hydration has a false-positive rate of 10% or higher, which leads to larger numbers of work-ups with negative results. A combination of Hemoccult II Sensa and HemeSelect (SmithKline Diagnostics) provides better results than Hemoccult II; however, this combination is more expensive, and may not be practical in routine clinical settings.

3. Evaluate the fecal occult blood test results.

One or more positive results in any of these six samples is considered a positive test for occult blood that cannot be ignored. After a race, marathon runners may have a positive fecal occult blood test. If a retrospective history of use of therapeutic nonsteroidal anti-inflammatory agents during the collection period is elicited, discontinue the agents, and perform another set of fecal occult blood tests after 3 weeks.

4. Evaluate every asymptomatic individual with a positive fecal occult blood test by flexible sigmoidoscopy and double-contrast barium enema or full colonoscopy.

In the past, sigmoidoscopy with double-contrast barium enema was often used; however, full colonoscopy is the current procedure of choice.

Approximately 1 to 5% of unselected persons tested with fecal occult blood tests have positive test results. Of those with positive test results, approximately 10% have cancer, and 20 to 30% have adenomas. The remainder have either a benign source of bleeding (e.g., proctitis, anal fissure, hemorrhoid) or no detectable lesion. Some individuals with a positive fecal occult blood test result and normal gastrointestinal studies may have a lesion that was not detected. These individuals should be re-evaluated in the future.

5. In patients with colorectal cancer, the following blood test results may be increased:

- **Erythrocyte sedimentation rate** caused by inflammatory complications of the tumor
- **Lactate dehydrogenase** coming from the cancer
- **Carcinoembryonic antigen** coming from the cancer
- **Leukocytes** caused by inflammatory complications of the tumor
- **Creatine kinase** originating in the cancer

- **Alkaline phosphatase** that may be due to the Regan alkaline phosphatase isoenzyme

6. In patients with colorectal cancer, the following blood test results may be decreased:

- **Hemoglobin and hematocrit** caused by iron deficiency anemia due to blood loss
- **Potassium** when the cancer is associated with a villous adenoma
- **Ferritin** related to iron deficiency anemia

BIBLIOGRAPHY

Aaltonen LA, Peltomäki P, Leach FS, et al: Clues to the pathogenesis of familial colorectal cancer. Science 260:812, 1993.
A new mutant gene on chromosome 2 has been linked with hereditary nonpolyposis colorectal cancer.
Allison JE, Tekawa IS, Ransom LJ, et al: A comparison of fecal occult-blood tests for colorectal-cancer screening. N Engl J Med 334:155, 1996.
An improved testing strategy may be to confirm a positive Hemoccult II Sensa test with a HemeSelect test.
Bhattacharya I, Sack EM: Screening colonoscopy: The cost of common sense. Lancet 347:1744, 1996.
Advocates colonoscopy as the most sensitive screening procedure for colorectal cancer.
Bond JH, Greenberger NJ: Screening for colorectal cancer. Hosp Pract 32:59, 1997.
Reviews strategies for colorectal cancer screening.
Dominitz JA, McCormick LH, Rex DK: Colorectal cancer: Latest approaches to prevention and screening. Patient Care 30:124, 1996.
Reviews screening guidelines—start by separating the average-risk from the high-risk patient.
Eisner MS, Lewis JH: Diagnostic yield of a positive fecal occult blood test found on digital rectal examination: Does the finger count? Arch Intern Med 151:2180, 1991.
A positive test result should be followed up, even if the sample was obtained by digital rectal examination.
Fleming JL, Ahlquist DA, McGill DB, et al: Influence of aspirin and ethanol on fecal blood levels as determined by using the HemoQuant assay. Mayo Clin Proc 62:159, 1987.
Discussion of the effects of two heavily used drugs, aspirin and ethanol, on tests for fecal occult blood.
Fuchs CS, Giovannucci EL, Colditz GA, et al: A prospective study of family history and the risk of colorectal cancer. N Engl J Med 331:1169, 1994.
A positive family history nearly doubles the risk of colon cancer.
Giovannucci E, Rimm EB, Stampfer MJ, et al: Aspirin use and the risk for colorectal cancer and adenoma in male health professionals. Ann Intern Med 121:241, 1994.
Giovannucci E, Egan KM, Hunter DJ, et al: Aspirin and the risk of colorectal cancer in women. N Engl J Med 333:609, 1995.
Many years of regular aspirin use appear to reduce the incidence of colorectal cancer.
Gomez JA, Diehl AK: Admission stool guaiac test: Use and impact on patient management. Am J Med 92:603, 1992.
Routine admission fecal occult blood testing seldom is useful.
Gopalswamy N, Stelling HP, Markert RJ, et al: A comparative study of eight fecal occult blood tests and HemoQuant in patients in whom colonoscopy is indicated. Arch Fam Med 3:1043, 1994.
Consider fecal occult blood tests as adjuncts to the history and physical examination in diagnosing gastrointestinal disease.
Griffiths EK, Schapira DV: Serum ferritin and stool occult blood and colon cancer screening. Cancer Detect Prev 15:303, 1991.

The sensitivity of low serum ferritin for detecting colon cancer was greater than that of fecal occult blood.

Levin B, Hess K, Johnson C: Screening for colorectal cancer: A comparison of 3 fecal occult blood tests. Arch Intern Med 157:970, 1997.
Of the three alternatives tested, nonhydrated Hemoccult had the best positive predictive value.

Mandel JS, Bond JH, Church TR, et al: Reducing mortality from colorectal cancer by screening for fecal occult blood. N Engl J Med 328:1365, 1993.
Solid evidence that screening reduces mortality from colorectal cancer.

Marcus AJ: Aspirin as prophylaxis against colorectal cancer. N Engl J Med 333:656, 1995.
Aspirin reduces risk of colorectal cancer.

Marshall JB: Colorectal cancer screening: Present strategies and future prospects. Postgrad Med 99:253, 1996.
Reviews current and future screening strategies for colorectal cancer.

Murphy GP (ed): Colorectal cancer. CA Cancer J Clin 47, March/April, 1997.
Reviews the diagnosis and management of colorectal cancer, including clinical and molecular approaches to diagnosis.

Ransohoff DF, Lang CA: Improving the fecal occult-blood test. N Engl J Med 334:189, 1996.
At the present time, the best test is Hemoccult II without hydration.

Rozen P, Ron E, Fireman Z, et al: The relative value of fecal occult blood tests and flexible sigmoidoscopy in screening for large bowel neoplasia. Cancer 60:2553, 1987.
Discusses the yield in patients with positive fecal occult blood tests in terms of benign and malignant lesions.

Rustgi AK: Hereditary gastrointestinal polyposis and nonpolyposis syndromes. N Engl J Med 331:1694, 1994.
Reviews the hereditary forms of colon cancer and their genetic basis.

Schnell T, Aranha GV, Sontag SJ, et al: Fecal occult blood testing: A false sense of security? Surgery 116:798, 1994.
Relying solely on fecal occult blood testing to detect colorectal cancer misses a number of cancers, especially left-sided cancers.

Screening for colorectal cancer—United States, 1992–1993, and new guidelines. MMWR 45:107, 1996.
Only a minority of Americans are being screened for colon cancer.

Selby JV, Friedman GD, Quesenberry CP Jr, et al: Effect of fecal occult blood testing on mortality from colorectal cancer. Ann Intern Med 118:1, 1993.
Fecal occult blood testing reduces colorectal cancer mortality by 25 to 30%.

Selby JV, Friedman GD, Quesenberry CP Jr: A case-control study of screening sigmoidoscopy and mortality from colorectal cancer. N Engl J Med 326:653, 1992.
Levin B: Screening sigmoidoscopy for colorectal cancer. N Engl J Med 326:700, 1992.
Screening sigmoidoscopy is effective in reducing colorectal cancer deaths—once every 10 years may be enough.

Speights VO, Johnson MW, Stoltenberg PH, et al: Complete blood count indices in colorectal carcinoma. Arch Pathol Lab Med 116:258, 1992.
Most cases of colorectal cancer are diagnosed in patients with normal hemoglobin and normal erythrocyte mean cell volume and red cell distribution width values.

Thomas WM, Pye G, Hardcastle JD, et al: Screening for colorectal carcinoma: An analysis of the sensitivity of Haemoccult. Br J Surg 79:833, 1992.
In spite of its limited sensitivity, the fecal occult blood test can identify individuals at high risk of asymptomatic carcinoma or adenoma.

Toribara NW, Sleisenger MH: Screening for colorectal cancer. N Engl J Med 332:861, 1995.
Reviews the pathophysiology and screening strategies for colorectal cancer.

Truszkowski J, Summers RW: Colorectal neoplasms. Postgrad Med 98:97, 1995.
Reviews screening, diagnosis, and therapy of colorectal neoplasms.

Van Dam J, Bond JH, Sivak MV Jr: Fecal occult blood screening for colorectal cancer. Arch Intern Med 155:2389, 1995.
Fecal occult blood screening can reduce mortality from colorectal cancer.

Wagner JL, Herdman RC, Wadhwa S: Cost effectiveness of colorectal cancer screening in the elderly. Ann Intern Med 115:807, 1991.
Concludes that screening for colorectal cancer in persons 65 to 85 years of age is cost-effective.

DIGITAL RECTAL EXAMINATION, PROSTATE-SPECIFIC ANTIGEN, AND PROSTATE CANCER

Recommendations for screening for prostate cancer using serum prostate-specific antigen (PSA) are from the American Cancer Society. The American Urological Association and the American College of Radiology endorse a similar approach. The National Cancer Institute, the U.S. Preventive Services Task Force, the Canadian Task Force on the Periodic Health Examination, and the Canadian Urological Association do not endorse screening with PSA. The College of American Pathologists endorses PSA testing only if digital rectal examination is performed. A reasonable compromise, which is recommended by the American College of Physicians, is to advise the patient of the issues and allow the patient to make an informed decision about being tested.

1. Offer both the prostate specific antigen blood test and the digital rectal examination annually, beginning at age 50, to men who have a life expectancy of at least 10 years and to younger men who are at high risk. Men in high risk groups, such as those with a strong familial predisposition (e.g., two or more affected first-degree relatives), or African Americans may begin at a younger age (e.g., 45 years).

Free PSA, PSA rate of change, PSA density, and PSA age-specific reference ranges are measurements that are being studied in an attempt to improve diagnostic sensitivity and specificity. Of these, free PSA seems to be the most useful.

Many authorities recommend wellness screening for prostate cancer using digital rectal examination; however, the American Cancer Society, the American Urological Association, and the College of American Pathologists believe that both serum PSA and digital rectal examination should be used. Among men, approximately 245,000 new cases of and 40,000 deaths from prostate cancer occur annually in the United States (less than lung cancer but more than colon cancer). Risk factors appear to include age, race, family history, vasectomy, and dietary fat intake. A newly detected gene, called hereditary prostate cancer 1, increases the risk of prostate cancer at age 80 from 50 to 88%. It probably accounts for no more than 3% of all cases of prostate cancer.

The role of screening with PSA and/or transrectal ultrasonography to detect prostate cancer is controversial. A recent study suggests that digital rectal examination plus serum PSA measurement detects significantly more prostate cancers than rectal examination alone, but others argue that many prostate cancers never cause clinical problems and that detecting these clinically silent cancers may expose patients to the risks of treatment without the potential for benefit. Moreover, approximately 30% of patients with benign prostatic hypertrophy have a high PSA concentration. Measuring the free (unbound) PSA and the rate of change in serum PSA and correlating the PSA concentration with prostatic volume (PSA density) may improve the diagnostic sensitivity and specificity of this tumor marker, but further study is necessary. Finasteride (Proscar), a drug for benign prostatic hypertrophy, can decrease PSA; men taking this drug should be followed with digital rectal examination as well as baseline and annual PSA measurements. A level of 5 ng/mL ($\geq$5 μg/L) or greater after 12 months of finasteride suggests prostate cancer.

2. If digital rectal examination of the prostate reveals an area of nodularity or induration, establish the diagnosis using PSA and a transrectal ultrasound (TRUS)–guided biopsy. Draw a blood specimen for determining serum PSA, and consider measuring serum prostatic acid phosphatase (PAP).

Definitive diagnosis is established by TRUS-guided biopsy and examination of prostate tissue under the microscope. Prostate biopsy but not digital rectal examination may increase PSA and PAP. TRUS alone does not increase the PSA in patients with prostate cancer or benign prostatic hypertrophy. It may, however, slightly increase PSA in patients with prostatitis. Extensive exercise should be avoided before measuring PSA because it can increase the level. Also, ejaculation can increase PSA for up to 2 days.

A PAP may be useful in differentiating serious disease in patients who have a normal PSA. An increased PAP and normal PSA have been observed in prostate cancer, polycythemia rubra vera, chronic myeloid leukemia, myeloproliferative syndrome, metastatic carcinoma (pancreatic, lung, colon, squamous cell), osteomyelitis, and tuberculosis. When monitoring patients with prostate cancer who are using hormone therapy, a PAP together with a PSA may be useful.

3. Evaluate the test results and obtain other appropriate studies: CBC, lactate dehydrogenase (LD), ALP, and hepatic and renal function studies.

PSA is a serum protease enzyme that circulates in the serum in two forms—free and bound. Moreover, at least five isoforms have been identified. Standardization of PSA assays is not a simple matter.

Reference Ranges

Test	Specimen	Conventional Units	International Units
Acid phosphatase: thymolphthalein monophosphate	Serum[1]	<0.8 U/L	<0.8 U/L
Prostate-specific antigen	Serum[2]	0–4 ng/mL	0–4 μg/L

[1]Automatic Clinical Analyzer (EI du Pont de Nemours & Co, Inc).
[2]Tandem-R PSA assay (Hybritech, Inc).

Most screening studies have used a PSA value of 4.0 ng/mL (4.0 μg/L) as the upper limit of the reference range. Assuming normal prevalence, the positive predictive value of PSA in conjunction with digital rectal examination is as follows:

POSITIVE PREDICTIVE VALUE OF PSA

Digital Rectal Examination	PSA Ranges (ng/mL [μg/L]*)		
	0.0–4.0	4.1–10	>10
Negative	9%	20%	31%
Positive	17%	45%	77%

$$\text{Positive predictive value} = \frac{\text{True positives}}{\text{True positives} + \text{False positives}}$$

*Tandem-R PSA assay (Hybritech, Inc.).
Source: Oesterling JE: Prostate-specific antigen: A valuable clinical tool. Oncology 5:112, 1991.

Prostate-Specific Antigen Density

The PSA density refers to a numerical ratio determined by dividing the PSA serum value by the volume of the prostate gland determined by TRUS. Because prostate cancer tissue produces more PSA per gram of tissue than does normal prostate tissue or benign prostatic hyperplasia, increased PSA density (>0.15) is suggestive of prostate cancer (>80% likelihood of detecting prostate cancer).

Prostate-Specific Antigen Velocity (Rate of Change of the Antigen with Time)

Prostate-specific antigen velocity refers to the rate of change in the PSA value over time. Patients whose PSA value increases more than 0.75 ng/mL (0.75 μg/L) per year should be regarded with a high degree of suspicion.

Prostate-Specific Antigen—Age-Specific Reference Ranges

Because benign prostatic hypertrophy occurs in practically every man and because this increased prostate volume is associated with higher serum PSA values, reference ranges increase with age as follows:

PROSTATE-SPECIFIC ANTIGEN AGE-SPECIFIC REFERENCE RANGES

	40–49 Years	50–59 Years	60–69 Years	70–79 Years
Oesterling JE, et al	0.0–2.5 ng/mL	0.0–3.5 ng/mL	0.0–4.5 ng/mL	0.0–6.5 ng/mL
Dalkin, et al	—	0.0–3.5 ng/mL	0.0–5.4 ng/mL	0.0–6.3 ng/mL
Crawford, et al	0.0–2.3 ng/mL	0.0–3.3 ng/mL	0.0–5.0 ng/mL	0.0–6.0 ng/mL

Source: Oesterling JE, Jacobsen SJ, Cooner WH: The use of age-specific reference ranges for serum prostate specific antigen in men 60 years old or older. J Urol 153:1160–1163, 1995.

Use of these age-specific ranges may increase the rate of cancer detection in younger men and decrease the number of biopsies in older patients.

Serum Free and Bound Prostate-Specific Antigens

Free PSA appears promising for ruling out carcinoma in patients with PSA values between 4.1 to 10 ng/mL (4.1 to 10 µg/L). Because men with cancer have lower free PSA, in a recent study, a free PSA cutoff of 24% or lower detected at least 95% of cancers and eliminated 13% of men without cancer. Some experts advocate measuring free PSA levels in men with PSA values of 2.5 or 3 to 4 ng/mL (2.5 or 3 to 4 µg/ L) in order to find more early cancers. Measuring free PSA in men whose total values are between 3 and 10 ng/mL can potentially detect men with prostate cancer while simultaneously eliminating many unnecessary negative biopsies.

Although not affected by digital rectal examination, the serum PSA level may increase 2-fold with prostate massage, 4-fold with cytoscopy, and more than 50-fold with needle biopsy or transurethral resection of the prostate. After any of these procedures, clinicians should wait at least 6 weeks before measuring serum PSA. Serum PSA is increased in patients with prostate cancer, benign prostate hypertrophy, and prostatitis. Some investigators believe that with a PSA level less than 10 ng/mL (<10 µg/L), the risk of having already mestastasized to bone is only about 1%. A PSA concentration greater than 10 ng/mL (>10 µg/ L) is highly suspicious for cancer, and the higher the PSA, the greater is the likelihood of advanced disease (e.g., lymph node metastases are present in two thirds of patients with a PSA concentration greater than 25 ng/mL [>25 µg/L]). PSA values may be unreliable in patients on antiandrogen therapy. It is wise to measure baseline PSA because this measurement will be useful for comparing with future measurements of PSA to determine adequacy of surgical removal of the cancer or recurrence.

Although serum PAP is rarely increased when the cancer is confined to the gland, approximately 80% of patients with locally invasive or metastatic cancer have sustained high values. In addition to prostate cancer, serum PAP may be increased secondary to prostatitis, prostate infarct, prostate surgery or biopsy, Gaucher's disease, Niemann-Pick disease, some benign and malignant hematologic disorders, and other miscellaneous conditions. Prostate massage may increase serum PAP for 72 hours, but routine digital examination appears to have no effect. Values are increased in some patients with benign hypertrophy, prostatitis, or retention of urine. It is not possible to determine whether such patients also have subclinical cancer of the prostate.

Serum ALP may be high because of osteoblastic bone metastases or cholestatic liver metastases. These high ALP values may occur in individuals who have an increased or normal PAP level. In patients with metastatic cancer who have a normal PAP level, a high ALP level can suggest the presence of metastatic disease, and a CBC can detect secondary anemia. A high serum urea nitrogen and creatinine concentration and an abnormal urinalysis can detect renal dysfunction such as obstructive uropathy. Serum LD, specifically LD-5, may increase secondary to the tumor mass.

A recent study indicated that normal serum acid and alkaline phosphatase levels and absence of bone pain in patients with newly diagnosed prostate cancer have a negative predictive value for bone metastases of 99% (i.e., bone scan may be omitted in such patients).

4. If the prostate biopsy is negative for cancer, the patient is probably free of disease, but remember that false-negative biopsy and test results can occur.

Approximately 50% of prostate nodules felt on rectal examination are confirmed as cancer. The sensitivity of a single biopsy to detect existing prostate cancer is approximately 80%. With repeated attempts, the sensitivity increases to 90%.

Up to 90% of patients with prostate cancer metastatic to bone have an increased serum ALP level because of osteoblastic activity. Liver metastases can also cause an increased ALP level that is secondary to cholestasis.

A negative chemistry and hematology screen—including normal serum PSA and PAP test results—does not completely exclude prostate cancer.

5. Grade and stage the tumor using test results in the context of clinical findings and radiographic data.

Prostate cancer should be histologically graded and clinically staged so that appropriate therapy can be chosen.

6. In addition to standard clinical procedures, use PSA to monitor the response of prostate cancer to treatment.

7. In men with prostate cancer, the following additional blood test results may be increased:

- **Erythrocyte sedimentation rate,** which indicates a worse prognosis
- **Carcinoembryonic antigen** originating in the tumor
- **Creatine kinase** coming from the tumor

8. In men with prostate cancer, the following additional blood test results may be decreased:

- **Hemoglobin and hematocrit**

BIBLIOGRAPHY

American College of Physicians: Screening for prostate cancer: Clinical Guideline Part III. Ann Intern Med 126:480, 1997.
Advocates allowing the patient to make an informed decision about being tested.
Anderson JR, Strickland D, Corbin D, et al: Age-specific reference ranges for serum prostate-specific antigen. Urology 46:54, 1995.
Oesterling JE, Jacobsen SJ, Cooner WH: The use of age-specific reference ranges for serum prostate-specific antigen in men 60 years old or older. J Urol 153:1160, 1995.
Gives reference ranges for PSA according to age.
Angier N: Scientists zero in on gene tied to prostate cancer. The New York Times, November 22, 1996, p A10.
The gene called HPC1, for hereditary prostate cancer 1, sits on the bottom half of chromosome 1.
Bangma CH, Kranse R, Blijenberg BG, et al: The value of screening tests in the detection of prostate cancer. Part I: Results of a retrospective evaluation of 1,726 men. Urology 46:773, 1995.
Free PSA adds little to present strategy for diagnosing prostate cancer.
Bruskewitz R, Carbone PP: Management dilemmas in prostate cancer. Hosp Pract 31:79, 1996.
Good discussion of the management issues in prostate cancer—especially screening.
Cantor SB, Spann SJ, Volk RJ, et al: Prostate cancer screening: A decision analysis. J Fam Pract 41:33, 1995.
When quality of life is the main issue, prostate cancer screening is not worth doing.
Catalona WJ, Hudson MA, Scardino PT, et al: Selection of optimal prostate-specific antigen cut-offs for early detection of prostate cancer. J Urol 152:2037, 1994.
Despite age-related changes, a PSA cut-off of 4.0 ng/mL (4.0 µg/L) should be used for any age group.
Catalona WJ, Smith DS, Wolfert RL, et al: Evaluation of percentage of free serum prostate-specific antigen to improve specificity of prostate cancer screening. JAMA 274:1214, 1995.
Free PSA is a promising test to improve specificity of prostate cancer screening for men with elevated total serum PSA levels.
Flood AB, Wennberg JE, Nease RF Jr: The importance of patient preference in the decision to screen for prostate cancer. J Gen Intern Med 11:342, 1996.
Because informed patient choices vary, PSA screening decisions should incorporate individual preferences.
Fowler JE, Pandey P, Braswell NT, et al: Prostate-specific antigen progression rates after radical prostatectomy or radiation therapy for localized prostate cancer. Surgery 116:302, 1994.
Discusses the use of PSA to monitor patients after radical prostatectomy or radiation therapy.

Frazier HA, Robertson JE, Humphrey PA, et al: Is prostate-specific antigen of clinical importance in evaluating outcome after radical prostatectomy? J Urol 149:516, 1993.
Although a postoperative elevated PSA may reflect residual tumor, its significance should be evaluated together with other clinical findings.

Frydenberg M, Stricker PD, Kaye KW: Prostate cancer diagnosis and management. Lancet 349:1681, 1997.
Good review of prostate cancer: screening, diagnosis, and treatment.

Gambino SR: Standardization of prostate-specific antigen tests. Lab Report Physicians 16:75, 1994.
Standardization of PSA tests is not a simple matter.

Gambino SR: An elevated PAP level, in the presence of a normal PSA level, usually indicates serious non-prostatic disease. Lab Report Physicians 16:70, 1994.
Lloyd AJI, Formby MR: Conditions associated with normal levels of prostate-specific antigen and elevation of prostatic acid phosphatase. Am J Clin Oncol 15:487, 1992.
An increased PAP and normal PSA have been described in prostate cancer and several serious non-prostatic diseases.

Garnick MB, Fair WR: Prostate cancer: Emerging concepts, Part I. Ann Intern Med 125:118, 1996; and Prostate cancer: Emerging concepts, Part II. Ann Intern Med 125:205, 1996.
Despite earlier detection, the optimal therapy for the early form of the disease is still enigmatic.

Gerber G, Chodak GW: Assessment of value of routine bone scans in patients with newly diagnosed prostate cancer. Urology 37:418, 1991.
Establishes that bone scans are unnecessary in newly diagnosed patients with normal chemistry test results and absence of bone pain.

Gittes RF: Carcinoma of the prostate. N Engl J Med 324:236, 1991.
Excellent review of pathogenesis, diagnosis, and management of prostate cancer.

Glenski WJ, Malek RS, Myrtle JF, et al: Sustained, substantially increased concentration of prostate-specific antigen in the absence of prostatic malignant disease: An unusual clinical scenario. Mayo Clin Proc 67:249, 1992.
Non-malignant conditions may occasionally be associated with very high PSA levels.

Gormley GJ, Stoner E, Ng J, et al: Effect of finasteride on prostate-specific antigen density. Urology 43:53, 1994.
Serum PSA of 10 ng/mL (10 µg/L) or greater before finasteride or 5 ng/mL (5 µg/L) or greater after 12 months of finasteride suggests prostate cancer.

Handley MR, Stuart ME: The use of prostate-specific antigen for prostate cancer screening: A managed care perspective. J Urol 152:1689, 1994.
A larger health maintenance organization concludes that PSA screening for cancer is not effective or cost-efficient.

Hayward RSA, Steinberg EP, Ford DE, et al: Preventive care guidelines: 1991. Ann Intern Med 114:758, 1991.
Authoritative recommendations for wellness screening for prostate cancer.

Hughes HR, Penney MD, Gryan P, et al: Serum prostatic specific antigen: *In vitro* stability and the effect of ultrasound rectal examination *in vivo*. Ann Clin Biochem 24 (suppl): SI206, 1987.
Reports the effects of transrectal ultrasonography on serum PSA.

Internal Medicine Clinic Research Consortium: Effect of digital rectal examination on serum prostate-specific antigen in a primary care setting. Arch Intern Med 155:389, 1995.
Digital rectal examination causes a statistically significant but clinically insignificant increase in PSA levels.

Jacobsen SJ, Klee GG, Lija H, et al: Stability of serum prostate-specific antigen determination across laboratory, assay, and storage time. Urology 45:447, 1995.
Compares the Tandem-R PSA assay (Hybritech) and the IMX assay (Abbott).

Johansson J-E, Sigurdsson T, Holmberg L, et al: Erythrocyte sedimentation rate as a tumor marker in human prostate cancer. Cancer 70:1556, 1992.
A high erythrocyte sedimentation rate indicates a worse prognosis in prostate cancer.

Kabalin JN: Screening for prostate cancer today. West J Med 162:272, 1995.
Cher ML, Carroll PR: Screening for prostate cancer. West J Med 162:235, 1995.
Reviews the pros and cons of screening for prostate cancer.

Meigs JB, Barry MJ, Oesterling JE, et al: Interpreting results of prostate-specific antigen testing for early detection of prostate cancer. J Gen Intern Med 11:505, 1996.
Discusses likelihood ratios for PSA test result interpretation.

Mettlin C, Littrup PJ, Kane RA, et al: Relative sensitivity and specificity of serum prostate-specific antigen level compared with age-referenced PSA, PSA density, and PSA change. Cancer 74:1615, 1994.
A simple elevation of PSA is the best indicator of prostate cancer.

Moul JW, Sesterhenn IA, Connelly RR, et al: Prostate-specific antigen values at the time of prostate cancer diagnosis in African-American men. JAMA 274:1277, 1995.
As a group, African-American men with newly diagnosed prostate cancer have higher PSA values at initial diagnosis than white men.

Neal DE Jr, Clejan S, Sarma D, et al: Prostate specific antigen and prostatitis: I. Effects of prostatitis on serum PSA in the human and nonhuman primate. Prostate 20:105, 1992.
Prostatitis increases serum PSA.

Oesterling JE: Age-specific reference ranges for serum PSA. N Engl J Med 335:345, 1996.
Morgan TO, Jacobsen SJ, McCarthy WF, et al: Age-specific reference ranges for serum prostate-specific antigen in black men. N Engl J Med 335:304, 1996.
Describes age-specific reference ranges for black men and discusses various PSA strategies designed to increase diagnostic sensitivity and specificity.

Oesterling JE: Prostate-specific antigen: A valuable clinical tool. Oncology 5:107, 1991.
Discussion from the Mayo Clinic on the role of PSA for screening, diagnosis, and management.

Oesterling JE, Jacobsen SJ, Clute CG, et al: Serum prostate-specific antigen in a community-based population of healthy men: Establishment of age-specific reference ranges. JAMA 270:860, 1993.
Age-specific reference ranges may decrease false-positive and false-negative PSA results.

Oesterling JE, Rice DC, Glenski WJ, et al: Effect of cystoscopy, prostate biopsy, and transurethral resection of prostate on serum prostate-specific antigen concentration. Urology 42:276, 1993.
Delay measuring PSA until 6 weeks after prostate biopsy or transurethral resection. Simple cystoscopy does not affect the PSA.

Oremek GM, Seiffert UB: Physical activity releases prostate-specific antigen from the prostate gland into blood and increases serum PSA concentrations. Clin Chem 42:691, 1996.
Extensive physical activity should be avoided before a serum PSA measurement.

Pienta KJ, Esper PS: Risk factors for prostate cancer. Ann Intern Med 118:793, 1993.
Risk factors for prostate cancer appear to include age, race, positive family history, vasectomy, and dietary fat intake.

Randrup E, Baum N: Prostate-specific antigen testing for prostate cancer: Practical interpretation of values. Postgrad Med 99:227, 1996.
Reviews several different PSA-based strategies for detecting prostate cancer.

Riehmann M, Rhodes PR, Cook TD, et al: Analysis of variation in prostate-specific antigen values. Urology 42:390, 1993.
Significant variability in PSA levels occurs that cannot be attributed to laboratory imprecision.

Smith JR, Freije D, Carpten JD, et al: Major susceptibility locus for prostate cancer on chromosome 1 suggested by a genome-wide search. Science 274:1371, 1996.
The data provide strong evidence of a major prostate cancer susceptibility locus on chromosome 1.

Thomson RD, Clejan S: Digital rectal examination: Associated alterations in serum prostate-specific antigen. Am J Clin Pathol 97:528, 1992.
Established that digital rectal examination does not significantly increase serum PSA and mentions that the American Urological Association endorses screening using digital rectal examination and PSA.

Vashi AR, Oesterling JE: Percent free prostate-specific antigen: Entering a new era in the detection of prostate cancer. Mayo Clin Proc 72:337, 1997.
Reviews the use of free PSA for detecting prostate cancer.

Wolf AMD, Nasser JF, Wolf AM, et al: The impact of informed consent on patient interest in prostate-specific antigen screening. Arch Intern Med 156:1333, 1996.
Recommends informed consent for PSA screening.

Woolf SH: Screening for prostate cancer with prostate-specific antigen: An examination of the evidence. N Engl J Med 333:1401, 1995.
Reviews the evidence for screening for prostate cancer with prostate-specific antigen.

ALCOHOL ABUSE

Recommendations for detecting alcohol abuse center on questionnaires. Of these, the CAGE questionnaire has been one of the most effective. Laboratory test results tend to be corroborative. The U.S. Preventive Services Task Force and other medical groups recommend screening for alcohol abuse.

1. To detect individuals with alcohol abuse, ask the CAGE questions. Laboratory tests may be more appropriate for assessing organ damage and monitoring therapy. Other questionnaires, such as the Michigan Alcoholism Screening Test (MAST), may also be used.

The Joint Committee of the National Council on Alcoholism and Drug Dependence and the American Society of Addiction Medicine define alcoholism as a primary, chronic disease with genetic, psychosocial, and environmental factors influencing its development and manifestations. The disease is often progressive and fatal. It is characterized by impaired control over drinking, preoccupation with the drug alcohol, use of alcohol despite adverse consequences, and distortions in thinking, most notably denial. Each of these symptoms may be continuous or periodic.

In the United States, alcohol causes about 100,000 deaths yearly, about half from trauma. Also, about half of motor vehicle deaths are related to alcohol. It costs society about $100 billion to $130 billion yearly.

When directly questioned about their drinking habits, individuals who abuse alcohol frequently underreport the quantity of alcohol they consume. The CAGE questions are designed to detect alcohol abuse in a less confrontational way. Sometimes individuals deny drinking altogether. In this circumstance, laboratory test results and other clues such as unexplained bruises and frequent ingestion of antacids for gastritis become more important. A history of trauma can signal the presence of alcohol abuse. Also, alcoholics often smoke and abuse other drugs. Exercise and physical fitness are frequently neglected. Hypertension, cardiomyopathy, cardiac arrhythmias, and myopathy are additional clues. Women are more susceptible than men to alcoholic cardiomyopathy and myopathy. Any patient with an odor of alcohol probably has a problem with alcohol. Some experts say that consuming five or more drinks at one sitting constitutes abusive drinking, and if this happens on five or more occasions over a period of 30 days it constitutes a drinking problem. Another definition of binge drinking based on the World Health Organization criteria is the number of times the patient has had six or more drinks on one occasion in the past 3 months. Canadian researchers suggest these guidelines for moderate drinking (below which alcohol-related problems are unlikely): maximum of 4 drinks per day and 16 per week for men and 3 per day and 12 per week for women. The U.S. Department of Agriculture and the National Institute of Alcohol and Drug Abuse recommend these safe limits of drinking: up to seven drinks per week for women and up to 14 drinks per week for men.

Helpful tests for alcohol abuse include a blood alcohol measurement; a complete blood count; red blood cell indices; examination of a Wright-stained blood smear for macrocytic red cells; and liver function tests, including serum GGT. It may be worthwhile to obtain a biochemical profile and a urinalysis because alcohol abuse affects so many analytes. Concerning blood alcohol, the mean rate of elimination is about 20 mg/dL/h (4.3 mmol/L/h). Urinary alcohol determinations on daily samples collected for at least 1 week have been recommended as an effective screening test for occult alcohol abuse. Serum fatty acid ethyl esters may be a good marker for recent alcohol ingestion; and serum carbohydrate-deficient transferrin determination is a promising test to detect alcohol abuse. High concentrations of carbohydrate-deficient transferrin occur in individuals drinking more than 50 to 80 g of alcohol per day for at least 1 week (one drink equals approximately 10 to 15 g of alcohol). The high values normalize slowly during abstinence, with a half-life of approximately 15 days.

The following alcohol-related disorders are divided into three levels: level 1 = strongly suggestive; level 2 = suggestive; and level 3 = consistent with the diagnosis of alcoholism.

LEVELS OF ALCOHOL-RELATED DISORDERS

Level 1	Pancreatitis; alcoholic hepatitis; cirrhosis; ascites without tumor; spontaneous bacterial peritonitis; alcoholic ketoacidosis; macrocytosis; Wernicke's encephalopathy; alcohol blood level; hepatorenal syndrome
Level 2	Gastritis; ethylene glycol intoxication; methylene intoxication; rhabdomyolysis; diabetes due to chronic pancreatitis; folic acid deficiency; thrombocytopenia; coagulopathy; hypersplenism; peripheral neuropathy without apparent cause; subdural hematoma; multiple skeletal fractures; gunshot or stab wound; hypophosphatemia; cerebral atrophy unrelated to age
Level 3	Esophagitis; esophageal carcinoma; hemorrhoids; atrial fibrillation (transient); unexplained cardiomyopathy; aspiration pneumonia; lung abscess; tuberculosis; hypocalcemia; impotence; iron deficiency anemia; seizure disorder; autonomic insufficiency without apparent cause; acute delirium without known drug cause; depression; suicide attempt; strong family history of liver disease; hypomagnesemia; pancreatic calcifications; low blood nitrogen level

Source: Mehler PS, McClellan MD, Lezotte D, et al: Improving identification of and intervention for alcoholism. West J Med 163:335–340, 1995. Reprinted by permission of Western Journal of Medicine.

The CAGE acronym focuses on Cutting down, Annoyance by criticism, Guilt feelings, and Eye-openers. The questions are as follows and the more positive answers, the greater the probability of alcohol abuse.

C: Have you ever felt you ought to cut down on your drinking?
A: Have people annoyed you by criticizing your drinking?
G: Have you ever felt bad or guilty about your drinking?
E: Have you ever had a drink first thing in the morning to steady your nerves or get rid of a hangover (eye-opener)?

CAGE Questionnaire

In a recent study on alcohol abuse, likelihood ratios were developed for alcoholism for the CAGE questionnaire. The gold standard was the revised criteria of the *Diagnostic and Statistical Manual of Mental Disorders—III*. The likelihood ratios were 0.14 for no positive answers, 1.5 for one positive answer, 4.5 for two positive answers, 13 for three positive answers, and 100 for four positive answers. These likelihood ratios were used to construct a table of pretest (prior) probabilities and posttest (posterior) probabilities as follows:

CAGE SCORES, PRIOR PROBABILITIES, AND ASSOCIATED POSTERIOR PROBABILITIES FOR ALCOHOLISM IN A GENERAL MEDICINE POPULATION

CAGE SCORE	Posterior Probabilities According to Prior Probabilities					
	10%	*15%*	*20%*	*24%*	*36%*	*63%*
0	2%	2%	3%	4%	7%	19%
1	14%	21%	27%	32%	46%	72%
2	33%	44%	53%	59%	72%	88%
3	59%	70%	76%	81%	88%	96%
4	92%	95%	96%	97%	98%	99%

Source: Buchsbaum DG, Buchanan RG, Centor RM, et al: Screening for alcohol abuse using CAGE scores and likelihood ratios. Ann Intern Med 115:776, 1991.

Using likelihood ratios to interpret CAGE scores enables the clinician to stratify patients along a continuum of risk for alcohol abuse. This is better than simply regarding two or more positive CAGE responses as positive and no or one positive CAGE response as negative for alcoholism. The problem with this approach is the difficulty in assigning prior probabilities in actual patient care situations. Intuitively, clinicians may be able to assign a prevalence factor to a particular population of patients as high, medium, or low for alcohol abuse.

Another method of detecting alcohol abuse is based on the blood alcohol concentration under different circumstances.

U.S. NATIONAL COUNCIL ON ALCOHOLISM CRITERIA FOR ALCOHOL ABUSE

Blood Alcohol Concentration	Findings
>100 mg/dL (>22 mmol/L)	At the time of routine examination by a physician
>150 mg/dL (>33 mmol/L)	Without gross evidence of intoxication
>300 mg/dL (>66 mmol/L)	At any time

2. If the answers to the CAGE questions and the laboratory test results are consistent with alcohol abuse, the diagnosis is supported with a level of confidence that depends on the number of consistent answers and positive test results. The CAGE questions are probably better than laboratory tests for detecting alcohol abuse.

Once ingested, ethanol is rapidly cleared from the blood, and after 24 hours it is completely gone. Changes in hematologic values, liver enzymes, and serum lipid concentrations persist for longer periods of time. Interestingly, individuals taking H_2-receptor antagonists (ranitidine and cimetidine) achieve significantly higher blood alcohol concentrations for a given number of alcoholic drinks consumed—probably because these drugs interfere with the metabolism of alcohol by alcohol dehydrogenase in the gastric mucosa.

Even without laboratory tests, a history of heavy drinking, appropriate clinical findings, and consistent answers to the CAGE questions may allow you to make the diagnosis. If laboratory test results are positive, they lend support to the diagnosis. An increased red cell mean corpuscular volume, increased GGT, and increased liver enzymes are consistent with alcohol abuse. Although the CAGE questions and laboratory tests are sensitive for alcohol abuse, they are not completely specific. Occasionally positive answers and test results occur in patients who are not alcoholics. With the CAGE questions, two positive answers are usually recommended for identifying alcohol abuse; three positive answers are highly predictive for the diagnosis. Also, there are other causes for an increased GGT value such as therapy with phenytoin sodium (Dilantin) or phenobarbital and other causes for increased transaminase and alkaline phosphatase values such as drug-related or viral hepatitis.

3. If the answers to the CAGE questions are negative and the laboratory test results are normal, the diagnosis of alcohol abuse is not supported by objective data.

Because the sensitivity of the CAGE questions and laboratory tests for alcohol abuse is less than 100%, negative answers and normal test results do not exclude the disorder with complete confidence. If clinical suspicion of alcohol abuse continues to exist, the CAGE questions and laboratory tests should be repeated in the future.

4. If you wish to monitor an alcoholic who is in a treatment program, measure GGT, AST, and ALT. If there is an odor of alcohol, measure blood alcohol.

When a patient is in a treatment program, a measurable level of blood or urinary alcohol provides evidence of failure to abstain from drinking. Indeed, regular determination of urinary alcohol is a convenient way to follow these patients—the only potential false positives are diabetics with a urinary tract infection by a fermentor such as *Candida albicans*. Another way to detect a drinking relapse is to measure GGT, AST, and ALT. An increase in the serum activity of any of these enzymes—GGT of 20% or more, AST of 40% or more, and ALT of 20% or more—above an individual's baseline values after 4 weeks of abstinence indicates a return to drinking. Of the three, the GGT is probably the most sensitive.

5. In the alcoholic patient, the following additional blood test results may be increased (* = abnormal test results that are "red flags" for alcohol abuse):

- **Prothrombin time (PT)** due to decreased hepatic synthesis of coagulation factors
- **Activated partial thromboplastin time,** less frequent than increased PT
- **Alcoholic pH changes;** respiratory alkalosis
- **Uric acid** (often >7 mg/dL [>416 μmol/L])*
- **Creatine kinase** caused by myopathy, rarely myoglobinemia, and myoglobinuria*
- **Lactate dehydrogenase**
- **Amylase and lipase** in patients with pancreatitis
- **Abnormal liver function tests** caused by fatty liver, alcoholic hepatitis, and/or cirrhosis; AST:ALT = >1*
- **HDL cholesterol,** which returns to baseline after 1 or 2 weeks of abstinence
- **Triglycerides** caused by increased hepatic production, often greater than 180 mg/dL (>2.06 mmol/L)*
- **Cortisol** after an alcoholic binge
- **Inhibition of vasopressin** at rising alcohol concentrations and the opposite at falling concentrations so that most alcoholics are often slightly overhydrated
- **Carcinoembryonic antigen** in patients with alcoholic liver disease

- **Alpha-fetoprotein** in chronic alcoholic patients consuming more than 60 g of alcohol per day
- **Serum osmotic pressure** when measured by a freezing point osmometer but not a vapor pressure osmometer; provided that other osmotically active substances such as methanol or mannitol are not present in the serum, the serum ethanol concentration can be calculated, based on the osmotic gap, as follows:

$$\text{Estimated blood alcohol (mg/dL)} = \text{Osmotic gap} \times \frac{100}{22} \text{ or}$$

$$\text{estimated blood alcohol mmol/L} = \text{Osmotic gap}$$

where osmotic gap equals measured osmolality minus calculated osmolality (all units in mOsm/kg) (see section "Classifying Acid-Base, Fluid Volume, Osmolality, and Electrolytes by Laboratory Tests" in Chapter 10).

6. In the alcoholic patient, the following additional blood test results may be decreased (* = abnormal test results that are "red flags" for alcohol abuse):

- **Anemia** from a variety of causes (e.g., iron or folate deficiency). Macrocytes may be present.*
- **Leukocytes** from bone marrow suppression*
- **Platelets** from bone marrow suppression*
- **Alcoholic pH changes,** metabolic acidosis
- **Glucose** in fasting patients because of suppression of gluconeogenesis by alcohol (as little as one or two drinks can cause this effect in any person)
- **Urea nitrogen** in severe liver diseases
- **Sodium**
- **Potassium**
- **Calcium**
- **Magnesium***
- **Phosphorus***
- **Thyroxine** (modestly) and a marked decrease in serum triiodothyronine; return to normal after several weeks of abstinence.
- **Testosterone**

BIBLIOGRAPHY

Adams WL, Barry KL, Fleming MF: Screening for problem drinking in older primary care patients. JAMA 276:1964, 1996.
Asking questions on the quantity and frequency of drinking in addition to administering the CAGE increases the number of problem drinkers detected.
American Medical Association Council on Scientific Affairs: Alcoholism in the elderly. JAMA 275:797, 1996.
Physicians need to become more active in the prevention, diagnosis, and treatment of alcoholism and alcohol-related problems in the elderly.

Angell M, Kassirer JP: Alcohol and other drugs: Toward a more rational and consistent policy. N Engl J Med 331:537, 1994.
Alcohol causes a large number of deaths and carries a huge cost to society.

Beresford TP, Blow FC, Hill E, et al: Comparison of CAGE questionnaire and computer-assisted laboratory profiles in screening for covert alcoholism. Lancet 336:482, 1990.
CAGE questions are probably better than laboratory tests for detecting alcohol abuse.

Bradley KA: Screening and diagnosis of alcoholism in the primary care setting. West J Med 156:166, 1992.
A good discussion of criteria for detecting alcoholic patients.

Brennan DF, Betzelos S, Reed R, et al: Ethanol elimination rates in an ED population. Am J Emerg Med 13:276, 1995.
The anticipated mean rate of ethanol elimination is 19.6 mg/dL/h (4.3 mmol/L/h), with only small effects of various factors on this elimination rate.

Buchsbaum DG: Quick, effective screening for alcohol abuse. Patient Care 29:56, 1995.
Suggestion for identifying problem drinkers.

Buchsbaum DG, Buchanan RG, Centor RM, et al: Screening for alcohol abuse using CAGE scores and likelihood ratios. Ann Intern Med 115:774, 1991.
Developed likelihood ratios for stratifying the posttest probability of alcohol abuse based on how many CAGE questions are answered affirmatively.

Callahan CM, Tierney WM: Health services use and mortality among older primary care patients with alcoholism. J Am Geriatr Soc 43:1378, 1995.
Alcohol problems in older patients often escape detection.

Christiansen M, Andersen JR, Torning J, et al: Serum alpha-fetoprotein and alcohol consumption. Scand J Clin Lab Invest 54:215, 1994.
Serum alpha-fetoprotein is increased in chronic alcoholics.

Conigrave KM, Saunders JB, Reznik RB, et al: Prediction of alcohol-related harm by laboratory test results. Clin Chem 39:2266, 1993.
Elevated values for serum GGT, AST, and erythrocyte mean cell volume identify patients at risk for the medical complications of alcohol abuse.

Crowley TJ: Alcoholism: Identification, evaluation, and early treatment. West J Med 140:461, 1984.
Discusses the use of CAGE questions and the Brief Michigan Alcoholism Test to detect alcohol abuse.

De Marchi S, Cecchin E, Basile A, et al: Renal tubular dysfunction in chronic alcohol abuse: Effects of abstinence. N Engl J Med 329:1927, 1993.
Outlines the electrolyte and acid-base disorders in alcoholics.

DiPadova C, Roine R, Frezza M, et al: Effects of ranitidine on blood alcohol levels after ethanol ingestion: Comparison with other H_2-receptor antagonists. JAMA 267:83, 1992.
Describes the increased blood alcohol values that occur in individuals taking H_2-receptor antagonists.

Doyle KM, Cluette-Brown JE, Dube DM, et al: Fatty acid ethyl esters in the blood as markers for ethanol intake. JAMA 276:1152, 1996.
Measurement of fatty acid ethyl esters in the blood may be a more sensitive indicator of ethanol ingestion than the measurement of blood ethanol.

Figueredo VM: The effects of alcohol on the heart: Detrimental or beneficial? Postgrad Med 101:165, 1997.
Drinking at least 80 g (5 oz) of alcohol per day (6 beers, a pint of whiskey, or a bottle and a half of wine) for more than 10 years puts a person at risk for cardiomyopathy.

Fink A, Hays RD, Moore AA, et al: Alcohol-related problems in older persons: Determinants, consequences, and screening. Arch Intern Med 156:1150, 1996.
Research is needed on the consequences of lower levels of alcohol consumption and the physical and psychosocial health of older individuals and on methods for distinguishing alcohol-related from age-related problems.

Friedman GD, Klatsky AL: Is alcohol good for your health? N Engl J Med 329:1882, 1993.
Moderate consumption of alcohol exerts a protective effect against coronary heart disease.

Gambino SR: Screening for occult alcoholism. Lab Report Physicians 2:42, 1980.
Urinary alcohol measurements are effective for detecting alcoholism.

Gaziano JM, Buring JE, Breslow JL, et al: Moderate alcohol intake, increased levels of

high-density lipoprotein and its subfractions and decreased risk of myocardial infarction. N Engl J Med 329:1829, 1993.
Alcohol decreases risk of myocardial infarct by increasing the level of HDL cholesterol.

Gilbert S: Doctors found to fail in diagnosing addictions. The New York Times, February 14, 1996, p B9.
Most doctors fail to ask patients about their alcohol and drug habits.

Hayward RSA, Steinberg EP, Ford DE, et al: Preventive care guidelines: 1991. Ann Intern Med 114:758, 1991.
Authoritative recommendations about programs to encourage the appropriate use of alcohol.

Irwin M, Baird S, Smith TL, et al: Use of laboratory tests to monitor heavy drinking by alcoholic men discharged from a treatment program. Am J Psychiatry 145:595, 1988.
Describes a way to use GGT, AST, and ALT tests to monitor abstinence.

Kitchens JM: Does this patient have an alcohol problem? JAMA 272:1782, 1994.
Describes three screening tests for an alcohol problem: the CAGE questionnaire, the Michigan Alcoholism Screening Test, and the Alcohol Use Disorders Identification Test questions.

Klatsky AL: Can a "drink a day" keep a heart attack away? Patient Care 29:39, 1995.
Light drinking protects against coronary artery disease and probably ischemic stroke. Three or more drinks a day are associated with medical problems.

Magarian GJ, Lucas LM, Kumar KL: Clinical significance in alcoholic patients of commonly encountered laboratory test results. West J Med 156:287, 1992.
Discusses abnormal test results that can occur in the alcoholic patient.

Marmot M: A not-so-sensible drinks policy. Lancet 346:1643, 1995.
The British Government's policy on alcohol, as stated in The Health of the Nation, has been to reduce the proportion of people drinking above the sensible limits (21 units a week for men and 14 for women).

Morse RM, Flavin DK, for the Joint Committee of the National Council on Alcoholism and Drug Dependence and the American Society of Addiction Medicine: The definition of alcoholism. JAMA 268:1012, 1992.
Establishes a precise definition of alcoholism.

Samet JH, Rollnick S, Barnes H: Beyond CAGE: A brief clinical approach after detection of substance abuse. Arch Intern Med 156:2287, 1996.
Positive response to the CAGE questions deserves further assessment such as clarification about adverse consequences, inquiry about loss of control, determination of the patient's perception of the substance use, and an assessment of the patient's readiness to change behavior.

Sanchez-Craig M, Wilkinson A, Davila R: Empirically based guidelines for moderate drinking: 1-year results from three studies with problem drinkers. Am J Public Health 85:823, 1995.
Canadian researchers recommend drinking thresholds for men and women below which alcohol-related problems are unlikely.

Spivak JL: Medical complications of alcoholism. *In* Spivak JL, Barnes HV (eds): Manual of Clinical Problems in Internal Medicine, 4th ed. Boston, Little, Brown & Co, 1990, p 533.
Summarizes alcohol's effects on many laboratory tests and includes annotated key references.

Urbano-Márquez A, Estruch R, Fernández-Solá J, et al: The greater risk of alcoholic cardiomyopathy and myopathy in women compared with men. JAMA 274:149, 1995.
Alcohol abuse places women at greater risk than men for cardiomyopathy and myopathy.

Wenrich MD, Paauw DS, Carline JD, et al: Do primary care physicians screen patients about alcohol intake using the CAGE questions? J Gen Intern Med 10:631, 1995.
Less than half of primary care physicians correctly diagnose alcohol abuse.

Wolf PL: Do discrepancies exist in serum osmolal gaps and calculated serum alcohol concentrations? Arch Pathol Lab Med 120:619, 1996.
Osterloh JD, Kelly TJ, Khayam-Bashi H, et al: Discrepancies in osmolal gaps and calculated alcohol concentrations. Arch Pathol Lab Med 120:637, 1996.
The use of osmolal gap for calculating low-molecular-weight, ingested exogenous substances, such as ethanol, is only a clinical guide and a first approximation.

Wrenn KD, Slovis CM, Minion GE, et al: The syndrome of alcoholic ketoacidosis. Am J Med 91:119, 1991.
Describes acid-base disturbances and other abnormal laboratory test results after an alcoholic binge.

DRUG ABUSE

Recommendations for drug abuse are from the medical literature. The U.S. Preventive Services Task Force believes that evidence is insufficient to recommend for or against routine screening.

1. If an individual shows clinical findings of drug abuse, if you wish to screen for drug abuse, or if you wish to monitor a known drug abuser, obtain a urine specimen collected by a reliable observer, request appropriate tests, and maintain a chain of custody. Consult the laboratory director or supervisor for information on anabolic steroid testing.

According to the National Institute on Drug Abuse, about 74 million Americans have used at least one illicit drug in their lifetime and 13 million have used an illicit drug in the last month.

Screening for drug abuse is practiced by the federal government and many private industries. The value of workplace screening has not been determined. Some authorities have recommended education and counseling for drug abuse in the context of a routine check-up.

Clinical findings of drug abuse include mental changes (delirium, dementia, depression); school difficulties, behavior problems, or unexplained medical problems in adolescents or young adults; and a newly developing psychosis or unexpected deterioration in occupational or social functioning. Known drug abusers should be tested to determine the specific drug or drugs of abuse.

The Rost drug questionnaire (similar to the CAGE questionnaire for alcohol abuse) can be used to screen for drug abuse by giving the individual a list of drugs of abuse and asking the following questions:

1. Have you misused one of these drugs more than five times in your life? ("Misused" means use of any listed drug without a prescription, use of more drug than was prescribed, or use of any drug for pleasure, that is, "to get high.")
2. Have you ever found that you needed to increase your use of a drug in order to get the same effect?
3. Have you ever had emotional or psychological problems from using drugs—like feeling crazy or paranoid or uninterested in things?

Blood is not a good specimen for drug abuse screening. The sensitivities of laboratory methods for detecting drugs in blood are not as good as in urine. Usually the drugs that can be detected in blood are limited to aspirin, acetaminophen, anticonvulsants, barbiturates, diazepam, and volatiles such as alcohol.

A critical issue in forensic drug abuse testing is observation of collection of the urine specimen by a reliable observer to ensure that the specimen truly belongs to the subject being tested. Collection personnel can inspect the urine color and measure its temperature, pH, and specific gravity to verify specimen validity. The specimen should be accurately labeled and refrigerated and a chain of custody maintained. A chain of custody involves documentation of every person who had custody of the specimen from the time it was collected to the time it was tested. Moreover, every person who had custody must have kept the specimen in a secure manner so that no one could have tampered with it.

Appropriate tests for drug abuse should include those for agents most prevalent in the group or class to which the individual belongs. Screening by thin-layer chromatography (TLC) is capable of detecting a wide spectrum of drugs. In contrast, screening by immunoassay detects only the individual agents included in the screening profile.

Because different drugs of abuse have different half-lives (e.g., cocaine, 40 to 80 minutes; amphetamines, 6 to 12 hours; marijuana or tetrahydrocannabinol [THC], 4 to 6 weeks), different screening schedules are necessary to detect different drugs as follows:

DETECTION LIMITS FOR URINE TESTING*

Drug	Dose (mg)	Detection Time	Screening Frequency
Amphetamines	30	1–120 hr	1–2/wk
Barbiturates			
Short-acting	100	6–24 hr	1–2/wk
Phenobarbital	30	At least 4 1/2 days	1–2/wk
Benzodiazepines			
Long-acting (diazepam)	10	7 days	1/wk
Short-acting (triazolam)	0.5	24 hr	2–3/wk
Cocaine	250	8–48 hr	2–3/wk
Methadone	40	7.5–56 hr	2–3/wk
Methaqualone	150	60 hr	1–2/wk
Morphine opiates (IV)	10	84 hr	1/wk
THC metabolites	†	7–34 days	1/mo
	‡	6–81 days	1/mo

*Detection time is the length of time the substance can be detected in the urine after a given dose. Screening frequency is the suggested number of times per week or per month that urine testing would be required to detect repeated use of a given drug.

†Weekly marijuana use.

‡Daily marijuana use.

Source: Saxon AJ, Calsyn DA, Haver VM, et al: Clinical evaluation and use of urine screening for drug abuse. West J Med 149:297, 1988.

2. Evaluate the test results.

Choose the most reputable laboratory available. You may wish to inquire about the laboratory's performance on outside proficiency surveys.

Laboratories use two types of tests, screening and confirmatory, for detecting and confirming drugs in urine. Initially a screening test is performed. A confirmatory test—using a more specific method—should be done to verify a positive screening test. The confirmatory test should be based on a different principle of analysis and be at least as sensitive as the screening test. Enzyme immunoassay (EIA), fluorescence polarization immunoassay, and radioimmunoassay are generally preferred for screening. TLC may also be used for screening. Gas chromatography and high-performance liquid chromatography are currently used for confirmatory analysis; however, gas chromatography–mass spectrometry (GC-MS) is the best confirmatory test.

3. Interpret test results in the context of clinical findings.

In drug abuse testing, as with all quantitative laboratory test results, decisions must be made about the threshold for a positive test result. In marijuana screening, for example, most laboratories use 0.05 µg/ml (0.05 mg/L) as a decision level that best discriminates between users and nonusers. A combination of EIA screening and GC-MS confirmation yields virtually 100% accuracy in detection of marijuana abuse.

Remember that, in contrast to ethanol, no established correlation exists between concentrations of drugs of abuse in body fluids and clinical impairment.

BIBLIOGRAPHY

Davis KH, Hawks RL, Blanke RV: Assessment of laboratory quality in urine drug testing: A proficiency testing pilot study. JAMA 260:1749, 1988.
  Survey of the quality of laboratory testing for drugs.
Everett WD, Linder M: Drug testing in the workplace: What primary care physicians need to know. Postgrad Med 91:287, 1992.
  Guidelines for testing procedures and interpretations of results in the workplace.
Farrar HC, Kearns GL: Cocaine: Clinical pharmacology and toxicology. J Pediatr 115:665, 1989.
  Reviews the pharmacology, detection, and management of cocaine intoxication.
Gerson B (ed): Clinical toxicology I and II. Clin Lab Med 10: June and September, 1990.
  Two volumes, totaling 647 pages, extensively covering the field.
Giannini AJ, Miller NS: Drug abuse: A biopsychiatric model. Am Fam Physician 40:173, 1989.
  Explains how different drugs exert their effects and provides a rationale for intervention.
Gilbert S: Doctors found to fail in diagnosing addictions. The New York Times, February 14, 1996, p B9.
  Most doctors fail to ask patients about their alcohol and drug habits.
Haverkos HW, Stein MD: Identifying substance abuse in primary care. Am Fam Physician 52:2029, 1995.
  Suggests a strategy for detecting drug abuse in primary-care patients.

McNagny SE, Parker RM: High prevalence of recent cocaine use and the unreliability of patient self-report in an inner-city walk-in clinic. JAMA 267:1106, 1992.
Cocaine abuse continues in epidemic proportions throughout the United States.

Moyer TP, Palmen MA, Johnson P, et al: Marijuana testing: How good is it? Mayo Clin Proc 62:413, 1987.
Demonstrates the accuracy of properly performed drug tests for marijuana.

Rost K, Burnam MA, Smith GR: Development of screeners for depressive disorders and substance disorder history. Med Care 31:189, 1993.
Developed the Rost drug questionnaire.

Samet JH, Rollnick S, Barnes H: Beyond CAGE: A brief clinical approach after detection of substance abuse. Arch Intern Med 156:2287, 1996.
Suggests a clinical approach for the management of patients with an alcohol or drug abuse problem.

Saxon AJ, Calsyn DA, Haver VM, et al: Clinical evaluation and use of urine screening for drug abuse. West J Med 149:296, 1988.
Good overview of detecting drug abuse.

Spivak JL: Medical complications of opiate and cocaine use. *In* Spivak JL, Barnes HV (eds): Manual of Clinical Problems in Internal Medicine, 4th ed. Boston, Little, Brown & Co, 1990, p 537.
Focuses on effects of opiates and cocaine and includes annotated key references.

Zwerling C, Ryan J, Orav EJ: Costs and benefits of preemployment drug screening. JAMA 267:91, 1992.
Presents a method for analyzing the costs and benefits of a pre-employment drug screening program.

HEMOCHROMATOSIS

Recommendations for hemochromatosis are from the College of American Pathologists.

1. Consider screening adults for hemochromatosis using fasting serum transferrin saturation—measure serum iron, transferrin, and percent transferrin saturation. If the transferrin saturation is greater than 60%, repeat the measurement using a fasting sample following an overnight fast. If the repeat transferrin saturation is greater than 60%, measure serum ferritin.

Approximately 3 to 5 persons of European descent per 1000 are homozygous for hemochromatosis, and the carrier frequency is 1 in 10 to 1 in 15. African-Americans are affected less frequently. Increasingly, individuals with hemochromatosis are being discovered with few or no clinical findings. Iron overload may be due to hereditary hemochromatosis or secondary to other causes such as ineffective erythropoiesis (e.g., β-thalassemia, sideroblastic anemia, aplastic anemia), in which iron absorption is increased and transfusions are frequent; chronic liver disease (e.g., alcoholic cirrhosis, conditions secondary to portacaval anastomosis, porphyria cutanea tarda); or ingestion of excessive iron. Hereditary hemochromatosis is caused by an abnormal gene on the short arm of chromosome 6, closely linked to the HLA-A locus. Recently, a new non–HLA-linked iron overload syndrome has been described in which transferrin saturation is normal. Increased iron (ferritin > 200 ng/mL [200 µg/L]) has been implicated as a risk factor for coronary heart disease.

Excessive iron deposits in the heart, liver, pancreas, adrenal glands, pituitary, hypothalamus, and joints result in congestive heart failure, arrhythmias, cirrhosis, hepatocellular carcinoma, insulin-dependent diabetes, hypogonadism, hypoaldosteronism, arthralgia, and arthritis. The disease is underdiagnosed because of lack of consideration, lack of recognition, confusion with other diseases, minimal clinical findings, and incomplete phenotypic expression of the hereditary variety in some persons. Although expert clinicians skilled in the clinical findings of hemochromatosis may identify these patients, many patients risk not being diagnosed except by laboratory tests. The tragedy of missed diagnosis is that these patients are treatable by therapeutic phlebotomy. Individuals with hemochromatosis are at risk for infections with iron-using bacteria such as *Yersinia enterocolitica*, *Pasteurella pseudotuberculosis*, and *Vibrio vulnificus* (from eating raw oysters).

2. Interpret test results in the context of clinical findings.

If serum ferritin exceeds 400 ng/mL (400 µg/L) in men or postmenopausal women or 200 ng/mL (200 µg/L) in premenopausal women, further evaluation is indicated. Elevated serum ferritin levels should be interpreted in the context of other conditions, which can increase serum ferritin, such as chronic inflammation, hyperthyroidism, or malignancy. Additional disorders include alcohol-related liver disease and Gaucher's disease. A high serum ferritin is not equivalent to a diagnosis of hemochromatosis. Finding a serum ferritin of 1,000 ng/mL (≥1000 µg/L) or greater is associated with liver disease, renal disease, immunodeficiency virus infections, malignancies, chronic transfusion, and sickle cell syndromes.

The "gold standard" for diagnosis has been demonstration of excessive iron deposits in liver tissue obtained by biopsy. Hepatic concentration of iron ranging from 200 to 800 µmol/g dry weight correlates with hemochromatosis (normal, <35 µmol/g). Patients with alcoholic siderosis have hepatic content ranging from 40 to 100 µmol/g. One can also calculate the hepatic iron index (hepatic iron content in µmol/g divided by age in years); the value is usually greater than 2 in homozygotes and less than 2 in patients with alcoholic siderosis.

Recently, a DNA-based test has become available for the screening and diagnosis of hereditary hemochromatosis.

3. Monitor therapeutic phlebotomy for hemochromatosis using serial determinations of blood hemoglobin and serum iron and ferritin.

Therapeutic phlebotomy—at least weekly—should be continued until the hemoglobin level decreases and the serum iron and the serum ferritin levels fall to less than 20 ng/mL (<20 µg/L).

4. In individuals with hemochromatosis the following blood test results may be increased:

- Glucose
- Transaminase
- Thyrotropin

5. In individuals with hemochromatosis, the following blood test results may be decreased:

- Platelets
- Thyroxine
- Testosterone
- Follicle-stimulating hormone and luteinizing hormone

BIBLIOGRAPHY

Adams PC, Kertsez AE, Valberg LS: Clinical presentation of hemochromatosis: A changing scene. Am J Med 90:445, 1991.
Clinical findings of hemochromatosis are very subtle. A high index of suspicion is necessary.
Bacon BR: Causes of iron overload. N Engl J Med 326:126, 1992.
Discusses the spectrum of iron overload diseases.
Baer DM, Simons JL, Staples RL, et al: Hemochromatosis screening in asymptomatic ambulatory men 30 years of age and older. Am J Med 98:464, 1995.
Supports the screening of white men aged 30 or older for hemochromatosis.
Balan V, Baldus W, Fairbanks V, et al: Screening for hemochromatosis: A cost-effectiveness study based on 12,258 patients. Gastroenterology 107:453, 1994.
Screening for hemochromatosis is cost-effective.
Bulaj ZJ, Griffen LM, Jorde LB, et al: Clinical and biochemical abnormalities in people heterozygous for hemochromatosis. N Engl J Med 335:1799, 1996.
Complications due to iron overload alone in these heterozygotes are extremely rare.
Bullen JJ, Spalding PB, Ward CG, et al: Hemochromatosis, iron, and septicemia caused by *Vibrio vulnificus.* Arch Intern Med 151:1606, 1991.
The organism thrives in a high-iron environment.
Dale DC, Federman DD (eds): Distinguishing hemochromatosis from alcoholic siderosis. Sci Am Med Bull 20:7, 1997.
Discusses the hepatic iron values diagnostic for hemochromatosis.
Delfino M: Serum ferritin in hyperthyroidism. Ann Intern Med 119:249, 1993.
Serum ferritin values are elevated in hyperthyroidism.
Dooley J, Walker AP, Macfarlane B, et al: Genetic haemochromatosis. Lancet 349:1688, 1997.
Reviews the diagnosis and management of hemochromatosis.
Edwards CQ, Kushner JP: Screening for hemochromatosis. N Engl J Med 328:1616, 1993.
Recommends a protocol for hemochromatosis screening and treatment.
Fargion S, Mandelli C, Piperno A, et al: Survival and prognostic factors in 212 Italian patients with genetic hemochromatosis. Hepatology 15:655, 1992.
Patients treated by phlebotomy before developing cirrhosis had normal survival.
George PM, Conaghan C, Angus HB, et al: Comparison of histological and biochemical hepatic iron indexes in the diagnosis of genetic hemochromatosis. J Clin Pathol 49:159, 1996.
Biochemical hepatic iron is more accurate than histology for diagnosing hemochromatosis.
Lee MH, Means RT Jr: Extremely elevated serum ferritin levels in a university hospital: Associated diseases and clinical significance. Am J Med 98:566, 1995.
Discusses the significance of very high serum ferritin without iron overload.

Little DS: Hemochromatosis: Diagnosis and management. Am Fam Physician 53:2623, 1996.
Screening is recommended in affected families, and screening programs for wider populations are being evaluated.

Moirand R, Mortaji AM, Loréal O, et al: A new syndrome of liver iron overload with normal transferrin saturation. Lancet 349:95, 1997.
Describes a new, non–HLA-linked iron overload syndrome in which transferrin saturation is normal and there is close association with various metabolic disorders.

Powell LW, Jazwinska EC: Hemochromatosis in heterozygotes. N Engl J Med 335:1837, 1996.
Hemochromatosis is among the most common inherited diseases in individuals of European descent.

Rouault TA: Hereditary hemochromatosis. JAMA 269:3152, 1993.
Good discussion of diagnosis and treatment of patients with hemochromatosis.

Salonen JT, Nyyssönen K, Korpela H, et al: High stored iron levels are associated with excess risk of myocardial infarction in Eastern Finnish men. Circulation 86:803, 1992.
Reports a correlation between high iron levels and increased risk of acute myocardial infarction.

Sheeny TW: Hemochromatosis: Early recognition of the hallmark features. Mod Med 60:61, 1992.
Suspicion is the key to early diagnosis of the disease.

Stipp D: Is Popeye doomed? Some experts sound warnings about ingesting too much iron. Wall Street Journal, January 17, 1992, p B1.
Warns that increasing iron supplementation of food is potentially dangerous for patients at risk for hemochromatosis.

Weintraub LR: The many faces of hemochromatosis. Hosp Pract 26:49, 1991.
Discusses the diagnosis and management of hemochromatosis.

CANCER SCREENING

Recommendations for cancer screening are from the American Cancer Society. These guidelines are more aggressive than those of the U.S. Preventive Services Task Force and others. Some areas of controversy include the use of annual prostate-specific antigen (PSA) testing for prostate cancer for men age 50 and over and mammography for breast cancer for women in their 40s. The National Cancer Institute, the American Medical Association, and the American College of Radiology have recently decided to support mammography for women in their 40s.

1. In wellness screening, consider following the American Cancer Society recommendations for the early detection of cancer in asymptomatic people.

Some cancer screening guidelines are controversial. Although consensus exists concerning the use of the Pap test for cervical cancer, disagreement remains about the use of PSA for prostate cancer screening and mammography for breast cancer screening in women in their 40s. Recently, support has been increasing for the American Cancer Society recommendation to offer mammography to women in their 40s. For colorectal cancer, some consensus exists regarding the use of fecal occult blood testing and sigmoidoscopy, but disagreement continues about the role of the digital rectal examination. Moreover, some experts have even recommended colonoscopy as the ultimate detection study for colorectal cancer.

SUMMARY OF AMERICAN CANCER SOCIETY RECOMMENDATIONS FOR THE EARLY DETECTION OF CANCER IN ASYMPTOMATIC PEOPLE

Site	Recommendation
Cancer-related checkup	A cancer-related checkup is recommended every 3 years for people age 20–40 and every year for people age 40 and older. This examination should include health counseling; and depending on a person's age, might include examinations for cancers of the thyroid, oral cavity, skin, lymph nodes, testes, and ovaries, as well as for some nonmalignant diseases.
Breast	Women 40 and older should have an annual mammogram and clinical breast exam (CBE) performed by a health care professional and should perform monthly breast self-examination. The CBE should be conducted close to the scheduled mammogram. Women ages 20–39 should have a CBE performed by a health care professional every 3 years and should perform monthly breast self-examination.
Colon and Rectum	Men and women age 50 or older should follow **one** of these examination schedules: • A fecal occult blood test every year and a flexible sigmoidoscopy every 5 years.* • A colonoscopy every 10 years.* • A double-contrast barium enema every 5 to 10 years.* *A digital rectal examination should be done at the same time as sigmoidoscopy, colonoscopy, or double-contrast barium enema. People who are at moderate or high risk for colorectal cancer should talk with a doctor about a different testing schedule.
Prostate	The American Cancer Society recommends that both the PSA blood test and the digital rectal examination be offered annually, beginning at age 50, to men who have a life expectancy of at least 10 years and to younger men who are at high risk. Men in high-risk groups, such as those with a strong familial predisposition (e.g., two or more affected first-degree relatives), or African Americans may begin at a younger age (e.g., 45 years).
Uterus	• Cervix: All women who are or have been sexually active or who are 18 and older should have an annual Pap test and pelvic examination. After three or more consecutive satisfactory examinations with normal

Table continued on following page

SUMMARY OF AMERICAN CANCER SOCIETY RECOMMENDATIONS
FOR THE EARLY DETECTION OF CANCER IN
ASYMPTOMATIC PEOPLE *Continued*

Site	Recommendation
Uterus	findings, the Pap test may be performed less frequently. Discuss the matter with your physician. • Endometrium: Women at high risk for cancer of the uterus should have a sample of endometrial tissue examined when menopause begins.

Source: Cancer Facts & Figures, 1998. Reprinted by permission of the American Cancer Society, Inc.

2. For additional information, see discussions of the Pap test and cervical cancer; occult fecal blood testing and colorectal cancer; and digital rectal examination, prostate-specific antigen, and prostate cancer elsewhere in this chapter.

BIBLIOGRAPHY

American College of Physicians: Screening for ovarian cancer: Recommendations and rationale. Ann Intern Med 121:141, 1994.
Carlson KJ, Skates SJ, Singer DE: Screening for ovarian cancer. Ann Intern Med 121:124, 1994.
Doesn't recommend general screening with ultrasonography or CA 125.
Bhattacharya I, Sack EM: Screening colonoscopy: The cost of common sense. Lancet 347:1744, 1996.
Advocates colonoscopy as the most sensitive screening procedure for colorectal cancer.
Brett AS: The mammography and prostate-specific antigen controversies: Implications for patient-physician encounters and public policy. J Gen Intern Med 10:266, 1995.
Analyzes the implications of the mammography and PSA controversies for the patient-physician encounter and public policy.
Czaja R, McFall SL, Warnecke RB, et al: Preferences of community physicians for cancer screening guidelines. Ann Intern Med 120:602, 1994.
Many physicians favor more aggressive screenings for cancer than are recommended by major advisory groups.
Einhorn N, Sjövall K, Knapp RC, et al: Prospective evaluation of serum CA 125 levels for early detection of ovarian cancer. Obstet Gynecol 80:14, 1992.
CA 125 screening for ovarian cancer is not recommended.
Fletcher SW: Whither scientific deliberation in health policy recommendations? N Engl J Med 336:1180, 1997.
Discusses the controversy about guidelines for mammography for women in their 40s.
Helzsouer KJ, Bush TL, Alberg AJ, et al: Prospective study of serum CA 125 levels as markers of ovarian cancer. JAMA 269:1123, 1993.
Serum CA 125 testing by itself is not useful for detecting ovarian cancer.
Jacobs I, Davies AP, Bridges J, et al: Prevalence screening for ovarian cancer in post-menopausal women by CA 125 measurement and ultrasonography. BMJ 306:1030, 1993.
Measuring serum CA 125 in postmenopausal women can detect early-stage ovarian cancer. The impact on mortality needs further study.

Kolata G: Another group's reversal on mammogram frequency. The New York Times, March 28, 1997, p A15.

The National Cancer Institute said that women in their 40s should have breast mammography every 1 or 2 years.

Mettlin C, Smart CR: Breast cancer detection guidelines for women aged 40 to 49 years: Rationale for the American Cancer Society reaffirmation of recommendations. CA Cancer J Clin 44:248, 1994.

Available data do not exclude a benefit for screening mammography for women under 50.

Meyers FJ: Screening for cancer: Is it worth it? West J Med 163:166, 1995.

McPhee SJ: Screening for cancer: Useful despite its limitations. West J Med 163:169, 1995.

Discusses the pros and cons of cancer screening.

Schapira MM, Matchar DB, Young MJ: The effectiveness of ovarian cancer screening: A decision analysis model. Ann Intern Med 118:838, 1993.

Routine screening for ovarian cancer using serum CA 125 and transvaginal sonography is not recommended.

Smart CR, Hendrick RE, Rutledge JH, et al: Benefit of mammography screening in women ages 40 to 49 years: Current evidence from randomized controlled trials. Cancer 75:1619, 1995.

Harris R, Leininger L: Clinical strategies for breast cancer screening: Weighing and using the evidence. Ann Intern Med 122:539, 1995.

Sickles EA, Kopans DB: Mammographic screening for women aged 40 to 49 years: The primary care practitioner's dilemma. Ann Intern Med 122:534, 1995.

Sox HC Jr: Screening mammography in women younger than 50 years of age. Ann Intern Med 122:550, 1995.

Mammographic screening is beginning to look beneficial for 40- to 49-year-old women.

Stacey-Clear A, McCarthy KA, Hall DA, et al: Breast cancer survival among women under age 50: Is mammography detrimental? Lancet 340:991, 1992.

Mammography may benefit women under 50.

Trends in cancer screening—United States, 1987 and 1992. MMWR 45:57, 1995.

Screening rates lag behind the national goals.

2

General and Miscellaneous Problems

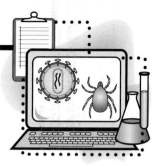

- Human Immunodeficiency Virus Infection and AIDS
- Lyme Disease
- Sexually Transmitted Disease
- Acute Food Poisoning
- Cerebrospinal Fluid Analysis
- Synovial Fluid Analysis
- Arthritis

HUMAN IMMUNODEFICIENCY VIRUS INFECTION AND AIDS

Recommendations for human immunodeficiency virus infection (HIV) and acquired immunodeficiency syndrome (AIDS) are from the medical literature. The Centers for Disease Control and Prevention and other medical groups recommend HIV testing for persons at increased risk.

1. For patients with clinical findings of AIDS or to screen for infection with HIV in persons at increased risk, request an enzyme-linked immunosorbent assay (ELISA) for HIV antibodies and confirm positive test results with a Western blot analysis, which identifies antibodies to specific viral proteins.

In the United States more than 500,000 individuals have acquired AIDS, and 62% of these have died. Worldwide, about 1.3 million people have AIDS and 21 million adults are infected with the virus—about 42% are women. At least several million children are infected. Without treatment, AIDS occurs approximately 10 years after the initial infection, and death usually ensues approximately 2 years after the development of AIDS. Women and older people who become infected with HIV develop AIDS sooner than young men.

There are two HIV viruses: HIV-1 and HIV-2. The main agent is HIV-1. HIV-1 is transmitted by intimate sexual contact, by blood-borne contamination, and vertically from mother to child. The risk of acquiring HIV-1 after receiving one unit of blood is about 1 in 500,000. Primary infection with HIV ranges from asymptomatic seroconversion to a severe symptomatic illness resembling infectious mononucleosis that can result in hospitalization.

2. Evaluate the tests.

Currently HIV infection is detected by a positive ELISA test and is confirmed by a positive Western blot analysis. At the Ohio State University Medical Center we use an ELISA test that detects HIV-1 and HIV-2 antibodies and a Western blot confirmation test that detects HIV-1 antibodies. A person is classified and notified as being HIV-1 seropositive only after blood sample test results are positive in three tests—two successive ELISAs and one confirmatory Western blot. Because antibodies may not appear in the serum for at least 6 weeks, other techniques are required to diagnose acute infection. Of these techniques, the p24 antigen test is widely used. Although it is specific, it is not considered to be completely sensitive; that is, a negative test result does not preclude the possibility of infection with HIV-1. Also, a rapid serum test to detect antibodies to HIV-1 is now available (Single Use Diagnostic System [SUDS] HIV-1, Murex Corporation).

In addition to standard HIV clinical laboratory tests, there are a variety of different in-home HIV-testing systems.

- Home-test kits using finger-stick blood (Confide from Johnson & Johnson or Home Access from Home Access Health Corporation)
- Home-test kit using oral secretions (OraSure HIV-1 Oral Specimen Collection Device from Epitope, Inc.)
- Home-test kit using urine (Sentinel HIV-1 Urine EIA from Seradyn, Inc.)

The home blood tests are generally accurate, but the "gold standard" is two successive clinical laboratory ELISA tests followed by a confirmatory positive Western blot test.

3. If the ELISA test and Western blot analysis are positive, consider the patient to be infected with HIV. Do not diagnose HIV infection solely on the basis of a positive ELISA test.

The sensitivity and specificity of the ELISA test is greater than 98%. When persons come from a clinical class with a low prevalence of HIV infection, false-positive results are more likely to occur. To exclude false-positive results, every positive ELISA test should be confirmed by a second ELISA test and a Western blot analysis. Indeterminant Western blot tests should be repeated monthly. Indeterminant patterns fall into three categories: (1) those in the early stages of HIV-1 infection; (2) those infected with a closely related retrovirus, HIV-2; and (3) truly false-positive results, that is, healthy people who are not infected with HIV-1. If the diagnosis is in doubt, other tests are available, such as the polymerase chain reaction (PCR).

4. If the ELISA test is negative, conclude that the patient is probably, but not necessarily, free of HIV infection.

With the ELISA test, occasional persons infected with HIV are negative for the antibody. There is a period of 6 to 8 weeks (sometimes up to 1 year or more) during a primary HIV infection when an HIV-infected person is seronegative. Some of these patients may have an acute febrile illness resembling influenza or infectious mononucleosis. When the suspicion for infection is high, the ELISA test should be repeated periodically for at least 1 year.

Patients with a variety of other diseases may have "AIDS-like" clinical findings, including abnormal laboratory test results such as depressed helper/suppressor T-cell ratios and polyclonal gammopathy. Do not automatically conclude that these patients are infected with HIV. If they are seronegative, they probably are not infected.

5. In patients with HIV infection, measure plasma HIV-1 ribonucleic acid (RNA) concentration and CD4 lymphocytes at baseline and periodically thereafter to monitor the course of the disease. Request additional tests based on clinical findings.

Plasma HIV-1 RNA concentrations can be measured by three different techniques:

- PCR
- Branched DNA (bDNA)
- Nucleic acid sequence-based amplification (NASBA)

Quantification of HIV-1 RNA in plasma provides a measure of actual virus replication. HIV-1 RNA in plasma is contained within circulating virus particles or viruses, each virion containing two copies of HIV-1 genomic RNA.

A high level of correlation exists between the level of CD4 lymphocytes and the progress of the disease—the lower the count, the worse the prognosis. Although in the past the CD4 lymphocyte count was the "gold standard" for monitoring the disease, it appears that the quantitative plasma HIV-1 RNA concentration is an earlier and better marker. Further, it appears that the concentration may be decreased by appropriate drug therapy and that the reduced concentration may correlate with slowing the course of the disease.

Patients with viral copies greater than 100,000/mL within 6 months from seroconversion are 10 times more likely to progress to AIDS over a 5-year period than those with less than 100,000 copies/mL. Moreover, fewer than 30% of patients with less than 10,000 copies/mL died within 10 years, whereas more than 70% of those with more than 10,000 copies/mL progressed to AIDS and died in a 10-year period.

A suggested laboratory evaluation includes the following: complete blood count, platelet count, liver function studies, baseline chest radiograph, CD4T cell testing, plasma level of HIV-1 RNA, purified protein derivative skin testing with controls, *Toxoplasma gondii* serologic testing, cytomegalovirus serologic testing, hepatitis B virus serologic testing, and *Treponema pallidum* serologic testing.

The complications of HIV infection at various CD4 lymphocyte counts are as follows:

CD4 Cell Count	Complications
>500/μL (>500 × 10^6/L)	Acute retroviral syndrome,* *Candida* vaginitis, persistent generalized lymphadenopathy
200–500/μL (200–500 × 10^6/L)	Pneumococcal and other bacterial pneumonia,* tuberculosis (pulmonary),* herpes zoster,* thrush. *Candida* esophagitis, cryptosporidiosis (self-limited), B-cell lymphoma
<200/μL (<200 × 10^6/L)	*Pneumocystis carinii* pneumonia,* disseminated chronic herpes simplex infection,* toxoplasmosis,* cryptococcosis,* disseminated histoplasmosis and coccidioidomycosis,* cryptosporidiosis (chronic), microsporidiosis, tuberculosis (miliary/extrapulmonary)*
<50/μL (<50 × 10^6/L)	Disseminated cytomegalovirus infection,* disseminated *Mycobacterium avium* complex*

*Associated with fever.

Most complications occur with increased frequency at lower CD4 cell counts.

Source: Adapted from Sullivan M, Feinberg J, Bartlett JG: Fever in patients with HIV infection. Infect Dis Clin North Am 10:149, 1996.

6. In patients with HIV infection, the following blood test results may be increased:

- **Potassium** due to effect of pentamidine on renal tubule
- **Abnormal liver function tests**
- **Amylase** from the pancreas
- **Lactate dehydrogenase (LD)** with lung infections
- **Triglycerides**
- **Erythrocyte sedimentation rate**
- **Glucose**
- **Cortisol**
- **Gamma globulins** (IgG, IgA, IgM, IgD) and circulating immune complexes
- **Lupus anticoagulant**
- **Positive Venereal Disease Research Laboratory (VDRL) test**— some may be false positive

7. In patients with HIV infection, the following blood test results may be decreased:

- **Hemoglobin and hematocrit** due to normochromic, normocytic anemia

- **Leukocytes** and decreased lymphocytes with decreased CD4 lymphocytes
- **Cholesterol**
- **Cortisol and aldosterone** due to primary adrenocortical insufficiency
- **Platelets,** either immune thrombocytopenic purpura or thrombotic thrombocytopenic purpura
- **Glucose**
- **Sodium** in up to 50% of hospitalized patients and 20% of ambulatory patients
- **Blastogenesis** (phytohemagglutinin or con A)
- **Vitamin B$_{12}$**

8. In patients with HIV infection with neurologic disorders, the following cerebrospinal fluid results may be increased:

- **Lymphocytes**
- **Protein**

HIV infection often involves the central nervous system (CNS), causing dementia in 40 to 60% of patients—usually those in advanced stages. An associated encephalitis may be present. CNS mass lesions may also occur in decreasing order of frequency as follows: toxoplasmosis, primary lymphoma, progressive multifocal leukoencephalopathy, other opportunistic infections, and cerebral infarctions. HIV-positive patients should be evaluated for neurosyphilis.

BIBLIOGRAPHY

Bayer R: Home testing for HIV: Has its time come? Patient Care 29:66, 1995.
   Discusses the potential role of home HIV testing.
Binderow SR, Cavallo RJ, Freed J: Laboratory parameters as predictors of operative outcome after major abdominal surgery in AIDS- and HIV-infected patients. Am Surg 59:754, 1993.
   Low serum albumin predicts poor operative outcome in HIV-infected patients.
Chalmers AC, Aprill BS, Shephard H: Cerebrospinal fluid and human immunodeficiency virus: Findings in healthy, asymptomatic, seropositive men. Arch Intern Med 150:1538, 1990.
   Even asymptomatic HIV-positive persons may show CSF pleocytosis, high protein levels, oligoclonal bands, and positive HIV culture.
Charache P, Cameron JL, Maters AW, et al: Prevalence of infection with human immunodeficiency virus in elective surgery patients. Ann Surg 214:562, 1991.
   Does not support screening before elective surgery.
Coodley GO, Coodley MK, Thompson AF: Clinical aspects of HIV infection in women. J Gen Intern Med 10:99, 1995.
   Reviews the similarities and differences of HIV infection in women versus men.
Cordes RJ, Ryan ME: Pitfalls in HIV testing: Application and limitations of current tests. Postgrad Med 98:177, 1995.
   Delineates the causes of false-positive, false-negative, and indeterminant HIV tests by ELISA and Western blot.
Craven DE, Steger KA, La Chapelle R, et al: Factitious HIV infection: The importance of documenting infection. Ann Intern Med 121:763, 1994.

The lesson is clear: Providers should document HIV positivity unequivocally before initiating treatment.

Darby SC, Ewart DW, Giangrande PLF, et al: Importance of age at infection with HIV-1 for survival and development of AIDS in UK haemophilia population. Lancet 347:1573, 1996.

Older people who become infected with HIV-1 develop AIDS sooner than younger patients.

De La Maza LM: Determining the number of copies of HIV-1 RNA in plasma: Applying this new test to management of patients. West J Med 167:35, 1997.

Gives prognostic information based on the number of viral copies per milliliter at baseline.

Feinberg MB: Changing the natural history of HIV disease. Lancet 348:239, 1996.

Discusses the impact of quantifying plasma HIV-1 RNA levels on choosing better therapies to contain and perhaps eliminate the infection.

Frank AP, Wandell MG, Headings MD, et al: Anonymous HIV testing using home collection and telemedicine counseling. Arch Intern Med 157:309, 1997.

Stryker J, Coates TJ: Home access HIV testing: What took so long? Arch Intern Med 157:261, 1997.

Home HIV testing proves accurate.

Freedberg KA, Malabanan A, Samet JH, et al: Initial assessment of patients infected with human immunodeficiency virus: The yield and cost of laboratory testing. J Acquir Immune Defic Syndr 7:1134, 1994.

Describes a panel of laboratory tests useful for assessing patients infected with HIV.

Gallo D, George JR, Fitchen JH, et al: Evaluation of a system using oral mucosal transudate for HIV-1 antibody screening and confirmatory testing. JAMA 277:254, 1997.

Overall, using oral secretions, the system correctly identified the presence of HIV antibodies in 99.9% of infected participants.

Grinspoon SK, Bilezikian JP: HIV disease and the endocrine system. N Engl J Med 327:1360, 1992.

Adrenal insufficiency is the most important abnormality, but a number of other abnormalities may occur.

Hughes MD, Stein DS, Gundacker HM, et al: Within-subject variation in CD4 lymphocyte count in asymptomatic human immunodeficiency virus infection: Implications for patient monitoring. J Infect Dis 169:28, 1994.

At least two CD4 measurements are needed to determine a true CD4 count with confidence.

Irwin K, Olivo N, Schable CA, et al: Performance characteristics of a rapid HIV antibody assay in a hospital with a high prevalence of HIV infection. Ann Intern Med 125:471, 1996.

The rapid enzyme assay (Genie HIV-1/HIV-2) done in the routine hospital laboratory was accurate for detecting HIV infection in an unselected hospital population.

Jacobson K, Jordan GW: Primary human immunodeficiency virus infection: Will you miss the diagnosis? West J Med 156:68, 1992.

Suggests an approach to diagnosing acute HIV infection.

Kassirer JP, Kopelman RL: Case 21—Interpreting negative test results, and Case 61—Learning clinical reasoning from examples. *In* Learning Clinical Reasoning. Baltimore, Williams & Wilkins, 1991, pp 130, 303.

Describes the clinical reasoning in two cases of patients with HIV infection.

Kleyman TR, Roberts C, Ling BN: A mechanism for pentamidine-induced hyperkalemia: Inhibition of distal nephron sodium transport. Ann Intern Med 122:103, 1995.

Because pentamidine is eliminated through urinary excretion, this renal tubular effect provides a mechanism for pentamidine-induced hyperkalemia.

Kreisberg R: We blew it. N Engl J Med 332:945, 1995.

Discusses the differential diagnosis of liver disease in a patient with AIDS.

Lackritz EM, Satten GA, Aberle-Grasse J, et al: Estimated risk of transmission of the human immunodeficiency virus by screened blood in the United States. N Engl J Med 333:1721, 1995.

Discusses transmission of HIV by transfused blood.

Landesman SH, Burns D: Quantifying HIV. JAMA 275:640, 1996.

Plasma HIV quantitative measurements may become important in managing HIV-positive patients.

Lipton SA, Gendelman HE: Dementia associated with the acquired immunodeficiency syndrome. N Engl J Med 332:934, 1995.
One third of adults and one half of children with AIDS have neurologic complications.

Mellors JW, Rinaldo CR Jr, Gupta P, et al: Prognosis in HIV-1 infection predicted by the quantity of virus in plasma. Science 272:1167, 1996.

Galetto-Lacour A, Yerly S, Perneger TV, et al: Prognostic value of viremia in patients with long-standing human immunodeficiency virus infection. J Infect Dis 173:1388, 1996.
Suggests that PCR measurement of plasma HIV RNA is a more powerful prognostic indicator than CD4 lymphocyte counts.

Melnick SL, Sherer R, Louis TA, et al: Survival and disease progression according to gender of patients with HIV infection: The Terry Beirn Community Programs for Clinical Research on AIDS. JAMA 272:1915, 1994.
Women have a greater risk of dying of HIV infection than do men.

Mocroft AJ, Johnson MA, Sabin CA, et al: Staging system for clinical AIDS patients. Lancet 346:12, 1995.
Suggests a staging system for managing AIDS patients.

Murthy UK, DeGregorio F, Oates RP, et al: Hyperamylasemia in patients with the acquired immunodeficiency syndrome. Am J Gastroenterol 87:332, 1992.
Pancreatic hyperamylasemia occurs frequently in AIDS patients.

Nuwayhid NF: Laboratory tests for detection of human immunodeficiency virus type 1 infection. Clin Diagn Lab Immunol 2:637, 1995.
Discusses the screening and confirmatory tests for detecting human immunodeficiency virus infection.

Owens DK, Holodniy M, Garber AM, et al: Polymerase chain reaction for the diagnosis of HIV infection in adults. Ann Intern Med 124:803, 1996.
The PCR assay is not sufficiently accurate to be used for the diagnosis of HIV infection without confirmation.

Owens DK, Nease RF Jr, Harris RA: Cost-effectiveness of HIV screening in acute care settings. Arch Intern Med 156:394, 1996.
Examines the cost and benefits of a voluntary HIV screening program in acute care settings.

Paltiel O, Falutz J, Veillieux M, et al: Clinical correlates of subnormal vitamin B_{12} levels in patients infected with human immunodeficiency virus. Am J Hematol 49:318, 1995.
Low serum vitamin B_{12} levels in HIV-positive patients.

Peckham C, Gibb D: Mother-to-child transmission of the human immunodeficiency virus. N Engl J Med 333:298, 1995.
If women and their infants are to benefit from current interventions, such as zidovudine treatment, and to receive optimal medical care, counseling and voluntary antenatal HIV testing must be encouraged and made more widely available.

Poznansky MC, Coker R, Skinner C, et al: HIV positive patients first presenting with an AIDS-defining illness: Characteristics and survival. BMJ 311:156, 1995.
Earlier detection of HIV infection may not prolong life.

Quinn TC: Global burden of the HIV pandemic. Lancet 348:99, 1996.
By the year 2000, the World Health Organization projections are that 26 million people will be infected with HIV, more than 90% of whom will be in developing countries.

Quist J, Hill AR: Serum lactate dehydrogenase in *Pneumocystis carinii* pneumonia, tuberculosis, and bacterial pneumonia. Chest 108:415, 1995.
Diagnostic value of serum lactate dehydrogenase in HIV-associated lung infections.

Schacker T, Collier AC, Hughes J, et al: Clinical and epidemiologic features of primary HIV infection. Ann Intern Med 125:257, 1996.
Primary HIV infection causes a recognizable clinical syndrome that is often underdiagnosed, even in persons enrolled in a program of routine surveillance for HIV infection.

Shor-Posner G, Basit A, Lu Y, et al: Hypocholesterolemia is associated with immune dysfunction in early human immunodeficiency virus-1 infection. Am J Med 94:515, 1993.
Low cholesterol as marker of disease progression in HIV-1 infection.

Update: HIV-2 infection among blood and plasma donors—United States, June 1992–June 1995. MMWR 44:603, 1995.
HIV-2 is still extremely rare in the United States but is now endemic in western Africa.

LYME DISEASE

Recommendations for Lyme disease are from the medical literature. The Centers for Disease Control and Prevention recommend a two-step testing algorithm.

1. In patients with clinical findings of Lyme disease, request a serum Lyme antibody test. Do not request this test in the absence of clinical findings.

Many infectious diseases are transmitted by ticks, including babesiosis, erlichiosis, Rocky Mountain spotted fever, tick paralysis, tularemia, and Lyme disease. Lyme disease is a multisystem disorder caused by the spirochete *Borrelia burgdorferi*, which is transmitted by tiny ixodid ticks. The size of the nymph tick form is 1 to 2 mm, and the adult tick is a little larger. More than 18,000 cases were reported in 1996, a 41% increase from 1995. Lyme disease typically occurs from May to August, and cases are concentrated in well-established areas in northeastern, north-central, and Pacific-coast states. Exposure exists when the patient was in an incidence area less than 30 days before the onset of erythema chronicum migrans (ECM); a history of tick bite is not essential. ECM is an enlarging annular rash with a red border and a clear center. Lyme disease has three stages:

Stage	Length	Symptoms
1	Lasting approximately 4 weeks	Flu-like illness or meningitis-like illness
2	Lasting days to months	Cardiac conduction disturbances and neurologic abnormalities
3	Lasting months to years	Chronic arthritis and chronic neurologic and skin abnormalities

The diagnosis of Lyme disease can be made either in the presence of ECM or with involvement of other organ systems and a history of exposure.

2. Evaluate the tests.

Establish the diagnosis using the ELISA or the immunofluoresence assay (IFA). In general, ELISA is preferable. All positive tests should be confirmed with a Western blot assay. Difficult cases may sometimes be diagnosed using the PCR on joint fluid. Usually not enough organisms are present in the blood to be detected by PCR.

3. A positive ELISA test and Western blot test establish the diagnosis of Lyme disease. A very small number of false positives in both assays may occur. The VDRL test, the rheumatoid factor test, and tests for antinuclear antibodies are usually negative.

Only 50% of the patients with early Lyme disease and ECM have positive serologic test results. Essentially 100% of patients with later disease and such complications as carditis, neuritis, and arthritis, as well as patients in remission, have positive serologic test results. It takes about 6 to 8 weeks following a tick bite for seroconversions to occur.

Sera from patients with other spirochetal diseases such as syphilis, yaws, pinta, leptospirosis, relapsing fever, periodontal disease, and some cases of HIV infection, infectious mononucleosis, rheumatic arthritis, and systemic lupus erythematosus may give false-positive ELISA results.

4. If the serologic test for Lyme disease is negative, rely on clinical findings to make the diagnosis.

Because a positive antibody response may not occur for weeks to several months after infection, some patients in the early stage of the disease may test negative. Patients with a negative test result and presumptive or clinical findings of Lyme disease should receive prompt antibiotic treatment without waiting for laboratory confirmation or convalescent specimens. Patients who have a compatible systemic illness without ECM or a known tick bite should have paired acute and convalescent serum samples tested. Seronegative Lyme disease has been reported.

5. In patients with Lyme disease, the following blood test results may be increased (especially in stage 1):

- **Erythrocyte sedimentation rate**—moderate
- **Total IgM.** Persistent increase is a predictor of later disease manifestations
- **Leukocyte count** with left shift in differential
- **Aspartate aminotransferase** in patients with prominent systemic symptoms, generally returning to normal several weeks after disease onset

6. In patients with Lyme disease, the following abnormal urine test results may occur:

- **Transient microscopic hematuria and mild proteinuria** in a few patients. Renal function usually is normal

7. In patients with Lyme disease with meningitis, the following abnormal cerebrospinal fluid (CSF) test results may occur:

- **IgM and IgG antibodies** to *B. burgdorferi* in the CSF
- **Normal to low glucose**

- **Increased cells,** 25 to 450/μL (25 to 450 cells × 10^6/L), mostly lymphocytes
- **Normal to high protein**

8. In patients with Lyme disease with arthritis, the following synovial fluid test results may occur:

- **Increased cells,** 500 to 110,000/μL (500 to 110,000 × 10^6/L), of which most are polymorphonuclear leukocytes
- **Biopsy findings** of fibrin deposits, synovial hypertrophy, vascular proliferation, and marked infiltration by lymphocytes and plasma cells
- **Protein,** 3 to 6 g/dL (30 to 60 g/L)

BIBLIOGRAPHY

Aguero-Rosenfeld ME, Horowitz HW, Wormser GP, et al: Human granulocytic ehrlichiosis: A case series from a medical center in New York state. Ann Intern Med 125:904, 1996. *The illness associated with human granulocytic ehrlichiosis in these patients from the northeastern United States was milder than that originally described in reports from the midwestern United States.*

Barron J: A plan to eliminate Lyme disease. The New York Times, July 29, 1997, p A14. *A significant increase in the number of cases of Lyme disease from 1995 to 1996.*

Centers for Disease Control: Lyme Disease—United States, 1994. JAMA 274:111, 1995. *Reviews statistics for Lyme disease.*

Centers for Disease Control: Recommendations for test performance and interpretation from the second national conference on serologic diagnosis of Lyme disease. MMWR 44:590, 1995.
    Association of State and Territorial Public Health Laboratory Directors and the Centers for Disease Control—Recommendations. *In* Proceedings of the Second National Conference on Serologic Diagnosis of Lyme Disease (Dearborn, MI). Washington, DC, Association of State and Territorial Public Health Laboratory Directors, 1995, pp 1–5.
    Still MM, Ryan ME: Pitfalls in diagnosis of Lyme disease: What you need to know about serologic testing. Postgrad Med 102:65, 1997. *The Centers for Disease Control and Prevention–sponsored conference recommends using a two-step testing algorithm to diagnose Lyme disease. The first test is an ELISA test, which, if positive, should be confirmed by a second test, a Western blot test.*

Conaty SM, Dattwyler RJ: Lyme disease: 10 questions physicians often ask. Consultant 36:2252, 1996. *All specimens submitted for testing should be evaluated in two steps: If results of ELISA or IFA testing are negative, no further testing is needed. If results are borderline or positive, Western blot analysis is needed to confirm the diagnosis.*

Kalish R, Persing DH, Segreti J, et al: How to recognize and treat tick-borne infections. Patient Care 31:184, 1997. *Practical discussion of the diagnosis and management of tick-borne infections.*

Ley C, Davila IH, Mayer NM, et al: Lyme disease in northwestern coastal California. West J Med 160:534, 1994. *It appears that Lyme disease is being overdiagnosed in this area.*

Lyme disease—United States, 1994. MMWR 44:459, 1995. *The incidence of Lyme disease was up in 1994.*

Rahn DW, Malawista SE: Lyme disease. West J Med 154:706, 1991. *Excellent general review of Lyme disease.*

Rees DHE, O'Connell S, Brown MM, et al: The value of serological testing for Lyme disease in the United Kingdom. Br J Rheumatol 34:132, 1995. *The ELISA test is a useful screening test, but its lack of specificity requires using immunoblot to confirm positive results.*

Sigal LH: The Lyme disease controversy. Arch Intern Med 156:1493, 1996.

The financial cost of the overdiagnosis and overtreatment of Lyme disease includes expenses related to testing and therapy and those of side effects and toxic effects of these treatments.

Sigal LH: Summary of the first 100 patients seen at a Lyme disease referral center. Am J Med 88:577, 1990.

Reports that of the first 100 patients referred to the Lyme Disease Center, only 37 had Lyme disease. Approximately half of the 91 courses of antibiotic therapy were probably unwarranted.

Steere AC: Lyme disease. N Engl J Med 321:586, 1989.

Thorough review of Lyme disease by the investigator who first detected it.

Steere AC, Taylor E, McHugh GL, et al: The overdiagnosis of Lyme disease. JAMA 269:1812, 1993.

Lyme disease is often overdiagnosed in patients with chronic malaise or myalgia.

Tick paralysis—Washington, 1995. MMWR 45:325, 1996.

The symptoms of tick paralysis begin after an embedded tick has fed for several days.

Vartiovaara I: Living with Lyme. Lancet 345:842, 1995.

A tragic story of failure to diagnose Lyme disease.

Verdon ME, Sigal LH: Recognition and management of Lyme disease. Am Fam Physician 56:427, 1997.

Lyme disease is a clinical diagnosis, and laboratory tests should be used only to clarify diagnostic issues. The current standard for laboratory diagnosis includes a two-step approach using an initial immunoassay with a confirmatory Western blot test.

Weinstein RS: Human ehrlichiosis. Am Fam Physician 100:1971, 1996.

Human monocytic ehrlichiosis is caused by Ehrlichia chaffeensis. *Human granulocytic ehrlichiosis is caused by an organism closely related to* Ehrlichia equi.

Wormser GP: A vaccine against Lyme disease? Ann Intern Med 123:627, 1995.

Prevention may soon be possible.

Zoschke DC: Is it Lyme disease? How to interpret results of laboratory testing. Postgrad Med 91:46, 1992.

Guidelines for resolving problems with currently available tests.

SEXUALLY TRANSMITTED DISEASE

Recommendations for sexually transmitted disease (STD) are from the medical literature. The Centers for Disease Control and Prevention (CDC) and other medical groups recommend testing for syphilis for pregnant women and syphilis and gonorrhea for persons at increased risk.

1. For patients with clinical findings of STD, perform appropriate tests, depending on the type of lesion. Regardless of the specific STD, consider screening for HIV with an ELISA test and for syphilis with either a VDRL test or an RPR test.

STD represents about 85% of the infectious diseases reported to the CDC. The annual incidence of selected STDs in 1994 is staggering.

STD	Cases
Chlamydia	4 million
Trichomoniasis	3 million
Pelvic inflammatory disease	1 million
Gonorrhea	800,000
Human papillomavirus	500,000–1 million

Table continued on following page

STD	Cases
Genital herpes	200,000–500,000
Syphilis	100,000
Acquired immunodeficiency syndrome	80,000
Hepatitis B	53,000
Chancroid	3,500
Congenital syphilis	3,400

Source: Adapted with permission from The Hidden Epidemic: Confronting Sexually Transmitted Diseases. Copyright 1997 by the National Academy of Sciences. Courtesy of the National Academy Press, Washington, D.C.

Several authorities recommend against general wellness screening for STDs but endorse selective wellness screening for individuals at increased risk. Physicians should be more proactive in taking sexual histories. HIV and syphilis counseling and testing for persons with STD are important parts of an HIV prevention program because patients who have acquired an STD have demonstrated the potential risk for acquiring HIV and syphilis. A positive HIV ELISA test should be repeated and confirmed with a Western blot test. A positive VDRL or RPR (nontreponemal) test should be confirmed with a treponemal test—either the microhemoagglutination *Treponema pallidum* assay or the fluorescent treponemal-antibody absorption test. Although the VDRL and RPR tests are equally valid, RPR titers are not equivalent to VDRL titers and are often slightly higher than VDRL titers. Both the VDRL and RPR tests can be carried out as qualitative and quantitative procedures; however, the titers are not interchangeable. Although there are many infectious and noninfectious causes for false-positive VDRL and RPR tests, only a small number cause false-positive treponemal tests (i.e., Lyme disease, leprosy, malaria, infectious mononucleosis, relapsing fever, leptospirosis, systemic lupus erythematosus). Both non-treponemal and treponemal tests may become negative after treatment; thus, negative test results do not necessarily exclude past syphilis infection.

2. In patients with genital ulcers or regional lymphadenopathy, consider the following:

Diseases/Agents	Clinical Findings	Tests
Herpes simplex virus infection	Painful, multiple, superficial ulcers; early lesions are vesicular	Tzanck smear and culture for herpes simplex virus
Syphilis	Painless, clean-based, indurated ulcer with painless regional lymphadenopathy	Darkfield examination, serology

Diseases/Agents	Clinical Findings	Tests
Chancroid	Painful, often multiple genital ulcers with painful inguinal lymphadenopathy	Smear and culture
Granuloma inguinale	Mildly painful ulcer that follows a painless papule	Smear, biopsy
Lymphogranuloma venereum	Small papular lesion	Serology, biopsy

3. In patients with lesions affecting epithelial surfaces, consider the following:

Diseases/Agents	Clinical Findings	Tests
Gonococcal infections	Urethritis and/or pelvic inflammatory disease	Culture, DNA probe, ligase chain reaction
Chlamydial infections	Urethritis and/or pelvic inflammatory disease	Culture, DNA probe, ligase chain reaction
Genital warts	Exophytic genital and anal warts	Human papillomavirus tests and biopsy of atypical, pigmented, or persistent lesions

4. In patients with findings suggestive of bacterial STD syndromes, consider the following:

Agents	Clinical Findings	Tests
Chlamydia trachomatis, Ureaplasma urealyticum, Trichomonas vaginalis, and herpes simplex virus	Nongonococcal urethritis	Culture, DNA probe, ligase chain reaction for *C. trachomatis* Tzanck smear and culture for herpes simplex virus Wet mount for *T. vaginalis*

Table continued on following page

Agents	Clinical Findings	Tests
Neisseria gonorrhoeae, C. trachomatis, T. vaginalis, herpes simplex, and HPV	Mucopurulent cervicitis	Culture, DNA probe, ligase chain reaction for *N. gonorrhoea* and *C. trachomatis*
N. gonorrhoeae and *C. trachomatis*	Epididymitis	
N. gonorrhoeae, C. trachomatis, anaerobes, gram-negative rods, streptococci, *Mycoplasma,* and *Ureaplasma*	Pelvic inflammatory disease	Tzanck smear and culture for herpes simplex virus
N. gonorrhoeae, C. trachomatis, Campylobacter jejuni, Shigella, T. pallidum, and cytomegalovirus	Sexually transmitted enteric disease	Wet mount for *T. vaginalis* Test and biopsy for HPV Culture and serology for other organisms

5. In women with vaginal findings, consider the following:

Diseases/Agents	Clinical Findings	Tests
Bacterial vaginosis (*Gardnerella*)	Thin, gray-white discharge	pH >4.5, fishy odor, wet mount shows clue cells
Candidiasis	Curdy, white discharge, prominent itching, and vulvovaginal irritation	pH 4 to 4.5, KOH prep shows pseudohyphae
Trichomoniasis	Thin, yellow/green, frothy discharge and vulvovaginal irritation	pH 5 to 6.0, wet mount shows motile trichomonads and neutrophils

6. In patients with miscellaneous findings, consider the following:

Diseases/Agents	Clinical Findings	Tests
Viral hepatitis (hepatitis B, delta hepatitis, and probably hepatitis C)	Constitutional and gastrointestinal symptoms, with enlarged tender liver	Liver function tests; viral serologic tests

Diseases/Agents	Clinical Findings	Tests
Cytomegalovirus	Heterophile-negative mononucleosis	Culture virus in throat, blood buffy coat, or urine; serologic tests
Pediculosis pubis	Intense itching	Lice or eggs on pubic hair
Scabies	Severe itching; worse at night	Scrapings, skin biopsy

7. Remember that syphilis has a variety of clinical presentations and test result patterns.

Syphilis has a variety of presentations that can be divided into five stages: primary stage (chancre); secondary stage (rash appearing in 1 to 4 months); latent stage (clearing of rash lasting 1 to many years); tertiary stage (gummas, neurosyphilis, cardiovascular syphilis); and congenital stage. Consult the references for additional information on diagnosing syphilis in these various stages.

BIBLIOGRAPHY

Adimora AA, Quinlivan EB: Human papillomavirus infection: Recent findings on progression to cervical cancer. Postgrad Med 98:109, 1995.
  Outlines recent advances in the diagnosis and management of HPV infection.
Andrews WW, Lee HH, Roden WJ, et al: Detection of genitourinary tract *Chlamydia trachomatis* infection in pregnant women by ligase chain reaction assay. Obstet Gynecol 89:556, 1997.
  Ligase chain reaction detected significantly more C. trachomatis *infections in both urine (16.9%) and cervical specimens (18.22%) than did cervical culture (6.1%).*
Cates W Jr, Hinman AR: Sexually transmitted diseases in the 1990's. N Engl J Med 325:1368, 1991.
  CDC experts emphasize the increased risk of HIV infection in individuals with other STDs, the rising incidence of syphilis, and the high prevalence of genital herpes simplex infections (one in six Americans) and human papillomavirus infections (one in three Americans).
Cohen MS: HIV and sexually transmitted diseases: The physician's role in prevention. Postgrad Med 98:52, 1995.
  Reviews the mechanisms of HIV transmission and discusses preventive strategies.
Ferris DG, Hendrich J, Payne PM, et al: Office laboratory diagnosis of vaginitis. J Fam Pract 41:575, 1995.
  The diagnosis of vaginitis by clinicians in the primary care setting is less than optimal.
Fox KK, Behets F: Vaginal discharge: How to pinpoint the cause. Postgrad Med 98:87, 1995.
  Reviews bacterial vaginosis, candidiasis, trichomoniasis, and other causes of vaginal discharge.
Gerbert B, Bleecker T, Bernzweig J: Is anybody talking to physicians about acquired immunodeficiency syndrome and sex? A national survey of patients. Arch Fam Med 2:45, 1993.
  Patients report that doctors neglect to take sexual histories.
Hart G, Rothenberg RB: Syphilis tests in diagnostic and therapeutic decision making. *In* Sox HC Jr (ed): Common Diagnostic Tests: Use and Interpretation, 2nd ed. Philadelphia, American College of Physicians, 1990, p 302.

Reviews the use of syphilis testing in the diagnosis and management of the disease.

Hayward RSA, Steinberg EP, Ford DE, et al: Preventive care guidelines: 1991. Ann Intern Med 114:758, 1991.
Authoritative recommendations for wellness screening for HIV, syphilis, gonorrhea, and chlamydial infection.

Hillier SL, Nugent RP, Eschenbach DA, et al: Association between bacterial vaginosis and preterm delivery of a low-birth-weight infant. N Engl J Med 333:1737, 1995.
Hauth JC, Goldenberg RL, Andrews WW, et al: Reduced incidence of preterm delivery with metronidazole and erythromycin in women with bacterial vaginosis. N Engl J Med 333:1732, 1995.
Bacterial vaginosis is associated with preterm delivery.

Hoffman IF, Schmitz JL: Genital ulcer disease: Management in the HIV era. Postgrad Med 98:67, 1995.
Discusses the differential diagnosis of genital ulcer disease.

Krieger JN, Jenny C, Verdon M, et al: Clinical manifestations of trichomoniasis in men. Ann Intern Med 118:844, 1993.
Physicians should not overlook trichomonas as a potential pathogen in men with mild urethritis.

Romanowski B, Sutherland R, Fick GH, et al: Serologic response to treatment of infectious syphilis. Ann Intern Med 114:1005, 1991.
After treatment, non-treponemal and treponemal tests may become negative.

Rusnak JM, Butzin C, McGlasson D, et al: False-positive rapid plasma reagin tests in human immunodeficiency virus infection and relationship to anticardiolipin antibody and serum immunoglobulin levels. J Infect Dis 169:1356, 1994.
Biologic false-positive RPR tests for syphilis occur in less than 1% of the general population but have been reported in up to 3.8% of subjects with HIV.

Safrin S: Sexually transmitted diseases: Ten questions physicians often ask. Consultant 36:2161, 1996.
Valuable diagnostic and therapeutic information about STD; for example, Trichomonas *can cause symptomatic infection in men.*

Schmid GP, Fontanarosa PB: Evolving strategies for management of the nongonococcal urethritis syndrome. JAMA 274:577, 1995.
Non-gonococcal urethritis is the most common STD that occurs in men.

1989 Sexually transmitted diseases treatment guidelines. MMWR 38:1, 1989.
Authoritative summary of guidelines for the management of sexually transmitted diseases.

Sobel JD: Vaginitis. N Engl J Med 337:1896, 1997.
Neither self-diagnosis nor diagnosis by a physician is reliable without laboratory confirmation.

Thomas DL, Rompalo AM, Zenilman J, et al: Association of hepatitis C virus infection with false-positive tests for syphilis. J Infect Dis 170:1579, 1994.
Hepatitis C infection may cause a false-positive RPR test.

Woods GL: Update on laboratory diagnosis of sexually transmitted diseases. Clin Lab Med 15:665, 1995.
Good discussion of miscellaneous tests for common STDs.

Woods ML II, McGee ZA: Sexually transmitted diseases: Highlights of the revised CDC management guidelines. Consultant 35:1298, 1995.
Discusses emergence of drug-resistant strains of causative organisms and stresses the risk of transmission of HIV.

Wooldridge WE: Syphilis: A new visit from an old enemy. Postgrad Med 89:193, 1991.
Discusses the upswing in syphilis rates, with guidelines for diagnosis and management.

Yinnon AM, Coury-Doniger P, Polito R, et al: Serologic response to treatment of syphilis in patients with HIV infection. Arch Intern Med 156:321, 1996.
Patients with syphilis who are HIV positive are less likely to experience serologic improvement after recommended therapy than are patients with syphilis who are HIV negative.

ACUTE FOOD POISONING

Recommendations for acute food poisoning following the ingestion of a meal are from the medical literature.

1. If an illness appears related to dining (i.e., occurring during or shortly after a meal), look for characteristic clinical findings and, when appropriate, obtain laboratory tests. Consult the state health laboratory for additional diagnostic support. See the discussion of acute diarrhea in Chapter 5 for additional recommendations, including testing for ova and parasites.

Illness related to dining is common. Usually, recognition of the characteristic findings, symptomatic therapy, and future avoidance of the offending agent are all that is required. Occasionally, laboratory tests are useful. The causes are classified as follows: food poisoning caused by an infectious agent, chemical food poisoning, food poisoning caused by toxins in seafood and mushrooms, and food hypersensitivity. Certainly, delayed diseases, such as hepatitis A, can be caused by contaminated food, but these delayed causes are not considered here.

2. To detect food poisoning caused by an infectious agent, consider the following:

Diseases/Agents	Clinical Findings	Tests
Bacillus cereus (toxin)	Nausea, vomiting, cramps, diarrhea 1–16 hr after ingestion, also liver failure	Culture food/stool; test for toxin.
Campylobacter jejuni (bacteria)	Fever and chills; rarely nausea, vomiting; cramps and diarrhea 2–10 days after ingestion, also Guillain-Barré syndrome	Culture stool, also serology.
Clostridium botulinum (toxin)	Afebrile, neurologic findings (visual problems, dysphagia, dysarthria, weakness, paralysis) and gastrointestinal findings (nausea, vomiting, cramps, diarrhea) 6 hr–8 days after ingestion—especially of home-processed fruits, vegetables, meats, and seafood	Culture food/stool; test for toxin.
Clostridium perfringens (toxin)	Cramps, diarrhea 8–24 hr after ingestion; nausea and vomiting much less common	Culture food/stool; test for toxin.
Escherichia coli (enterotoxigenic) causing traveler's diarrhea	Cramps and watery diarrhea 24–72 hr after ingestion; nausea and vomiting less common; contaminated seafood recently incriminated	
Escherichia coli 0157:H7 (bacteria)	Bloody diarrhea, hemorrhagic colitis, and hemolytic-uremic syndrome from eating contaminated hamburger, salami, unpasteurized milk/cider, lake water, lettuce, and from personal contact	Culture stool; test for toxin.

Table continued on following page

Diseases/Agents	Clinical Findings	Tests
Listeria monocytogenes	Sepsis and meningitis—especially in immunocompromised patients	Culture blood or spinal fluid.
Protozoa (spore-forming): *Cryptosporidia,* Microsporidia, *Isospora,* and *Cyclospora*	Diarrhea after ingestion of contaminated food or water; *Cyclospora* from raspberries	Acid-fast stains of stool specimens. Also wet-mount phase microscopy and epifluorescence microscopy.
Salmonella/Shigella (bacteria)	Fever and chills, nausea, vomiting, watery diarrhea, abdominal pain 8–48 hr after ingestion of contaminated food—especially insufficiently cooked eggs and domestic fowl, which are a source of *Salmonella*	Culture stool.
Staphylococcal food poisoning (toxin)	Nausea, vomiting, cramps, diarrhea 2–7 hr after ingestion	Culture food.
Vibrio cholerae (toxin)	Vomiting and mild to severe diarrhea 12–48 hr after ingestion of raw seafood; no cramps or fever	Culture stool.
Vibrio parahaemolyticus (bacteria)	Nausea, vomiting, cramps, and explosive watery diarrhea 4–96 hr after eating seafood	Culture stool.
Vibrio vulnificus (bacteria)	Septicemia and wound infections 24–48 hr after ingestion of raw oysters or sea water; patients with liver disease, low gastric acid, hemochromatosis, or immunodeficiency at risk	Culture blood, stool, and skin lesions.
Yersinia enterocolitica	Fever, headache, nausea, vomiting, and abdominal pains	Culture stool.

3. To detect chemical food poisoning, consider the following:

Diseases/Agents	Clinical Findings	Tests
Heavy metals: arsenic, cadmium, copper, tin, zinc, mercury, etc.	Vomiting, cramps, and diarrhea within hours of ingestion	Blood and urine for heavy metals
Monosodium glutamate (MSG)—the Chinese restaurant syndrome	Flushing, paresthesias, chest pain, facial pressure and burning, dizziness, sweating, headaches, palpitation, weakness, nausea, and vomiting shortly after MSG ingestion	
Seaweed	Nausea, vomiting, diarrhea, and burning sensation	

Diseases/Agents	Clinical Findings	Tests
Sodium nitrite—hot dog headache	Headache after ingesting smoked meats	
Sulfites	Flushing, bronchospasm, hypotension within minutes of ingesting sulfites (e.g., salads, shrimp, dried fruit, gelatin, pickles, sausage, cheese, wine, fruit juice)	
Wasabi (horseradish used with sushi)—the Japanese restaurant syndrome	Fainting, pallor, sweating, staggering, and confusion immediately after ingestion of wasabi	

4. To detect the food poisoning caused by toxins in seafood or mushrooms, consider the following:

Diseases/Agents	Clinical Findings	Tests
Ciguatera fish poisoning (ciguatoxin) resulting from contamination by dinoflagellates and blue-green algae	Nausea, vomiting, cramps, and diarrhea, with numbness, pruritus, paresthesias of lips a few minutes to 30 hr after ingesting toxic fish (e.g., barracuda, red snapper, amberjack, grouper, mullet)	Immunoassays exist but are not widely available. A rapid-stick immunoassay has been developed.
Dungeness crab (from eating internal organs) and mussel poisoning resulting from contamination by domoic acid, a toxin produced by marine plankton	Nausea, cramps, and diarrhea; in severe cases headache, dizziness, facial grimace, disorientation, memory loss, excessive bronchial secretions, breathing problems, and even death within 48 hr	
Mushroom poisoning (amatoxin and phalloidin)	Fever, abdominal pain, nausea, vomiting, and diarrhea in 6–24 hr; then hepatic and renal dysfunction in 24–48 hr; then cardiomyopathy, coagulopathy, coma, and possibly death after ingestion of *Amanita* mushrooms	Obtain complete blood count, coagulation tests, biochemical profile, including hepatic and renal function tests, and urinalysis; gastric aspirate, vomitus, or stool can be analyzed for toxins by thin-layer chromatography.
Paralytic shellfish poisoning (PSP); saxitoxin resulting from contamination by toxic red tides of algae of the North Atlantic and Pacific coasts and brevetoxin in the Gulf of Mexico	Paresthesias and numbness with nausea, vomiting, diarrhea, muscle paralysis, and even death 30 min–2 hr after eating shellfish; PSP most common between April and October	

Table continued on following page

Diseases/Agents	Clinical Findings	Tests
Scombroid fish poisoning (histamine); most common cause of fish poisoning. Toxins formed by bacteria	Flushing, headache, dizziness, nausea, vomiting, cramps, and diarrhea (histamine-like reaction) beginning minutes to hours after ingesting fish (e.g., scombroid fish [tuna, mackerel, skipjack, bonito] and non-scombroid fish [mahi mahi, bluefish, amberjack, herring, sardines, anchovies]) or cheese; persons receiving isoniazid at risk	

5. To detect food hypersensitivity, consider the following:

Diseases/Agents	Clinical Findings	Tests
Food allergy (IgE mediated)	Anaphylactic reaction minutes–2 hr after ingesting food allergin (e.g., peanuts, walnuts, eggs, fish, crustaceans, and milk)	Positive skin test or radioallergosorbent test to offending food
Tartrazine (yellow dye)	Urticaria or angioedema and/or acute bronchospasm 1–several hours after ingesting tartrazine; sometimes a history of urticarial or bronchospastic aspirin intolerance	

6. Interpret any test results in the context of clinical findings, and treat the patient symptomatically unless specific therapy is available.

Treatment options include the following: symptomatic therapy, emptying the gastrointestinal tract of the offending agent, antibiotics, antitoxins, hemodialysis, and chelating agents.

BIBLIOGRAPHY

Bacillus cereus food poisoning associated with fried rice at two child day care centers—Virginia, 1993. MMWR 43:177, 1994.
   Bacillus cereus *can be transmitted by rice.*
Barton ED, Tanner P, Turchen SG, et al: Ciguatera fish poisoning—a Southern California epidemic. West J Med 163:31, 1995.
   A rapid-stick enzyme immunoassay using horseradish and peroxidase-labeled sheep anti-ciguatera toxin antibody has been developed by Hawaii Chemtect International

(Ciguatect) for detecting ciguatera toxins and toxins associated with diarrheic shellfish poisoning.

Besser RE, Lett SM, Weber JT, et al: An outbreak of diarrhea and hemolytic uremic syndrome from *Escherichia coli* 0157:H7 in fresh-pressed apple cider. JAMA 269:2217, 1993.
Escherichia coli *0157:H7 may be transmitted by apple cider.*

Bolton CF: The changing concepts of Guillain-Barré syndrome. N Engl J Med 333:1415, 1995.
Rees JH, Soudain SE, Gregson NA, et al: *Campylobacter jejuni* infection and Guillain-Barré syndrome. N Engl J Med 333:1374, 1995.
C. jejuni *is the chief precipitant of the Guillain-Barré syndrome.*

Boyce TG, Swerdlow DL, Griffin PM: *Escherichia coli* 0157:H7 and the hemolytic-uremic syndrome. N Engl J Med 333:364, 1995.
In the United States, E. coli *0157:H7 causes more than 20,000 infections and up to 250 deaths each year.*

Buchanan RL, Ericsson CD, Hull AE, et al: The rising tide of foodborne and waterborne infections. Patient Care 31:30, 1997.
Good review of foodborne illness.

Escherichia coli 0157:H7 outbreak linked to commercially distributed dry-cured salami—Washington and California, 1994. MMWR 44:157, 1995.
Escherichia coli *0157:H7 may be found in salami.*

FDA says eating type of crab poses danger. The New York Times, December 29, 1991, p Y11.
Describes hazards of eating viscera of Dungeness crab contaminated by the toxin domoic acid.

Foodborne outbreak of diarrheal illness associated with *Cryptosporidium parvum*—Minnesota, 1995. MMWR 45:783, 1996.
Add cryptosporidiosis to your list of possible causes of suspected foodborne gastroenteritis.

Geller RJ, Olson KR, Senécal PE: Ciguatera fish poisoning in San Francisco, California, caused by imported barracuda. West J Med 155:639, 1991.
Describes 12 cases of ciguatera fish poisoning.

Goodgame RW: Understanding intestinal spore-forming protozoa: Cryptosporidia, microsporidia, isospora, and cyclospora. Ann Intern Med 124:429, 1996.
Spore-forming protozoa can cause gastroenteritis in normal as well as immunodeficient patients.

Greenwald DA, Brandt LJ: Recognizing *E. coli* 0157:H7 infection. Hosp Pract 32:123, 1997.
Discusses the various clinical presentations and their diagnosis and management.

Herwaldt BL, Ackers M-L, Cyclospora Working Group: An outbreak in 1996 of cyclosporiasis associated with imported raspberries. N Engl J Med 336:1548, 1997.
Describes a large outbreak that occurred in North America.

Hughes JM, Potter ME: Scombroid fish poisoning: From pathogenesis to prevention. N Engl J Med 324:766, 1991.
Good discussion of scombroid fish poisoning and other causes of food poisoning. Millions of cases of food poisoning are estimated to occur in the United States annually.

Koenig KL, Mueller J, Rose T: *Vibrio vulnificus:* Hazard on the half shell. West J Med 155:400, 1991.
Highlights the serious risk of eating raw oysters. The infection can also be secondary to contamination of a wound in brackish waters.

Lake-associated outbreak of *Escherichia coli* 0157:H7—Illinois, 1995. MMWR 45:437, 1996.
E. coli *0157:H7 may be transmitted by lake water.*

Levine WC, Griffin PM, Gulf Coast Vibrio Working Group: Vibrio infections on the Gulf Coast: Results of first year of regional surveillance. J Infect Dis 167:479, 1993.
Infections with Vibrio *species may be due to eating contaminated Gulf Coast finfish or shellfish.*

Mahler H, Pasi A, Kramer JM, et al: Fulminant liver failure in association with the emetic toxin of *Bacillus cereus.* N Engl J Med 336:1142, 1997.
Food poisoning with Bacillus cereus *can cause liver failure.*

Mahon BE, Mintz ED, Greene KD, et al: Reported cholera in the United States, 1992–1994: A reflection of global changes in cholera epidemiology. JAMA 276:307, 1996.

Cholera—still rare in the United States—is increasing in incidence.

Mead PS, Finelli L, Lambert-Fair MA, et al: Risk factors for sporadic infection with *Escherichia coli* 0157:H7. Arch Intern Med 157:204, 1997.

Hamburgers prepared at home are an important source of E. coli *0157:H7 infections.*

Outbreak of cryptosporidiosis at a day camp—Florida, July–August, 1995. MMWR 45:442, 1996.

If you suspect a diagnosis of cryptosporidiosis, you should specifically request testing for this organism.

Outbreak of gastrointestinal illness associated with consumption of seaweed—Hawaii, 1994. MMWR 44:724, 1995.

Consumption of seaweed can cause gastroenteritis.

Outbreaks of *Cyclospora cayetanensis* infection—United States, 1996. MMWR 45:549, 1996. Update: Outbreaks of *Cyclospora cayetanensis* infection—United States and Canada, 1996. MMWR 45:611, 1996.

Cyclospora *can be diagnosed by identifying oocytes in stool, but the procedures (wet-mount phase microscopy, acid-fast staining, and epifluorescence microscopy) are not routine in most clinical laboratories.*

Outbreaks of *Salmonella enteritidis* gastroenteritis—California, 1993. MMWR 42:793, 1993.

Salmonella *may be transmitted by raw eggs.*

Paralytic shellfish poisoning: Massachusetts and Alaska, 1990. MMWR 40:157, 1991.

Points out a hazard of eating shellfish.

Perl TM, Bédard L, Kosatsky T, et al: An outbreak of toxic encephalopathy caused by eating mussels contaminated with domoic acid. N Engl J Med 322:1775, 1990.

Teitelbaum JS, Zatorre RJ, Carpenter S, et al: Neurologic sequelae of domoic acid intoxication due to the ingestion of contaminated mussels. N Engl J Med 322:1781, 1990.

Documents domoic acid intoxication from eating mussels.

Preliminary report: Foodborne outbreak of *Escherichia coli* 0157:H7 infections from hamburgers—western United States. MMWR 42:85, 1993.

Physicians should consider Escherichia coli *0157:H7 infection in patients with gastroenteritis and the hemolytic-uremic syndrome.*

Sampson HA, Metcalfe DD: Food allergies. JAMA 268:2840, 1992.

Discusses the pathophysiology, diagnosis, and therapy of food allergies.

Su C, Brandt LJ: *Escherichia coli* 0157:H7 infection in humans. Ann Intern Med 123:698, 1995.

Reviews the clinical relevance of this increasingly common infection.

Vibrio vulnificus infections associated with eating raw oysters—Los Angeles, 1996. MMWR 45:621, 1996.

Immunocompromised patients or those with liver disease should be advised of the hazards of eating raw seafood, particularly oysters.

CEREBROSPINAL FLUID ANALYSIS

Recommendations for CSF analysis are from the medical literature.

1. In patients with appropriate clinical indications, perform lumbar puncture and analyze the CSF.

Appropriate indications and contraindications for performing lumbar puncture follow. A guideline used by some experienced clinicians is that if you think of a lumbar puncture during a work-up, you should do it! In a recent article, the authors suggest that we may be doing too many lumbar punctures in children with orbital and periorbital cellulitis.

Diagnostic Indications	Therapeutic Indications	Contraindications
Known or suspected meningitis and encephalitis • Acute: bacterial, viral • Subacute: tuberculous, syphilitic, fungal, neoplastic • Chronic: syphilitic, granulomatous, neoplastic Intracranial or intraspinal hemorrhage if computed tomography (CT) or magnetic resonance imaging (MRI) is not available Multiple sclerosis Acute polyneuropathy Suspected benign intracranial hypertension (pseudotumor) only if CT or MRI is negative	Intrathecal administration of antimicrobial or chemotherapeutic agents CSF drainage in patient with benign intracranial hypertension or communicating hydrocephalus	Intracranial hypertension due to mass lesion or obstructive hydrocephalus (suggest funduscopic examination before lumbar puncture) Bleeding diathesis Local skin or epidural infections

Source: Victor JD: Neurologic diagnostic procedures. *In* Bennett JC, Plum F (eds): Cecil Textbook of Medicine, 20th ed. Philadelphia, WB Saunders, 1996, p 1960.

With the patient in the lateral recumbent position and before CSF is withdrawn, measure CSF pressure (normal, 90 to 180 mm). If CSF pressure is high (>180 mm) or low (<90 mm), remove only 1 mL of fluid and remeasure CSF pressure (carefully exclude increased intracranial pressure—a marked fall in pressure should cause concern). If CSF pressure is normal with no marked fall in pressure with removal of 1 mL, 10 to 20 mL of CSF may slowly be removed. Divide the CSF sample into three sterile tubes: (1) for chemistry and immunology (protein, glucose, LD, serology), (2) for microbiology (Gram stain; bacterial, fungal, and viral cultures; India ink preparation; antigen tests), and (3) for cell count and differential. Before the needle is removed, record opening pressure, closing pressure, and amount of fluid removed.

2. Interpret test results in the context of clinical findings.

TYPICAL CSF FINDINGS IN VARIOUS CONDITIONS

Condition	Pressure (mm CSF)	Gross Appearance	WBC/μL (WBC × 10⁶/L)	Protein (mg/dL) (g/L)	Glucose (mg/dL) (mmol/L)
Normal	50–200	Clear, colorless	0–10 (0–10) lymphocytes and monocytes	<45 (<0.45)	50–80 (2.78–4.44) or 2/3 blood glucose
Acute bacterial meningitis	Increased to 200–500	Turbid, may clot	100–10,000 (100–10,000) polymorphonuclear leukocytes	50–500 (0.50–5.00)	Absent or very low
Tuberculous meningitis	Increased to 200–500	Turbid, pellicle common	10–500 (10–500) chiefly lymphocytes	50–500 (0.50–5.00)	Often under 40 (2.22)
Aseptic or viral meningitis	Increased to 200–500	Clear or slightly turbid	10–500 (10–500) chiefly lymphocytes	45–200 (0.45–2.00)	Normal
Multiple sclerosis	Normal	Clear, colorless	Normal or 10–50 (10–50) lymphocytes	Normal or 45–100 (0.45–1.00)	Normal
Cerebral thrombosis	Usually normal to slightly increased	Clear	Usually normal	Normal to 45–100 (0.45–1.00)	Normal
Cerebral hemorrhage	Usually normal	Bloody or xanthochromic	Increased red blood count (RBC)	Increased 45–100 (0.45–1.00)	Normal
Subarachnoid hemorrhage	Increased to 200–500	Bloody or xanthochromic	Increased RBC	Increased 50–1000 (0.50–10.00)	Normal
Brain tumor	Usually increased to 200–500	Clear or xanthochromic	Normal to 50 (50) lymphocytes	Normal or slightly increased	Normal or slightly decreased

Source: Bakerman S, Bakerman P, Strausbaugh P: ABC's of Interpretive Laboratory Data, 3rd ed. Myrtle Beach, SC, Interpretive Laboratory Data, Inc., 1994, p 137.

Meningitis

A Wright stain, Gram stain (sensitivity, approximately 60 to 80%), acid-fast stain (sensitivity, approximately 40%), and India ink preparation (sensitivity, approximately 25 to 50%) are valuable for determining the cause of an infectious process. Serum C-reactive protein may be used to distinguish bacterial meningitis (increased values) from viral meningitis. Antigen tests may also be helpful. Cultures are the "gold standard" for diagnosing the cause of infections (sensitivity, approximately 80 to 90%).

For syphilis, the CSF VDRL and CSF fluorescent treponemal antibody with absorption tests are appropriate.

Rarely, aseptic meningitis is drug induced (e.g., trimethoprim, sulfadiazine, ibuprofen, immune globulins, azathioprine). Results of lumbar puncture usually show an increased opening pressure and CSF pleocytosis. The condition rapidly resolves (24 to 48 hours) after cessation of the offending medication.

Neurologic Disorders

Besides its use for determining the white blood cell differential count, a Wright-stained preparation of CSF is useful to determine the presence of leukemia cells, tumor cells, and other elements.

The CSF IgG index [(CSF IgG level/CSF albumin level) ÷ (serum IgG level/serum albumin level)] is abnormal in multiple sclerosis (MS) in approximately 90% of patients. Increased values may also occur with many other CNS inflammatory conditions. CSF immunoelectrophoresis detects oligoclonal bands of IgG, which are found in patients with MS (sensitivity, 83 to 90%); however, they may also be present in other inflammatory and neoplastic conditions.

CSF lactate may be high with any condition associated with CNS anoxia. It is also increased in patients with bacterial, tuberculous, and fungal meningitis—more so than in viral meningitis.

Determination of CSF LD has been advocated during the first hours after a stroke: Significantly higher values occur in patients with stroke (40.9 ± 14.5 U/L) than in patients with transient ischemic attacks (11.8 ± 2.9 U/L).

BIBLIOGRAPHY

Aseptic meningitis: New York state and United States, weeks 1–36, 1991. MMWR 40:773, 1991.
Aseptic meningitis is on the rise.
Chaudhry HJ, Cunha BA: Drug-induced aseptic meningitis. Postgrad Med 90:65, 1991.
Highlights a rare cause of aseptic meningitis.
Ciarallo LR, Rowe PC: Children with periorbital and orbital cellulitis. J Pediatr 122:355, 1993.
Lumbar punctures may be overdone in children with orbital and periorbital cellulitis.

Elmore JG, Horwitz RI, Quagliarello VJ: Acute meningitis with a negative Gram's stain: Clinical and management outcomes in 171 episodes. Am J Med 100:78, 1996.
Patients may present with clinical acute meningitis with a negative Gram stain. A proven diagnostic cause was more likely in patients older than 60 years, those who presented during the winter months, and those with presence of comorbid disease.

Granter SR, Doolittle MH, Renshaw AA: Predominance of neutrophils in the cerebrospinal fluid of AIDS patients with cytomegalovirus radiculopathy. Am J Clin Pathol 105:364, 1996.
An increased number of neutrophils in the CSF of an AIDS patient without an identified infectious organism strongly suggests cytomegalovirus radiculopathy.

Hall CD, Snyder CR, Robertson KR, et al: Cerebrospinal fluid analysis in human immuno-deficiency virus infection. Ann Clin Lab Sci 22:139, 1992.
Reviews the CSF changes in 59 HIV-infected patients.

Hansson L-O, Axelsson G, Linné T, et al: Serum C-reactive protein in the differential diagnosis of acute meningitis. Scand J Infect Dis 25:625, 1993.
Results indicate that a discriminatory C-reactive protein level of 2 mg/dL (20 mg/L) for children under 6 years of age and 5 mg/dL (50 mg/L) for older patients can be used to distinguish between bacterial and viral meningitis, except when the illness does not last more than 12 hours.

Kjeldsberg CR, Knight JA: Body Fluids, 2nd ed. Chicago, American Society of Clinical Pathologists, 1986.
Contains excellent colored photographs of various kinds of Wright-stained cells in the CSF fluid.

Kleine TO, Hackler R, Meyer-Rienecker H: Classical and modern methods of cerebrospinal fluid analysis. Eur J Clin Chem Clin Biochem 29:705, 1991.
Reviews new developments in the analysis of CSF.

Knight JA: Advances in the analysis of cerebrospinal fluid. Ann Clin Lab Sci 27:93, 1997.
Discusses new tests that may be useful in the evaluation of patients with both primary and metastatic malignancies, Alzheimer's disease, Creutzfeldt-Jakob disease, global ischemia, various psychiatric disorders, and CSF otorrhea and rhinorrhea, and in the differential diagnosis of cortical versus lacunar stroke.

Lampl Y, Paniri Y, Eshel Y, et al: Cerebrospinal fluid lactate dehydrogenase levels in early stroke and transient ischemic attacks. Stroke 21:854, 1990.
Suggests CSF LD to distinguish a stroke from a transient ischemic attack.

Lampl Y, Paniri Y, Eshel Y, et al: LDH isoenzymes in cerebrospinal fluid in various brain tumors. J Neurol Neurosurg Psychiatry 53:697, 1990.
Suggests CSF LD-1:LD-2 ratio to distinguish primary brain tumors from metastatic brain tumors.

Sigurdardóttir B, Björnsson OM, Jónsdóttir KE, et al: Acute bacterial meningitis in adults: A 20-year overview. Arch Intern Med 157:425, 1997.
In adults, meningococci and pneumococci were the most common agents. Pneumococci and Listeria were most common in patients aged 45 years or older.

Whiting AS, Johnson LN: Papilledema: Clinical clues and differential diagnosis. Am Fam Physician 45:1125, 1992.
Papilledema is a sign of increased intracranial pressure.

• •

SYNOVIAL FLUID ANALYSIS

Recommendations for synovial fluid (SF) analysis are from the medical literature.

1. In patients with synovial effusion, obtain radiographic studies and consider an arthrocentesis. Request SF analysis, including Gram stain, cultures, crystal analysis, cell count, and differential.

The cause of acute monoarticular arthritis with synovial effusion can often be diagnosed by SF analysis, particularly when the arthritis is due to gout, pseudogout, or septic arthritis.

In 100 consecutive patients undergoing joint aspiration, the diagnoses were as follows:

Diagnosis	No. of Patients
Noninflammatory disease	
Osteoarthritis	14
Trauma	11
Inflammatory disease	
Rheumatoid arthritis	11
Crystal-induced arthritis	25
Septic arthritis*	8
Miscellaneous diagnoses†	5
No diagnosis	26

*Includes five patients with probable septic arthritis.

†Includes two patients with sickle cell anemia and one patient each with systemic lupus erythematosus, mixed connective tissue disease, and hepatitis B.

Source: Shmerling RH, Delbanco TL, Tosteson ANA, et al: Synovial fluid tests: What should be ordered? JAMA 264:1009–1014, 1990. Copyright 1990, American Medical Association.

Record the total volume and appearance of the removed SF, and estimate viscosity by allowing the SF to form a string when dripping from a syringe with the needle removed (normal SF forms a 4- to 6-cm string). Strings less than 3 cm indicate low viscosity because of depolymerization of hyaluronate, which is compatible with inflammatory conditions such as septic arthritis, gouty arthritis, and rheumatoid arthritis. A false-positive string test can occur with a rapid effusion after trauma. Alternatively, a poor mucin clot within 1 minute of adding a few drops of synovial fluid to 20 mL of 5% acetic acid indicates depolymerization of hyaluronate (Ropes test). Hemorrhagic effusions occur with trauma, fracture, neurotropic arthropathy, tumor, pigmented villonodular synovitis, hemorrhagic diathesis, and septic arthritis. Remember that more than one disease can occur simultaneously in the same joint (e.g., septic arthritis and lupus erythematosus; septic arthritis and gout; gout and rheumatoid arthritis; and septic arthritis and rheumatoid arthritis). Likewise, several different crystals can occur together (e.g., urate and pyrophosphate crystals; apatite and pyrophosphate crystals; and urate and apatite crystals). In patients with monoarticular effusions, consider bacterial infection (e.g., gonococcal arthritis or tuberculosis).

2. Interpret test results in the context of clinical findings.

With the exception of tests for crystals and infectious agents, most other studies are relatively non-specific. Therefore, it is particularly important that tests for crystals and infectious agents are done well.

Normal synovial fluid is clear and pale yellow in appearance, contains no abnormal elements, and has a white blood cell count of 0 to 200 μL (0 to 200 × 10^6/L), of which less than 10% are neutrophils.

CATEGORIES OF SYNOVIAL FLUID FINDINGS

Diagnosis	Appearance	Total White Cell Count per mm³*	Polymorphonuclear Cells	Miscellaneous
Normal	Clear, pale yellow	0–200	Less than 10%	—
Group I (noninflammatory)				
Osteoarthritis	Clear to slightly turbid	50–2000 (600)	Less than 30%	Cartilage fragments
Group II (mildly inflammatory)				
Systemic lupus erythematosus (SLE) Scleroderma	Clear to slightly turbid	0–9000 (3000)	Less than 20%	—
Group III (severely inflammatory)				
Gout	Turbid	100–160,000 (21,000)	Approximately 70%	Monosodium urate crystals
Pseudogout	Turbid	50–75,000 (14,000)	Approximately 70%	Calcium pyrophosphate dihydrate crystals
Rheumatoid arthritis	Turbid	250–80,000 (19,000)	Approximately 70%	—
Group IV (infectious)				
Acute bacterial	Very turbid	150–250,000 (80,000)	Approximately 90%	Culture positive
Tuberculosis	Turbid	2500–100,000 (20,000)	Approximately 60%	Culture often negative

*Averages in parentheses
Source: Arnold WJ, Ike RW: Specialized procedures in the management of patients with rheumatic diseases. *In* Wyngaarden JB, Smith LH, Bennett JC (eds): Cecil Textbook of Medicine, 19th ed. Philadelphia, WB Saunders, 1992, p 1504.

SYNOVIAL FLUID CRYSTALS

Crystal	Polarization Microscopy	Other Identification
Monosodium urate	Strong negative birefringence,* needle shaped, long	Uricase digestion X-ray diffraction
Calcium pyrophosphate dihydrate (CPPD)	Weak positive birefringence, rhomboid or small rods, pleomorphic	X-ray diffraction
Calcium phosphate (hydroxyapatite)	Not easily visualized	Electron microscopy X-ray diffraction
Cholesterol	Rhombic or platelike, notched corners, multicolored, occasionally small and needle-like	Chemical determination
Corticosteroids	Pleomorphic, variable birefringence	Follows intra-articular steroid treatment

*Birefringence refers to crystals that are doubly refractive in plane-polarized light.
Source: Cohen AS: Specialized diagnostic procedures in the rheumatic diseases. *In* Wyngaarden JB, Smith LH (eds): Cecil Textbook of Medicine, 18th ed. Philadelphia, WB Saunders, 1988, p 1994.

Septic Arthritis

The most important diagnosis to distinguish from other causes of arthritis is septic arthritis. Synovial fluid leukocyte count and percent neutrophils are the most accurate and useful tests for diagnosing the cause of joint effusions. Glucose and protein measurements are less useful. In more than 80% of cases, the synovial fluid leukocyte count and neutrophil percentage values are normal in non-inflammatory disease. A Gram stain is helpful but is not completely sensitive; cultures are usually positive in most cases of septic arthritis. Acid-fast stains for tuberculosis are not very sensitive; a biopsy may be helpful for rapid diagnosis.

BIBLIOGRAPHY

Gatter RA, Schumacher HR: A Practical Handbook of Joint Fluid Analysis, 2nd ed. Philadelphia, Lea & Febiger, 1991.
Practical monograph on joint fluid analysis.
Handy JR: Pyrophosphate arthropathy in the knees of elderly persons. Arch Intern Med 156:2426, 1996.
The joint fluid of acute pyrophosphate arthropathy has a white blood cell count of about 20,000/mm³ (20 × 10⁹/L) with 0.9 (90%) polymorphonuclear leukocytes, with calcium pyrophosphate dehydrate crystals usually being intracellular.
Kjeldsberg CR, Knight JA: Body Fluids, 2nd ed. Chicago, American Society of Clinical Pathologists, 1986.
Contains colored photographs of various kinds of Wright-stained cells in synovial fluid.
Kortekangas P, Aro HT, Lehtonen O-P: Synovial fluid culture and blood culture in acute arthritis. Scand J Rheumatol 24:44, 1995.
Confirms the reliability of culturing a single synovial fluid specimen by any of several methods.
Marino C, McDonald E: Diagnostic joint aspiration: When is it necessary? Emerg Med 24:67, 1992.
Acute monoarticular arthritis often needs aspiration—particularly to diagnose gout, pseudogout, and septic arthritis.

O'Duffy JD: Acute monoarthritis: Managing the swollen, painful joint. Consultant 36:431, 1996.
Discusses the differential diagnosis of septic and crystalline arthritis.
Rosenthal J: Acute monoarticular arthritis: Sleuthing out the cause. Postgrad Med 89:79, 1991.
Provides a strategy for diagnosing the cause of monoarticular arthritis.
Shmerling RH, Delbanco TL, Tosteson ANA, et al: Synovial fluid tests: What should be ordered? JAMA 264:1009, 1990.
Reviews the diagnostic yield of synovial fluid laboratory tests.
Stimmler MM: Infectious arthritis: Tailoring initial treatment to clinical findings. Postgrad Med 99:127, 1996.
Analysis and culture of synovial fluid can provide the definitive diagnosis in patients with infectious arthritis.
Towheed TE, Hochberg MC: Acute monoarthritis: A practical approach to assessment and treatment. Am Fam Physician 54:2239, 1996.
The most common causes are trauma, crystals (gout and pseudogout), and infection.

ARTHRITIS

Recommendations for arthritis are from the medical literature.

1. In patients with joint pain due to arthritis, consider the clinical findings, look for diagnostic clues, and request appropriate tests. This discussion does not address periarticular disorders related to injuries, fibromyalgia, polymyositis, and polymyalgia rheumatica.

These disorders may be approached as follows:

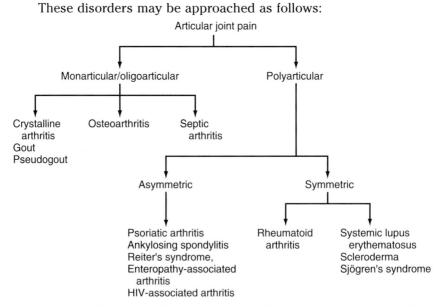

Source: Litman K: A rational approach to the diagnosis of arthritis. Am Fam Physician 53:1295–1310, 1996. Published with permission from the American Academy of Family Physicians.

Clinically, it is useful to assess whether the arthritis is monoarticular/oligoarticular or polyarticular. If the arthritis is monoarticular and acute and an effusion is present, consider aspirating fluid for laboratory studies, and refer to the discussion on synovial fluid analysis earlier in this chapter. If more than one joint is involved and findings of systemic disease are present, consider the diagnosis of rheumatic disease.

Rather than requesting "arthritis panels" of tests, it is better to perform a careful history and physical examination and consider specific tests based on the affected joints and diagnostic clues as follows:

DIAGNOSIS OF ARTHRITIS

Affected Joints	Diagnostic Clues	Test Considerations
Gout Large cool joints; first metatarsophalangeal joint, ankle, knee, elbow, wrist	Intermittent severe attacks; tophi (crystals in cartilage, tendons); history of increased alcohol use; high purine diet; renal stones or dysfunction Family history Male : female ratio: 2 to 7 : 1	Uric acid, joint aspirate crystal analysis, urinalysis (for hematuria)
Calcium pyrophosphate deposition disease (also called chondrocalcinosis and pseudogout) Similar to gout	Similar to gout without tophi or renal disease; attacks may be triggered by trauma or overuse	Joint aspirate crystal analysis; radiographs (may show calcification of menisci)
Osteoarthritis Weight-bearing or chronically stressed joints; spine, hip, knee, fingers, and toes (including DIP)	Pain with use, relief with rest; slowly progressive with exacerbations Family history	Radiographs; if diagnosis is unclear, consider ESR or CRP (usually normal) or joint aspiration.
Septic arthritis Knee, hip, sternum; any joint if associated with local infection or trauma	Fever common Gonococcal: young adults, female : male ratio: 2 : 1 Nongonococcal: any age; patient often immunocompromised or IV drug user; extra-articular source of infection	White blood cell count (elevated), joint aspirate cell count (elevated), Gram stain
Spondyloarthropathies (ankylosing spondylitis; Reiter's syndrome; psoriatic, enteropathy-associated arthritis; HIV-associated arthritis)		

Location	Clinical findings	Laboratory tests
Spine, large and small joints, tendon insertions	Reiter's syndrome: uveitis, urethritis, cervicitis; Psoriatic: skin plaques; Ankylosing spondylitis: sacroiliitis, decreased respiratory excursion; Enteropathy-associated: inflammatory bowel disease; HIV-associated: evidence of AIDS; Family history	ESR or CRP (elevated); radiographs of sacrum (ankylosing spondylitis); urethral or cervical smear (Reiter's syndrome); consider HLA-B27 assay if diagnosis unclear (low specificity when disease unlikely)
Rheumatoid arthritis Extremities, especially hands (sparing of DIPs)	Gelling (morning stiffness) for more than 1 hour; three or more joints involved; arthritis of hands; symmetric arthritis; rheumatoid nodules; positive for rheumatoid factor; radiologic findings of erosions of periarticular osteoporosis; four of seven needed for diagnosis; Family history	ESR or CRP (elevated); rheumatoid factor (usually elevated)
Systemic Lupus Erythematosus Extremities, especially hands, wrists, knees	Malar or discoid rash; photosensitivity; oral ulcers; nonerosive arthritis; serositis (pleuritis, pericarditis); renal disease (proteinuria, casts); hematologic disease (anemia, decreased white blood cells, decreased platelet count); neurologic disease (seizure, psychosis); immunologic (anti-DNA antibodies, anti-Smith antibodies) false-positive VDRL; positive ANA test; 4 of these 11 needed for diagnosis; Family history; Female:male ratio: 5:1	ANA (elevated), ESR or CRP (elevated); consider CBC, urinalysis, creatinine, specific ANA testing

ESR = erythrocyte sedimentation rate; CRP = C-reactive protein; DIP = distal interphalangeal joint; HIV = human immunodeficiency virus; AIDS = acquired immunodeficiency syndrome; ANA = antinuclear antibodies; CBC = complete blood count.

Source: Litman K: A rational approach to the diagnosis of arthritis. Am Fam Physician 53:1295–1310, 1996. Published with permission from the American Academy of Family Physicians.

2. Evaluate the tests.

The following blood tests may be useful:

- Complete blood count
- Erythrocyte sedimentation rate (ESR)
- C-reactive protein
- Complement
- Antinuclear antibody (ANA)
- Autoantibody profile
- Uric acid
- Rheumatoid factor
- HLA-B27 assay

3. Interpret test results in the context of clinical findings.

The radiographic features of osteoarthritis include joint space loss, subchondral increase in bone density, osteophyte formation, and subchondral cysts, whereas the features of rheumatoid arthritis include periarticular soft tissue swelling, juxta-articular osteoporosis, juxta-articular erosions, and joint space narrowing.

Laboratory test results in osteoarthritis are normal. In rheumatoid arthritis, the rheumatoid factor may be positive (80%) and the ANA may also be positive (50%—usually diffuse in immunofluorescence). Anemia of chronic disease, an increased ESR, and a hypergammaglobulinemia with polyclonal gammopathy are often present. There may be thrombocytosis.

Other diagnoses that should be ruled out include the spondyloarthropathies, systemic lupus erythematosus (SLE), systemic sclerosis, Lyme disease, and crystal-induced arthritis (gout and pseudogout).

In patients with SLE there may be hemolytic anemia, leukopenia, lymphocytopenia, and thrombocytopenia. ANA positivity occurs in about 95% of patients with SLE. Specific autoantibody testing may be helpful.

BIBLIOGRAPHY

Litman K: A rational approach to the diagnosis of arthritis. Am Fam Physician 53:1295, 1996.
Discusses the use of laboratory tests in the diagnosis of arthritis.
Peterson LS, Cohen MD: Rheumatic disease: How to use the laboratory in the workup. Consultant 36:1329, 1996.
Reviews the use of antibody tests to diagnose rheumatic disease.
Sanmartí R, Collado A, Gratacós J, et al: Reduced activity of serum creatine kinase in rheumatoid arthritis: A phenomenon linked to the inflammatory response. Br J Rheumatol 33:231, 1994.
The clinical significance of the reduced creatine kinase in rheumatoid arthritis is unknown.
Shmerling RH, Delbanco TL: How useful is the rheumatoid factor? An analysis of sensitivity, specificity, and predictive value. Arch Intern Med 152:2417, 1992.
Rheumatoid factor should be selectively ordered when rheumatic disease is suspected.

Slater CA, Davis RB, Shmerling RH: Antinuclear antibody testing: A study of clinical utility. Arch Intern Med 156:1421, 1996.
  More selective ordering of the ANA test might improve its clinical utility.
Thomas MJ, Adebajo A, Chapel HM, et al: The use of rheumatoid factors in clinical practice. Postgrad Med J 71:674, 1995.
  When this test is applied to general hospital or community populations, it performs poorly.
Wallendal M, Stork L, Hollister TR, et al: The discriminating value of serum lactate dehydrogenase levels in children with malignant neoplasms presenting as joint pain. Arch Pediatr Adolesc Med 150:70, 1996.
  A high LD level may be present in cancer patients.
Wolfe F, Michaud K: The clinical and research significance of the erythrocyte sedimentation rate. J Rheumatol 21:1227, 1994.
  Discusses guidelines for the interpretation of the ESR.

3

Cardiovascular Diseases

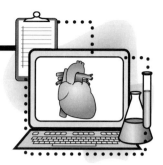

- Acute Myocardial Infarction
- Congestive Heart Failure
- Hypertension
- Digoxin Monitoring

ACUTE MYOCARDIAL INFARCTION

Recommendations for acute myocardial infarction (AMI) are from the medical literature. The American College of Cardiology, the American Heart Association, and the World Health Organization have made recommendations regarding the management of AMI.

1. For emergency department patients with typical clinical findings of AMI together with positive and unequivocal electrocardiographic (ECG) findings, admit the patient and measure creatine kinase-MB (CK-MB) and cardiac troponin I (cTnI) at baseline and repeat at 12 hours (Keffer, 1997).

Up to 7 million Americans have coronary artery disease. Of these, about 1.5 million suffer an AMI every year, and approximately 0.5 million die. Moreover, up to 25% of AMI's are silent; these silent or painless infarcts are more common in diabetics and after cardiac transplantation. A major problem is the correct diagnosis of AMI in the emergency department. On the one hand, about 75% of patients who do not have AMI are admitted to an expensive coronary care unit; conversely, every year approximately 30,000 patients with an AMI are sent home.

Clinical findings of AMI include crushing substernal chest pain or pressure, sweating, nausea/vomiting, dyspnea, pallor, and bradycardia/tachycardia. The diagnosis of AMI, as formally established by the World Health Organization, requires at least two of the following criteria: a history of characteristic chest pain, evolutionary changes on the electrocardiogram, and elevation of serial cardiac enzymes.

2. For emergency department patients with an atypical presentation of AMI and a negative or equivocal ECG, assay for cTnI and CK-MB as a baseline. If CK-MB is more than 4.0 ng/mL (4.0 µg/L [or equivalent by other mass assay]), then perform total CK and CK indexes. Repeat the CK-MB at 4, 8, and 12 hours after arrival at the emergency

department. Confirm the appearance or rise of CK-MB with concurrent and subsequent cTnI measurements. If the cTnI baseline is positive for an earlier AMI, then it is appropriate to monitor the patient with cTnI only (Keffer, 1997).

The differential diagnosis of chest pain follows:

Cardiac	Aortic stenosis, coronary artery disease, pericarditis, hypertrophic cardiomyopathy
Gastrointestinal	Biliary disease, esophageal motility disorders, esophageal reflux (esophagitis), hiatal hernia, Mallory-Weiss syndrome, pancreatitis, peptic ulcer disease
Vascular	Aortic dissection, pulmonary embolism, pulmonary hypertension
Pulmonary	Mediastinitis or mediastinal emphysema, pleuritis or pneumonia, pneumothorax, tracheobronchitis, tumor
Musculoskeletal	Arthritis of the shoulder or spine, herniated cervical disk, chest wall contusion or trauma, costochondritis (Tietze's syndrome), intercostal muscle cramps, myositis, rib fracture, subacromial bursitis
Other	Chest wall tumors, breast disorders, herpes zoster, psychological

Source: Moreyra E, Taheri H, Wasserman A: Chest pain: Is it life-threatening—or benign? Consultant 35:1820, 1995.

3. For clinical settings other than the emergency department, evaluate patients for possible AMI as follows:

In addition to the emergency department, there are several different settings in which cardiac markers are useful.

Noncardiac surgical group	cTnI at baseline and repeat testing at 6, 12, and 24 hours after operation
Cardiac surgical group	cTnI at baseline before operation and at time zero and 6 and 12 hours after removal of cross clamps
Cardiac trauma	cTnI at 4, 8, and 12 hours. Subsequent sampling at 12-hour intervals up to 48 hours to detect occult trauma
Postinfarction or extension group	cTnI or CK-MB daily for approximately 5 days

Source: Keffer JH: The cardiac profile and proposed practice guideline for acute ischemic heart disease. Am J Clin Pathol 107:398–408, 1997. Copyright © 1997 by the American Society of Clinical Pathologists. Reprinted with permission.

4. Evaluate the tests.

The following figure illustrates the evolution of various serum markers of myocardial damage after the occurrence of AMI.

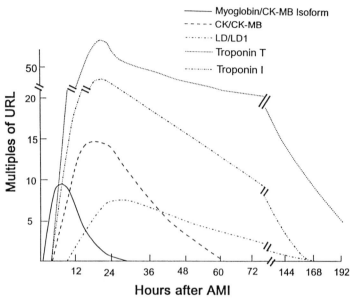

URL = Upper reference limit.
Source: Wong SS: Strategic utilization of cardiac markers for the diagnosis of acute myocardial infarction. Ann Clin Lab Sci 26:301–312, 1996. Copyright 1996 by the Institute for Clinical Science.

Myoglobin

Measurement of myoglobin has been advocated because it is significantly increased earlier than other markers. Nonspecificity is problematic because of increased myoglobin from skeletal muscle disease or trauma. The BB isoenzyme of glycogen phosphorylase has been recommended as an even earlier marker of AMI than myoglobin. In a European study of 271 patients with an AMI, it was the most sensitive marker of AMI during the first 4 hours after chest pain.

CK-MB Isoforms or Subforms

Although CK-MB isoforms are alleged to increase before CK-MB, it is unclear if this is true when CK-MB is properly measured by mass assay. Nevertheless, CK-MB isoforms continued to be recommended for the early diagnosis of AMI.

Troponins

Cardiac troponin T (cTnT) and cTnI assays, based on the use of monoclonal antibodies, are excellent tests of myocardial infarction. The cTnI assay may be better than the cTnT because cTnT is nonspecifically elevated in patients with chronic renal failure. Moreover, cTnT may be increased in patients with muscle trauma or rhabdomyolysis, as well as in patients with polymyositis/dermatomyositis. The more rapid performance of cTnI immunoassays makes them suitable for fast turnaround time testing. With additional studies, the comparative attributes of cTnI versus cTnT continues to evolve.

Creatine Kinase and Creatine Kinase-MB

CK and CK-MB are currently the standard markers for diagnosing AMI. A method of choice is CK-MB by mass immunoassay. Using single test results in the emergency department, the CK was elevated in only 38% and the CK-MB in only 34%. Therefore, serial measurements are necessary.

Interestingly, although serum CK and sometimes CK-MB are elevated in hypothyroidism, cTnI is not. Thus, in the setting of hypothyroidism and chest pain, cTnI is the superior marker of myocardial injury.

Lactate Dehydrogenase (LD) and LD Isoenzymes

LD and LD isoenzymes are currently measured at baseline and every 24 hours for 2 to 3 days. Recent studies suggest that LD studies are confirmatory, not always necessary, and required only if admission has been delayed more than 24 hours or if the CK studies fail to show an abnormality. Measurement of cTnI makes LD studies unnecessary.

5. Interpret test results in the context of clinical findings.

A thoughtful review of the entire presentation—clinically, electrocardiographically, biochemically, and by additional tests if necessary—allows for appropriate disposition of the patient.

6. In patients with AMI, the following blood test results may be increased:

- **Hematocrit** may show a small early increase related to decreased blood volume, followed by a small decrease later.
- **Leukocytes, increased erythrocyte sedimentation rate (ESR), and C-reactive protein** caused by the inflammatory response associated with the infarct. Leukocytosis appears within hours of onset of pain, persists for 1 to 2 weeks, and often reaches 12 to 15 $\times$ 10^3 cells/μL (12 to 15 $\times$ 10^9 cells/L). ESR rises more slowly than

leukocyte levels, peaks during the first week, and sometimes remains increased for 1 to 2 weeks.

- **Glucose** related to diabetes mellitus as a predisposing risk factor or simply secondary to the stress of the infarct. In stress hyperglycemia, hemoglobin A_{1c} is normal. In nondiabetics, mortality rate of 3.4% at admission glucose levels less than 120 mg/dL (<6.7 mmol/L) rises to 42.9% at levels greater than 180 mg/dL (>10.0 mmol/L).
- **Urea nitrogen and creatinine** related to decreased renal perfusion. Increased creatinine is associated with increased mortality.
- **Aspartate aminotransferase (AST)** from infarct and possibly from hepatic congestion
- **Alanine aminotransferase (ALT) and LD$_5$** may occur from congestion and poor perfusion of the liver secondary to heart failure. Thus, ALT is a good way to monitor congestive heart failure secondary to AMI.
- **Bilirubin** with severe heart failure from hepatic failure
- **Lactate** (>32 mg/dL [>3.6 mmol/L]) occurs in 60% of patients the day before the development of shock.
- **Triglycerides** peak at 3 weeks; increase may persist for 1 year.
- **Cholesterol,** which may constitute a predisposing risk factor for coronary heart disease. If cholesterol level can be measured within the first 24 hours of infarction, it is statistically the same as the preinfarction level.

7. In patients with AMI, the following blood test results may be decreased:

- **pH** with metabolic acidosis caused by tissue hypoxia
- **Partial pressure of oxygen** from cardiopulmonary dysfunction. Mild hypoxemia can occur even without complications.
- **Lymphocytopenia** is consistent with AMI.
- **Sodium**
- **Potassium** caused by either a high level of circulating catecholamines or previous diuretic therapy. Potassium value less than 3.6 mEq/L (<3.6 mmol/L) during admission is a risk factor for ventricular arrhythmia within 6 hours after admission.
- **Albumin** caused by hepatic congestion

BIBLIOGRAPHY

Adams JE III, Bodor GS, Dávila-Román VG, et al: Cardiac troponin I: A marker with high specificity for cardiac injury. Circulation 88:101, 1993.
Cardiac troponin I elevations occur rarely or not at all in patients without cardiac injury.
Adams JE III, Dávila-Román VG, Bessey PO, et al: Improved detection of cardiac contusion with cardiac troponin I. Am Heart J 131:308, 1996.
Serum cTnI is useful for the accurate diagnosis of cardiac injury in patients with blunt chest trauma, and it is easier to measure and less costly than echocardiography.
Adams JE III, Sicard GA, Allen BT, et al: Diagnosis of perioperative myocardial infarction with measurement of cardiac troponin I. N Engl J Med 330:670, 1994.

Cardiac troponin I is the most specific test for perioperative myocardial infarction.
Adams J, Trent R, Rawles J, et al: Earliest electrocardiographic evidence of myocardial infarction: Implications for thrombolytic treatment. BMJ 307:409, 1993.
The ECG is not likely to be helpful in determining whether patients should receive early thrombolytic therapy.
Apple FS: Acute myocardial infarction and coronary reperfusion: Serum cardiac markers for the 1990s. Am J Clin Pathol 97:217, 1992.
Reviews the use of cardiac markers for diagnosing AMI.
Apple FS: Glycogen phosphorylase BB and other cardiac proteins: Challenges to creatine kinase MB as the marker for detecting myocardial injury. Clin Chem 41:963, 1995.
Cardiac troponin I seems to be the troponin of choice for evaluating myocardial damage in patients with severe skeletal muscle injury.
Bellodi G, Manicardi V, Malavasi V, et al: Hyperglycemia and prognosis of acute myocardial infarction in patients without diabetes mellitus. Am J Cardiol 64:885, 1989.
Correlates increasing admission glucose values in non-diabetics with increasing mortality.
Bhayana V, Gougoulias T, Cohoe S, et al: Discordance between results for serum troponin T and troponin I. Clin Chem 41:312, 1995.
Li D, Keffer J, Corry K, et al: Nonspecific elevation of troponin T levels in patients with chronic renal failure. Clin Biochem 28:474, 1995.
Frankel WL, Herold DA, Ziegler TW: Cardiac troponin T is elevated in asymptomatic patients with chronic renal failure. Am J Clin Pathol 106:118, 1996.
Cardiac troponin I is more specific for AMI than cardiac troponin T.
Clausen TG, Brocks K, Ibsen H: Hypokalemia and ventricular arrhythmias in acute myocardial infarction. Acta Med Scand 224:531, 1988.
Hypokalemia during admission, whether spontaneous or diuretic induced, correlates with an increased incidence of ventricular arrhythmia.
Cohen LF, Mohabeer AF, Keffer JH, et al: Troponin I in hypothyroidism. Clin Chem 42:1494, 1996.
In the setting of hypothyroidism and chest pain, cTnI is the superior marker of myocardial injury.
Galvani M, Ottani F, Ferrini D, et al: Prognostic influence of elevated values of cardiac troponin I in patients with unstable angina. Circulation 95:2053, 1997.
Data indicate that cTnI is an important prognostic variable in patients with unstable angina. Elevations of cTnI predict an adverse short- and long-term prognosis.
Gambino SR: Cardiac troponin I and glycogen phosphorylase BB. Lab Report Physicians 17:65, 1995.
Cardiac troponin I is recommended as a replacement for CK-MB and glycogen phosphorylase BB as a replacement for myoglobin.
Gibler WB, Runyon JP, Levy RC, et al: A rapid diagnostic and treatment center for patients with acute chest pain in the emergency department. Ann Emerg Med 25:1, 1995.
In low- and medium-risk patients, cardiac markers at 3, 6, and 9 hours with continuous 12-lead ECG with ST-segment test monitoring for 9 hours are recommended. Echocardiography and graded exercise testing are performed at the end of 9 hours.
Guest TM, Ramanathan AV, Tuteur PG, et al: Myocardial injury in critically ill patients: A frequently unrecognized complication. JAMA 273:1945, 1995.
Serum troponin detects unrecognized myocardial injury in critically ill patients.
Hedges JR, Young GP, Henkel GF, et al: Serial ECGs are less accurate than serial CK-MB results for emergency department diagnosis of myocardial infarction. Ann Emerg Med 21:1445, 1992.
Serial CK-MB is better than serial ECGs, but the combination is better than each alone.
Hohnloser SH, Zabel M, Kasper W, et al: Assessment of coronary artery patency after thrombolytic therapy. Accurate prediction utilizing the combined analysis of three noninvasive markers. J Am Coll Cardiol 18:44, 1991.
Early peak CK predicts successful thrombolysis.
Ishikawa Y, Saffitz JE, Mealman TL, et al: Reversible myocardial ischemic injury is not associated with increased creatine kinase activity in plasma. Clin Chem 43:467, 1997.
Increased creatine kinase reflects myocardial necrosis.

Jaffe AS, Landt Y, Parvin CA, et al: Comparative sensitivity of cardiac troponin I and lactate dehydrogenase isoenzymes for diagnosing acute myocardial infarction. Clin Chem 42:1770, 1996.

Criteria based on cTnI should improve the accuracy of retrospective diagnoses of AMI.

Keffer JH: Myocardial markers of injury: Evolution and insights. Am J Clin Pathol 105:305, 1996.

Excellent review of markers of myocardial injury.

Keffer JH: The cardiac profile and proposed practice guideline for acute ischemic heart disease. Am J Clin Pathol 107:398, 1997.

Recommended testing strategies for a variety of clinical situations.

Lee TH, Goldman L: Serum enzyme assays in the diagnosis of acute myocardial infarction: Recommendations based on a quantitative analysis. *In* Sox HC Jr (ed): Common Diagnostic Tests: Use and Interpretation, 2nd ed. Philadelphia, American College of Physicians, 1990, p 35.

Reviews the use of serum enzymes for the diagnosis of AMI.

Lynch M, Hoffmann NV, Aroney CN: Thrombolytic treatment and proteinuria. Br Heart J 74:354, 1995.

Streptokinase and tissue plasminogen therapy may cause proteinuria.

Matts JP, Karnegis JN, Campos CT, et al: Serum creatinine as an independent predictor of coronary heart disease mortality in normotensive survivors of myocardial infarction. J Fam Pract 36:497, 1993.

An increased serum creatinine level is associated with increased coronary mortality and increased overall mortality.

Mavric Z, Zaputovic L, Zager D, et al: Usefulness of blood lactate as a predictor of shock development in acute myocardial infarction. Am J Cardiol 67:565, 1991.

In patients who were not in shock during admission, high blood lactate level correlated with risk of shock in the next 24 hours.

Montague C, Kircher T: Myoglobin in the early evaluation of acute chest pain. Am J Clin Pathol 104:472, 1995.

Evaluates the use of myoglobin in acute chest pain.

Moreyra E, Taheri H, Wasserman A: Chest pain: Is it life-threatening—or benign? Consultant 35:1819, 1995.

Discusses the differential diagnosis of chest pain.

Puleo PR, Meyer D, Wathen C, et al: Use of a rapid assay of subforms of creatine kinase MB to diagnose or rule out acute myocardial infarction. N Engl J Med 331:561, 1994.

Subforms of creatine kinase MB can be used to detect AMI within 6 hours after the onset of symptoms.

Rabitzsch G, Mair J, Lechleitner P, et al: Immunoenzymometric assay of human glycogen phosphorylase isoenzyme BB in diagnosis of ischemic myocardial injury. Clin Chem 41:966, 1995.

Glycogen phosphorylase isoenzyme BB was the most sensitive marker for detection of AMI during the first 4 hours of onset of chest pain.

Randall DC, Jones DL: Eliminating unnecessary lactate dehydrogenase testing. Arch Intern Med 157:1441, 1997.

Most US hospitals continue to include LDH testing in their panels to rule out myocardial infarction despite national guidelines recommending otherwise.

Ryan TJ, Anderson JL, Antman EM, et al: ACC/AHA guidelines for the management of patients with acute myocardial infarction. J Am Coll Cardiol 28:1328, 1996.

Two major cardiology groups issue joint guidelines for managing acute myocardial infarction.

Saxena S, Anderson DW, Kaufman RL, et al: Quality assurance study of cardiac isoenzyme utilization in a large teaching hospital. Arch Pathol Lab Med 117:180, 1993.

The results of the study show that physicians continue to order the CK and CK-MB tests inappropriately for most patients (62%).

Sullebarger JT, Greenland P: Myocardial infarction. *In* Panzer RJ, Black ER, Griner PF (eds): Diagnostic Strategies for Common Medical Problems. Philadelphia, American College of Physicians, 1991, p 55.

Recommends strategies for the diagnosis of myocardial infarction.

Thomson SP, Gibbons RJ, Smars PA, et al: Incremental value of the leukocyte differential and the rapid creatine kinase-MB isoenzyme for the early diagnosis of myocardial infarction. Ann Intern Med 122:335, 1995.

In the emergency department, an elevated rapid CK-MB and a decreased relative lymphocyte percentage gave a sensitivity of 44%, a specificity of 99.7%, and a positive predictive value of 97%.

Tucker JF, Collins RA, Anderson AJ, et al: Early diagnostic efficiency of cardiac troponin I and troponin T for acute myocardial infarction. Acad Emerg Med 4:13, 1997.

Cardiac troponin I, CK-MB, and myoglobin are significantly more specific for AMI than are CK and cTnT.

Udea S, Ikeda U, Yamamoto K, et al: C-reactive protein as a predictor of cardiac rupture after acute myocardial infarction. Am Heart J 131:857, 1996.

A persistently elevated serum C-reactive protein (>20 mg/dL [>200 mg/L]) is of predictive value for cardiac rupture after AMI.

Wong SS: Strategic utilization of cardiac markers for the diagnosis of acute myocardial infarction. Ann Clin Lab Sci 26:301, 1996.

Proposes a strategy for the utilization of cardiac markers.

Zalenski RJ, McCarren M, Roberts R, et al: An evaluation of a chest pain diagnostic protocol to exclude acute cardiac ischemia in the emergency department. Arch Intern Med 157:1085, 1997.

Discusses a diagnostic protocol, including serial measurements of CK-MB, ECG, and clinical assessments followed by exercise ECG for those with negative initial serial testing.

CONGESTIVE HEART FAILURE

Recommendations for congestive heart failure (CHF) are from the medical literature.

1. In patients with clinical findings of CHF, request a complete blood count (CBC), serum electrolytes (including magnesium), glucose, urea nitrogen, creatinine, albumin, sensitive thyrotropin (sTSH) (if patients have atrial fibrillation, evidence of thyroid disease, or older than age 65), liver function tests, arterial blood gas analysis, and a urinalysis. Other useful studies include chest radiography, ECG, echocardiography or radionuclide ventriculography, and exercise testing. Unless an obscure cause is suggested by clinical findings, measurement of vitamin levels, myocardial biopsy, and tests for lead, iron, cocaine, or other toxins are not warranted.

Each year CHF, a syndrome affecting approximately 1% of the North American population, develops in approximately 400,000 Americans. It is the only major cardiovascular disease with an increasing incidence. The leading cause is myocardial infarction. For individuals older than age 75, the prevalence of the syndrome rises to approximately 10%. Mortality risk for patients with CHF has been reported to be as high as 50% at 2 years following diagnosis. In the United States, $8 billion is spent annually to hospitalize patients with CHF.

Clinical findings include dyspnea on exertion, orthopnea, paroxysmal nocturnal dyspnea, jugular venous distention, third heart sound, fatigue, pulmonary edema, pedal edema, and ascites. A CBC is useful to detect anemia and an sTSH to detect thyroid dysfunction. Although serum electrolyte values are generally normal before treatment, diuretic therapy and sodium restriction can cause abnormalities. Reductions in renal blood flow can increase serum urea nitrogen and creatinine concentrations, and poor cardiac output with congestion of the liver can cause abnormal liver function test results. Congestion of the lungs can cause pulmonary edema and affect arterial blood gas values. Pleural and pericardial effusions may occur. Ascites is a late manifestation. Increased atrial natriuretic peptide is present in patients with CHF. The New York Heart Association has functionally classified CHF as follows:

Classification	Characteristics
Class I (asymptomatic)	No limitation; evidence of cardiac disease but no symptoms of heart failure, even with exercise
Class II (mild)	Slight limitation; symptoms of heart failure but only with exercise
Class III (moderate)	Marked limitation; symptoms of heart failure with mild exercise (e.g., walking)
Class IV (severe)	Inability to perform any physical activity; symptoms present at rest

Source: Mair FS: Management of heart failure. Am Fam Physician 54:245–254, 1996. Published with permission from the American Academy of Family Physicians.

It is important to distinguish CHF due to systolic dysfunction from that due to diastolic dysfunction, because the management may differ.

2. Interpret test results in the context of clinical findings.

Hyperglycemia is common, probably related to stress. Hypoglycemia may occur in the presence of severe, prolonged hepatic congestion and severely compromised cardiac output.

The serum urea nitrogen, creatinine, and uric acid values may be increased secondary to reductions in renal blood flow and glomerular filtration rate. Urea nitrogen values may be as high as 80 to 100 mg/dL (29 to 36 mmol/L) and are disproportionately high relative to those for creatinine. This prerenal azotemia is usually characterized by a urea:creatinine ratio greater than 15:1.

Prolonged rigid sodium restriction coupled with intensive diuretic therapy and the inability to excrete water may lead to hypervolemic hyponatremia, which occurs despite an increase in total body sodium in the context of an expanded extracellular fluid volume. Prolonged administration of kaliuretic diuretics such as thiazides or loop diuretics may cause hypokalemia. Hypokalemia is associated with a poor prognosis as a result of ventricular arrhythmias. Triamterene is often administered with thiazides for its potassium-sparing effect. In patients with terminal heart failure, hyperkalemia may occur. A serum potassium concentration greater than 5.5 mEq/L (>5.5 mmol/L) is a contraindication to therapy with angiotensin-converting enzyme inhibitors.

In failure of the right side of the heart, acute congestive hepatomegaly can cause a significant increase of serum AST and ALT values to several thousand units, which may resemble the findings with acute viral hepatitis. Low cardiac output is often present. A differential clue is that, in contrast to those with viral hepatitis, the increased transaminase values of heart failure can return to normal within 5 to 7 days of successful treatment. In a patient with AMI the AST level is increased, but in one with AMI with CHF both the AST and ALT levels are increased. Other liver function test results may be increased. They include serum alkaline phosphatase, lactate dehydrogenase (LD) (especially isoenzyme LD_5), and total and conjugated bilirubin. In fact, frank jaundice may occur. The prothrombin time may be prolonged. Rarely, acute hepatic decompensation can occur, with hepatic coma and an increased blood ammonia concentration.

In one study chronic CHF was categorized as mild, moderate, or severe. The mean values for the liver function test results in patients in the mild and moderate groups were normal or mainly normal. Patients in the severe group had significantly higher activities of AST (65 ± 83 U/L), ALT (77 ± 102 U/L), and LD (282 ± 91 U/L), and an increased total bilirubin concentration (1.7 ± 0.8 mg/dL [29 ± 14 μmol/L]). In patients with chronic congestive hepatomegaly, serum albumin may be decreased not only because of liver dysfunction, but also because of protein-losing enteropathy (a rare occurrence).

In failure of the left side of the heart with acute pulmonary edema, arterial blood gas determinations can help assess decreased oxygenation (decreased PO_2). Cyanosis is seen with greater than 5 g/dL (>50 g/L) of reduced hemoglobin.

Oliguria is characteristic of heart failure, and urinary specific gravity may be low. Mild albuminuria (<1 g/day) is common, and the urinary sediment may show isolated red blood cells, white blood cells, and casts (hyaline and granular). With acute oliguria, the urinary sodium concentration in a CHF patient is generally less than 20 mEq/L (<20 mmol/L), whereas in a patient with acute renal failure caused by intrinsic renal disease or postrenal obstruction, the urinary sodium concentration is typically greater than 40 mEq/L (>40 mmol/L).

3. In patients with CHF receiving drug therapy, monitor the patient for possible adverse effects of drugs.

For example, thiazides and loop diuretics can cause alkalosis and increased serum glucose, uric acid, calcium, total cholesterol, low-density lipoprotein cholesterol, triglycerides, and possibly plasma renin activity, and decreased serum potassium, magnesium, glomerular filtration rate, and lithium clearance (in patients receiving lithium therapy). The hypercholesterolemic effect of diuretics may abate with continued administration of the drug. Uncommon effects include inappropriate antidiuretic hormone secretion and decreased red blood cells, white blood cells, and platelets.

Potassium-sparing diuretics (e.g., triamterene) can cause megaloblastic anemia, increased potassium and plasma renin activity, and decreased glomerular filtration.

To determine which drug increases or decreases serum lipid values, wait until the patient has been taking the drug for at least 6 to 8 weeks before measuring lipids. See the discussion of serum cholesterol in Chapter 1 for a table of drug effects on serum lipids.

4. In patients with CHF, the following blood test results may be increased:

- **ESR**—this is of little clinical value
- **Magnesium** associated with worse prognosis related to severity of disease and poor organ function

5. In patients with CHF, the following blood test results may be decreased:

- **Hematocrit,** mild, even when red blood cell mass is increased
- **ESR**—this is of little clinical value
- **Magnesium** caused by anorexia, malabsorption, and excessive use of diuretic agents; when less than 1.6 mEq/L (<0.66 mmol/L), associated with worse prognosis related to ventricular arrhythmia and sudden death.
- **Cholesterol** with severe congestion of the liver

BIBLIOGRAPHY

Bales AC, Sorrentino MJ: Causes of congestive heart failure: Prompt diagnosis may affect prognosis. Postgrad Med 101:44, 1997.
   Good discussion of diagnostic tests.
Clark AJ, Coats AJS: Usefulness of arterial blood gas estimations during exercise in patients with chronic heart failure. Br Heart J 71:528, 1994.
   Patients with heart failure become breathless with exercise, but their arterial oxygen and carbon dioxide tensions and arterial oxygen saturation remain near normal.
Clinical Quality Improvement Network Investigators: Mortality risk and patterns of practice in 4606 acute care patients with congestive heart failure: The relative importance of age, sex, and medical therapy. Arch Intern Med 156:1669, 1996.
   Congestive heart failure constitutes a principal growth area in contemporary clinical cardiology.
Cohen JA, Kaplan MM: Left-sided heart failure presenting as hepatitis. Gastroenterology 74:583, 1978.
   Points out that liver enzyme values may be very high in CHF and may simulate hepatitis.
Fleg JL, Hinton PC, Lakatta EG, et al: Physician utilization of laboratory procedures to monitor outpatients with congestive heart failure. Arch Intern Med 149:393, 1989.
   Describes the most common tests that physicians use to monitor outpatients with CHF.
Gottlieb SS, Baruch L, Kukin ML, et al: Prognostic importance of the serum magnesium concentration in patients with congestive heart failure. J Am Coll Cardiol 16:827, 1990.
   Correlates hypomagnesemia and hypermagnesemia with a worse prognosis.
Haber HL, Leavy JA, Kessler PD, et al: The erythrocyte sedimentation rate in congestive heart failure. N Engl J Med 324:353, 1991.
   The ESR in patients with CHF may be high or low and is of limited clinical value.

Kubo SH, Walter BA, John DHA, et al: Liver function abnormalities in chronic heart failure: Influence of systemic hemodynamics. Arch Intern Med 147:1227, 1987.
Quantifies liver function test abnormalities based on the severity of liver dysfunction.

Lardinosis CK, Neuman SL: The effects of antihypertensive agents on serum lipids and lipoproteins. Arch Intern Med 148:1280, 1988.
Describes the adverse effects of diuretics in CHF.

Mair FS: Management of heart failure. Am Fam Physician 54:245, 1996.
Optimal treatment of CHF depends on accurate diagnosis.

Parmley WW, Chaterjee K, Francis GS, et al: Congestive heart failure: New frontiers. West J Med 154:427, 1991.
Good review of CHF.

Powers ER, Bergin JD: Recent advances in evaluating and managing congestive heart failure. Modern Med 60:54, 1992.
Discusses the diagnosis and management of patients with CHF.

Seager LH: Congestive heart failure: Considerations for primary care physicians. Postgrad Med 98:127, 1995.
Gives guidelines for managing patients with CHF.

Wilkins MR, Redondo J, Brown LA: The natriuretic-peptide family. Lancet 349:1307, 1997.
Plasma concentrations of atrial natriuretic peptide may be a useful marker of cardiac function.

HYPERTENSION

Recommendations for hypertension are from the Joint National Committee on Detection, Evaluation, and Treatment of High Blood Pressure and the medical literature.

1. For patients with newly discovered hypertension, request a CBC, measurements of serum glucose (fasting), urea nitrogen or creatinine, potassium, calcium, uric acid, cholesterol, high-density lipoprotein (HDL) cholesterol, a urinalysis, and an ECG. Do not routinely perform the following studies: chest radiography, intravenous pyelography, and plasma renin determinations.

About 50 million Americans have hypertension, with 90 to 95% of cases classified as essential hypertension. An early Cleveland Clinic study of nearly 5000 patients showed that 89% had primary or essential hypertension, 5% had secondary hypertension from renal parenchymal disease and 4% from renovascular disease. All other causes accounted for less than 2% of cases. The relatively high prevalence of secondary hypertension in the Cleveland Clinic study may be related to the referral center setting.

The revised classification for blood pressure in adults aged 18 and older is as follows:

	Blood Pressure (mm Hg)	
Category	*Systolic*	*Diastolic*
Normal	<130	<85
High normal	130–139	85–89

Category	Blood Pressure (mm Hg)	
	Systolic	*Diastolic*
Hypertension		
Stage 1—mild	140–159	90–99
Stage 2—moderate	160–179	100–109
Stage 3—severe	180–209	110–119
Stage 4—very severe	≥210	≥120

Reflects those who are not taking antihypertensive drugs and who are not acutely ill.

Source: Prisant LM: Hypertension. *In* Conn RB, Borer WZ, Snyder JW (eds): Current Diagnosis, 9th ed. Philadelphia, WB Saunders, 1997, p 350.

Since the mid-1960s, when the Veteran's Administration Cooperative Trials established less than 140/90 as the treatment standard, mortality rates have decreased for coronary artery disease and hypertension-related stroke. However, hypertension-related renal disease continued to increase. Now it is thought that, except for patients with contraindications such as coronary artery disease or a history of myocardial infarction, less than 130/85 may be a better goal to decrease the incidence of renal disease.

Hemoglobin and hematocrit values are useful in detecting anemia, which can stress the heart and be a clue to renal disease. Occasionally, erythrocytosis with an expanded blood volume may be present. A baseline leukocyte count and platelet count may be of assistance in monitoring drug therapy (e.g., thiazide diuretics and methyldopa can cause leukopenia and thrombocytopenia), and a fasting serum glucose level can be used to detect diabetes mellitus, which may be associated with accelerated atherosclerosis, renal vascular disease, and diabetic nephropathy. Additionally, hyperglycemia can signal the presence of adrenal hyperfunction, Cushing's syndrome, and pheochromocytoma. Glucose concentrations may also be affected by therapy. Serum determinations of urea nitrogen or creatinine and a urinalysis are useful for detecting renal disease and providing an index of baseline renal function. Absence of proteinuria virtually rules out renal parenchymal disease as a cause of hypertension. Urinary crystals may suggest a stone-forming tendency. Serum potassium measurements serve not only as a screen for mineralocorticoid-induced hypertension but also as a baseline measurement before initiating drug therapy. Serum uric acid concentration is often increased in patients with renal and essential hypertension and may be increased by thiazide treatment; it may be a predictor of gout (the level of uric acid exceeds 7 mg/dL [416 μmol/L] at some time in virtually all patients with gout). Increased serum cholesterol and decreased HDL cholesterol are important risk factors for accelerated atherosclerosis. Serum cholesterol may be increased by antihypertensive drugs such as thiazide diuretics. A serum calcium level serves to exclude hypercalcemia as a primary cause for hypertension.

Although a chest radiograph, intravenous pyelography, and plasma renin determinations were formerly considered part of the routine evaluation of newly discovered hypertensive patients, they are no longer recommended except under unusual circumstances.

2. Interpret test results in the context of clinical findings.

For most hypertensive patients, the laboratory evaluation at this point is complete. Baseline data are in place, and target organ damage is assessed. Patients with a high serum total cholesterol concentration and/or low HDL cholesterol concentration should be studied further to determine low-density lipoprotein cholesterol and triglyceride concentrations and whether the hypercholesterolemia is primary or secondary. Physicians may select additional tests, based on their clinical judgment. Type and frequency of repeated laboratory tests should be based on the severity of target organ damage and the effects of the selected treatment program. If a specific form of secondary hypertension is suspected because of certain clinical and laboratory clues, commence studies for coarctation, Cushing's syndrome, pheochromocytoma, primary aldosteronism, and renovascular hypertension. Remember that increased intracranial pressure and drugs and hormones can cause hypertension (e.g., alcohol, amphetamines, oral contraceptives, estrogens, non-steroidal anti-inflammatory drugs, cyclosporine, and excess steroid or thyroid hormone). Additional disorders associated with hypertension are pregnancy, anxiety, primary hyperparathyroidism, carcinoid syndrome, acromegaly, pancreatitis, and burns.

3. Additional diagnostic testing should be reserved for cases in which potentially correctable causes of hypertension are suspected.

This category includes patients whose age at onset is less than 30 years or more than 55 years and patients who respond poorly to aggressive medical treatment as well as patients with severe hypertension (diastolic blood pressure higher than 110 to 119 mm Hg) or abrupt onset of hypertension.

- **To diagnose coarctation of the aorta, look for greater systolic pressure between the right arm and legs, decreased pulses in the legs, left ventricular hypertrophy, and rib notching by chest radiography. Confirm the diagnosis with radiographic studies, that is, aortography.**
- **To diagnose Cushing's syndrome (hypertension, central obesity, glucose intolerance, weakness [hypokalemia], depression), measure a 24-hour urine free cortisol level or perform an overnight dexamethasone suppression test.**

The 24-hour urine free cortisol test is nearly 100% sensitive and specific for diagnosing Cushing's syndrome; false-negative test results are rare, and except when stress leads to an increased cortisol excretion or with chronic alcoholism, false-positive urine free cortisol values are seldom seen. Always refer to the reference range of the laboratory you use; in general, however, a 24-hour urine cortisol concentration less than 100 μg/24 hours (<276 nmol/24 hours) excludes the diagnosis, whereas a level greater than 150 μg/24 hours (>414 nmol/24 hours) strongly suggests the diagnosis.

Another approach is to perform the overnight dexamethasone suppression test by giving the patient an oral dose of 1 mg of dexamethasone at 10:00 P.M. and measuring the serum or plasma cortisol concentration at 8:00 A.M. the next morning. A level less than 5 μg/dL (<138 nmol/L)—typically 1 to 2 μg/dL (28 to 55 nmol/L),—is present in most normal patients, whereas a value greater than 10 μg/dL (>276 nmol/L) is typical of Cushing's syndrome. False-positive results are seen more commonly with the overnight dexamethasone suppression test than with urinary free cortisol and may be due to stress, anticonvulsants, estrogens, and unipolar depression.

- **To diagnose pheochromocytoma (hypertension, weight loss, glucose intolerance, "spells" of palpitations, perspiration, pounding headache, and pallor [the "four p's"], tremor, and nervousness), measure 24-hour urinary metanephrine excretion or a 12-hour overnight urine collection for metanephrine and creatinine.**

In unstressed patients, the 24-hour metanephrine test is nearly 100% sensitive and has almost no false-negative results. Increased values occur in times of severe stress, but results are usually normal when the test is repeated. Although the 24-hour urine test is preferable, the 12-hour metanephrine test is satisfactory when combined with a test for creatinine. A normal urinary metanephrine:creatinine ratio is less than 1.2 μg metanephrine/mg creatinine (<0.69 mmol/mol creatinine); patients with the disease have higher ratios. If spells are part of the clinical presentation, a 2-, 4-, or 6-hour urine collection for determining metanephrine and creatinine values during a spell should be done.

If the clinical findings are suggestive and the urinary metanephrine test results are normal or equivocal, consider measuring urinary vanillylmandelic acid or catecholamines or both. These measurements are more specific (fewer false-positive results) and less sensitive (more false-negative results) and more subject to drug interferences than metanephrine determinations. Measurement of plasma catecholamines may be helpful.

- **To diagnose primary hyperaldosteronism (hypertension and hypokalemia), determine whether the urinary potassium level is high when the serum potassium level is low. If this is the case, measure plasma renin activity (PRA).**

The two most common causes of hypokalemia are diuretic therapy and primary aldosteronism. Begin by measuring urinary potassium levels when the serum potassium level is low because a urinary potassium level less than 30 mEq/L (<30 mmol/L) excludes hyperaldosteronism. PRA is a good initial screening test for primary hyperaldosteronism. Low PRA is highly suggestive of primary hyperaldosteronism. Once low PRA has been found in a patient with hypokalemia caused by renal potassium wasting, aldosterone should be measured; it is typically found to be high.

- **To diagnose renovascular hypertension, perform renal scintigraphy after a 25-mg dose of captopril (higher dose in obese patients). A renal arteriogram is the diagnostic "gold standard."**

Consider renovascular hypertension in older, compliant patients if hypertension persists despite a well-tolerated two- or three-drug regimen. Other risk factors include onset of hypertension in a person under age 30 and hypertension associated with unexplained and progressive renal functional impairment. Renal scintigraphy with captopril has a sensitivity of 92% and a specificity of 80% in screening for renovascular hypertension.

- **To diagnose renal parenchymal disease, consider a 24-hour urine collection to calculate creatinine clearance and quantify proteinuria. Confirmatory tests include radiographic studies and a renal biopsy.**
- **To diagnose thyroid dysfunction, request an sTSH test. See the discussion of thyroid dysfunction in Chapter 8. Secondary hypertension may occur in patients with hyperthyroidism or hypothyroidism.**

4. In patients with hypertension who are on drug therapy, monitor the patients for possible adverse effects of drugs.

For example, beta blockers can cause increased serum potassium and triglyceride concentrations and decreased HDL cholesterol concentration, glomerular filtration rate, and PRA. A rare effect is a positive antinuclear antibody test. To assess the effects of a drug on serum lipid values, wait until the patient has been taking the drug for at least 6 to 8 weeks before measuring serum lipids.

5. In patients with hypertension, the following blood test results may be increased:*

- **Glucose** caused by diuretic use, diabetes mellitus, Cushing's syndrome, acromegaly, pheochromocytoma
- **Creatinine** caused by primary renal disease, acromegaly, ACE inhibitor use, renovascular hypertension. Avoid renally excreted drugs.
- **Uric acid** caused by gout, diuretics, chronic renal failure, polycythemia, hyperparathyroidism, hypothyroidism, polycystic kidney disease, toxemia of pregnancy
- **Potassium** caused by chronic renal failure, ACE inhibitor therapy,

---

*Source: Prisant LM: Hypertension. *In* Conn RB, Borer WZ, Snyder JW (eds): Current Diagnosis, 9th ed. Philadelphia, WB Saunders, 1997, p 355.

potassium-sparing diuretics, Type IV renal tubular acidosis, salt substitutes, potassium chloride supplement
- **Calcium** caused by thiazide diuretic use, hyperparathyroidism
- **Liver function tests** caused by ethanol abuse. Avoid hepatically metabolized drugs.
- **Cholesterol** primary lipid disorder, hypothyroidism, nephrotic syndrome, hyperparathyroidism, hypercortisolism, progestational agents, anabolic steroids
- **Triglycerides** caused by obesity, diabetes mellitus, chronic renal failure, liver disease, ethanol abuse, estrogen use, beta blocker use, diuretic use

6. In patients with hypertension, the following blood test results may be decreased:*

- **Potassium,** caused by diuretic use, primary hyperaldosteronism, Cushing's syndrome

BIBLIOGRAPHY

Adcock BB, Ireland RB Jr: Secondary hypertension: A practical diagnostic approach. Am Fam Physician 55:1263, 1997.
A practical discussion of when and how to diagnose secondary causes of hypertension.
Alderman MH: Which antihypertensive drugs first—and why˜ JAMA 267:2786, 1992.
Describes the impressive declines in coronary artery disease and stroke associated with aggressive detection and treatment of hypertension.
Cryer PE: Pheochromocytoma. West J Med 156:399, 1992.
Reviews the pathophysiology, diagnosis, and management of pheochromocytoma.
Elliot WJ, Martin WB, Murphy MD, et al: Comparison of two noninvasive screening tests for renovascular hypertension. Arch Intern Med 153:755, 1993.
Renal scintigraphy after captopril was better than plasma renin activity after captopril to screen for renovascular hypertension.
Gifford RW Jr: Evaluation of the hypertensive patient with emphasis on detecting curable causes. Milbank Q 47:170, 1969.
Most hypertensive patients have primary or essential hypertension.
Grimm RH Jr, Flack JM, Grandits GA, et al: Long-term effects on plasma lipids of diet and drugs to treat hypertension. JAMA 275:1549, 1996.
Various antihypertensive drugs differ in their long-term effects on blood lipids.
Héron E, Chatellier G, Billaud E, et al: The urinary metanephrine-to-creatinine ratio for the diagnosis of pheochromocytoma. Ann Intern Med 125:300, 1996.
Measurement of the metanephrine-to-creatinine ratio is a sensitive and specific test for pheochromocytoma.
Heyka RJ, Vidt DG: Hypertension: Pitfalls in diagnosis, pointers on finding the source. Consultant 36:226, 1996.
Recommendations for the diagnosis of primary and secondary hypertension.
Joint National Committee on the Detection, Evaluation, and Treatment of High Blood Pressure: The Fifth Report of the Joint National Committee on Detection, Evaluation, and Treatment of High Blood Pressure (JNC V). Arch Intern Med 153:154, 1993.
Weber MA, Laragh JH: Hypertension: Steps forward and steps backward. Arch Intern Med 153:149, 1993.
Advocates treating systolic hypertension in the elderly and suggests ambulatory blood

*Source: Prisant LM: Hypertension. *In* Conn RB, Borer WZ, Snyder JW (eds): Current Diagnosis, 9th ed. Philadelphia, WB Saunders, 1997, p 355.

pressure monitoring for selected patients with resistant, episodic, or "white coat" hypertension.

Lenders JWM, Keiser HR, Goldstein DS, et al: Plasma metanephrines in the diagnosis of pheochromocytoma. Ann Intern Med 123:101, 1995.
Krakoff LR: Searching for pheochromocytoma: A new and better test? Ann Intern Med 123:150, 1995.
Tests for plasma metanephrine are more sensitive than tests for plasma catecholamines or urinary metanephrines.
Levy D: Have expert panel guidelines kept pace with new concepts in hypertension? Lancet 346:1112, 1995.
Hypertension guidelines have steadily lowered the blood pressure thresholds for defining hypertension and those for initiating pharmacologic treatment.
Littenberg B: A practice guideline revisited: Screening for hypertension. Ann Intern Med 122:937, 1995.
All adults should periodically be offered sphygmomanometry in a case-finding setting.
Peaston RT, Lennard TWJ, Lai LC, et al: Overnight excretion of urinary catecholamines and metabolites in the detection of pheochromocytoma. J Clin Endocrinol Metab 81:1378, 1996.
Overnight measurement of urinary catecholamines and metabolites looks promising to diagnose pheochromocytoma.
Peplinski GR, Norton JA: The predictive value of diagnostic tests for pheochromocytoma. Surgery 116:1101, 1994.
This study indicates that the single best biochemical indicator of a pheochromocytoma is an elevated 24-hour urinary metanephrine level.
Perneger TV, Nieto FJ, Whelton PK, et al: A prospective study of blood pressure and serum creatinine. JAMA 269:488, 1993.
The optimal level of blood pressure to avoid renal insufficiency is the lowest level, and that blood pressure, even within the normal range, may be an important risk factor for incipient renal insufficiency.
Preston RA, Singer I, Epstein M: Renal parenchymal hypertension: Current concepts of pathogenesis and management. Arch Intern Med 156:602, 1996.
Hypertension is both a cause and consequence of renal disease, and it may be difficult to distinguish these clinically.
Ram CVS, Fierro G: Secondary hypertension: When to suspect—and how to diagnose—renal artery stenosis. Consultant 35:1454, 1995.
Rule out renal artery stenosis in older patients who do not respond to therapy, in onset of hypertension before age 30, and in hypertension with unexplained progressive renal functional impairment.
Randin D, Vollenweider P, Tappy L, et al: Suppression of alcohol-induced hypertension by dexamethasone. N Engl J Med 332:1733, 1995.
Heavy drinking may cause cardiovascular complications by provoking short-term increases in blood pressure and platelet aggregation. In the absence of illness related to alcohol use, the consumption of one or two drinks per day still seems a safe and advisable practice.
Reeves RA: Does this patient have hypertension? How to measure blood pressure. JAMA 273:1211, 1995.
Reviews techniques for measuring blood pressure.
Setaro JF, Moser M: Hypertension: What to include in a cost-effective office workup. Consultant 35:957, 1995.
Expert recommendations about what to include and what not to include in the routine evaluation of newly hypertensive patients.
Steigerwalt SP: Unraveling the causes of hypertension and hypokalemia. Hosp Pract 30:67, 1995.
Diuretic therapy and primary aldosteronism cause hypokalemia.

DIGOXIN MONITORING

Recommendations for digoxin monitoring are from the medical literature.

1. Monitor the serum concentration of digoxin in the following cir-

cumstances: to assess patient compliance, to tailor an optimal dosing schedule, and to confirm a clinical impression of toxicity. Routine measurement of serum digoxin concentration is inappropriate.

For monitoring digoxin, draw the sample at least 12 hours after the last dose and after four to five half-lives (6 to 7 days with normal renal function) after a dosage change. In a group of hospitalized patients receiving digoxin, the incidence of toxicity was approximately 15%, with another 3 to 5% of patients showing symptoms and clinical findings suggestive of toxicity. These findings include (1) ventricular arrhythmias, including ventricular tachycardia; accelerated junctional rhythms; atrial tachycardia with AV block; AV dissociation; progression of AV block; and (2) anorexia; nausea, vomiting; visual disturbances; weakness. Digoxin toxicity may occur after accidental ingestion of cardiac glycoside–containing plants, such as oleander.

2. Evaluate the test.

If the patient is receiving other digitalis preparations, determine whether they interfere with the test. After administration of Digibind (Fab antidigoxin antibody for treating digoxin overdose), total serum digoxin concentrations are no longer meaningful.

REFERENCE RANGE

Test	Specimen	Conventional Units	International Units
Digoxin	Serum trough (>12 hr after dose)	For CHF: 0.8–1.5 ng/mL	1.0–1.9 nmol/L
		For arrhythmias: 1.5–2.0 ng/mL	1.9–2.6 nmol/L
		Toxic: >2.5 ng.mL	>3.2 nmol/L

3. Interpret test results in the context of clinical findings.

Most patients experience the maximal increase in cardiac contractility at a serum concentration of 1.4 ng/mL (1.8 nmol/L), with little increase at higher serum values. Toxicity typically is associated with a serum concentration of at least 1 ng/mL (1.3 nmol/L). With serum concentrations approaching or above 2 ng/mL (2.6 nmol/L), the risk of toxicity becomes unacceptably high. Thus, the toxic-to-therapeutic ratio is narrow, and digoxin monitoring is quite helpful.

When serum concentrations of digitalis glycosides are excessive, consider these reasons.*

- A dose too large for the age group

*Source: Koren G, Soldin SJ: Cardiac glycosides. *In* Gerson B (ed): Therapeutic Drug Monitoring—II: Patient Care and Applications. Clin Lab Med 7:601, 1987.

- Improved bioavailability of a new product
- Renal insufficiency
- Interaction with other drugs: quinidine, verapamil, amiodarone, indomethacin
- Presence of endogenous digoxin-like factors
- Poisoning: accidental, children, elderly; suicide attempt; intentional (homicidal); or iatrogenic (medication error)
- Inappropriate sampling time

When determining individual sensitivity to digitalis, consider these factors:*

- Type and severity of underlying cardiac disease
- Serum electrolyte derangement
  Hypokalemia or hyperkalemia
  Hypomagnesemia
  Hypercalcemia
  Hyponatremia
- Acid-base imbalance
- Concomitant drug administration
  Anesthetics
  Catecholamines and sympathomimetics
  Antiarrhythmic agents
- Thyroid status
- Renal function
- Autonomic nervous system tone
- Respiratory disease

BIBLIOGRAPHY

Cauffield JS, Gums JG, Grauer K: The serum digoxin concentration: Ten questions to ask. Am Fam Physician 56:495, 1997.
  Effective interpretation of the digoxin concentration requires consideration of the patient's renal function and clinical status, possible drug interactions, time of the assay, and other variables.
The Digitalis Investigation Group: The effect of digoxin on mortality and morbidity in patients with heart failure. N Engl J Med 336:525, 1997.
  Packer M: End of the oldest controversy in medicine: Are we ready to conclude the debate on digitalis? N Engl J Med 336:575, 1997.
  Digoxin did not reduce overall mortality, but it reduced the rate of hospitalization both overall and for worsening heart failure.
Edner M, Ponikowski P, Jogestrand T: The effect of digoxin on the serum potassium concentration. Scand J Clin Lab Invest 53:187, 1993.
  Digoxin concentration after a 2-hour rest correlates better with the patient's clinical status. The serum potassium level is modestly higher.
Kelly DP, Fry ETA: Heart failure. *In* Woodley M, Whelan A (eds): Manual of Medical Therapeutics, 27th ed. Boston, Little, Brown & Co, 1992, p 105.
  Discusses the use of digoxin-specific Fab antibody fragments for managing digoxin intoxication.

*Source: Smith TW: Heart failure. *In* Wyngaarden JB, Smith LH, Bennett JC (eds): Cecil Textbook of Medicine, 20th ed. Philadelphia, WB Saunders, 1996, p 227.

Kelly RA, Smith TW: Use and misuse of digitalis blood levels. Heart Dis Stroke 1:117, 1992.
Recent guidelines for digoxin monitoring.

Keys PW, Stafford RW: Digoxin: Therapeutic use and serum concentration monitoring. *In* Taylor WJ, Finn AL (eds): Individualizing Drug Therapy: Practical Applications of Drug Monitoring, vol 3. New York, Gross, Townsend, Frank, 1981.
Good discussion of practical issues.

Koren G, Soldin SJ: Cardiac glycosides. *In* Gerson B (ed): Therapeutic Drug Monitoring—II: Patient Care and Applications. Clin Lab Med 7:587, 1987.
Resource for digoxin therapy in patient care.

Matzuk MM, Shlomchik M, Shaw LM: Making digoxin therapeutic drug monitoring more effective. Ther Drug Monit 13:215, 1991.
Emphasizes sampling at least 12 hours after the last dose and four to five half-lives after a dosage change.

Miller JJ, Straub RW Jr, Valdes R Jr: Digoxin immunoassay with cross-reactivity to digoxin metabolites proportional to their biological activity. Clin Chem 40:1898, 1994.
Different immunoassays react with digoxin metabolites in a variety of ways.

Mooradian AD: Digitalis: An update of clinical pharmacokinetics, therapeutic monitoring techniques, and treatment recommendations. Clin Pharmacokinet 15:165, 1988.
Useful theoretical and practical information.

Safadi R, Levy I, Amitai Y, et al: Beneficial effect of digoxin-specific Fab antibody fragments in oleander intoxication. Arch Intern Med 155:2121, 1995.
Digoxin-specific Fab antibody fragments are effective in patients with accidental ingestion of cardiac glycoside–containing plants.

Steiner JF, Robbins LJ, Hammermeister KE, et al: Incidence of digoxin toxicity in outpatients. West J Med 161:474, 1994.
The low rate of digoxin toxicity in outpatients parallels the decline in the incidence of toxicity observed in hospital-based studies.

4

Respiratory Diseases

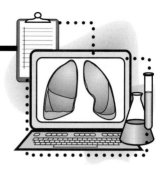

- Acute Pharyngitis
- Allergic Rhinitis
- Acute Bacterial Sinusitis
- Community-acquired Pneumonia
- Pulmonary Embolism
- Chronic Obstructive Pulmonary Disease
- Pleural Fluid Analysis

ACUTE PHARYNGITIS

Recommendations for acute pharyngitis are from the medical literature. For diagnosing streptococcal pharyngitis, the American Academy of Pediatrics and the American Heart Association recommend that a negative rapid antigen test be followed with a throat culture.

1. In adult patients (>18 years) with a sore throat, determine management by the presence or absence of four key clinical findings: (1) fever, (2) tonsillar exudate, (3) anterior tender cervical lymphadenopathy, and (4) lack of cough.

- When all four findings are present, treat immediately without a rapid antigen test or throat culture.
- When all four findings are absent, a rapid antigen test or throat culture is not required unless the patient has special risk factors.
- When some of these findings are present, obtain a rapid antigen test or throat culture.

For children (aged 3 to 18 years), obtain a rapid antigen test or throat culture. If the rapid antigen test is negative, obtain a throat culture.

Leukocyte count, C-reactive protein, erythrocyte sedimentation rate, antistreptolysin O titer, and other laboratory tests are not helpful.

Group A streptococcal pharyngitis usually occurs in children between 5 and 15 years but may occur in adults. When the probability of group A streptococcal infection is high (>30%), it is prudent to treat adult patients immediately with antibiotics. Relying on a rapid antigen test or throat culture test result in this group is inappropriate because false-negative test results may occur. On the other hand, in adult patients, when the probability of group A streptococcal infection is low, the risks of antibiotic therapy (drug reaction and fatal anaphylaxis) approximate the risks of streptococcal pharyngitis and its complications. In this situation it is appropriate to withhold antibiotics and obtain a rapid antigen test or throat culture. When the probability of group A streptococcal infection is very low (<3%), a rapid antigen test or throat culture is not required unless the patient has special risk factors.

In children, the clinical findings are more variable and the presence or absence of the organism must be documented. Early treatment with antibiotics can prevent acute rheumatic fever and may shorten the course of the illness, reducing fever and local and systemic symptoms. The presence of typical clinical findings of acute viral infection may dissuade the physician from considering acute streptococcal pharyngitis.

2. Acute pharyngitis may be caused by other microorganisms as well as group A streptococci, as indicated in the following table.

OROPHARYNGEAL MICROORGANISMS

Colonizing Organisms	Pharyngitis as Part of Systemic Infectious Disease	Pathogens in Acute Pharyngitis
Group A, B, C, and G streptococci	Epstein-Barr virus	Group A, B, C, and G streptococci
Oral anaerobes	Cytomegalovirus	Adenovirus
Streptococcus pneumoniae	*Mycoplasma pneumoniae*	Respiratory viruses
	Chlamydia pneumoniae	*Candida albicans*
Haemophilus influenzae	*Franciscella tularensis*	Herpes simplex
	Enteroviruses	*Neisseria gonorrhoeae*
Haemophilus parainfluenzae	Influenza A and B	
	Rubella	*Corynebacterium diphtheriae*
Staphylococcus aureus	Measles	
	Toxoplasma gondii	*Corynebacterium haemolyticum*
	Coxiella burnetii	
	Bordetella pertussis	

Source: Cunha BA: Acute pharyngitis. *In* Conn RB, Borer WZ, Snyder JW (eds): Current Diagnosis, 9th ed. Philadelphia, WB Saunders, 1997, p 292.

Consider the possibilities of mycoplasmal, gonococcal, or *Chlamydia trachomatis* pharyngitis in patients with persistent pharyngitis and a negative culture for group A streptococci or in patients with a positive culture who are not responding to penicillin. Consider infectious mononucleosis in patients with persistent systemic illness, lymphadenopathy, and splenomegaly. Consider diphtheria in unvaccinated populations, and look for a gray membrane that is firmly adherent to the tonsillar or pharyngeal mucosa. Specimens from both throat and nasopharynx should be submitted for culture confirmation of diphtheria. Pertussis should be considered in patients with pharyngitis, nonproductive cough, and lymphocytosis. Antibiotic therapy in patients with non-streptococcal pharyngitis is often inappropriate.

3. Use good technique when obtaining a throat culture and performing laboratory tests.

When obtaining a throat culture, use a Dacron swab (cotton fibers may inhibit *Neisseria*) and vigorously rub the posterior pharynx, the tonsils or tonsillar pillars, and areas of purulence, exudation, or ulceration. Using a tongue blade helps prevent contamination with buccal organisms. Use of a self-contained collection or transport system such as the Culturette (Becton Dickinson) makes collection and transport of throat cultures relatively simple and convenient. With good specimens and the proper procedure, the sensitivity for group A streptococci is approximately 95%. A recent study showed that a well-performed single-plate aerobic throat culture has a sensitivity of 96% and a specificity of 99.5%. With poor specimens and poor procedure, the sensitivity may be as low as 30%. If you suspect gonococcal pharyngitis or the meningococcal carrier state, the swab is best inoculated onto a previously warmed JEMBEC plate (or other suitable medium) as soon as the culture is obtained. Inoculated plates should be incubated overnight at 95°F (35°C) in an atmosphere of 5 to 10% carbon dioxide before shipment to a laboratory. Immediate shipment kills *Neisseria* if present. Another option when *Neisseria* is suspected is to place the swab in a transport medium before sending it to the laboratory. Perform a test for heterophil antibody (Monospot test) if you suspect infectious mononucleosis.

A positive rapid antigen test or throat culture for group A streptococci may reflect infection or an asymptomatic carrier state (false positive). In children the carrier rate can be up to 15%. At present there is no accurate way to distinguish between true streptococcal infection and the carrier state at the time of initial presentation. In infected patients the false-negative rate of a well-performed single throat culture is approximately 5%. A Gram stain of exudative material that shows gram-positive cocci in chains together with cellular debris and abundant neutrophils strongly suggests streptococcal infection.

4. Perform follow-up cultures in patients with persistent clinical findings or with unusually high risk of acute rheumatic fever.

Routine follow-up cultures are not required.

BIBLIOGRAPHY

Barnes HV: Streptococcal infections. *In* Spivak JL, Barnes HV (eds): Manual of Clinical Problems in Internal Medicine, 4th ed. Boston, Little, Brown & Co, 1990, p 460.
  Good discussion of diagnosis and management, with annotated key references.
Bisno AL: Group A streptococcal infections and acute rheumatic fever. N Engl J Med 325:783, 1991.
  Even today, physicians should be alert to the possibility of acute rheumatic fever.

Centor RM, Meier FA, Dalton HP: Throat cultures and rapid tests for diagnosis of group A streptococcal pharyngitis in adults. *In* Sox HC Jr (ed): Common Diagnostic Tests: Use and Interpretation, 2nd ed. Philadelphia, American College of Physicians, 1990, p 245.
Good review of group A streptococcal pharyngitis with recommendations for management.

Dippel DWJ, Touw-Otten F, Habbema JDF: Management of children with acute pharyngitis: A decision analysis. J Fam Pract 34:149, 1992.
Suggests using a rapid antigen test and prompt penicillin therapy in children with a high probability of streptococcal pharyngitis.

Hedges JR, Singal BM, Estep JL: The impact of a rapid screen for streptococcal pharyngitis on clinical decision making in the emergency department. Med Decis Making 11:119, 1991.
Rapid diagnostic tests have done little to improve the overall quality of care.

Komaroff AL: Sore throat in adult patients. *In* Panzer RJ, Black ER, Griner PF (eds): Diagnostic Strategies for Common Medical Problems. Philadelphia, American College of Physicians, 1991, p 186.
When key clinical findings are absent, the probability of streptococcal pharyngitis is very low (<3%) and a throat culture is unnecessary unless the patient has special risk factors.

Michel RS, Hayden GF, Hendley JO: Pharyngitis in children: When to culture, when to treat. Consultant 35:1469, 1995.
Throat culture is the diagnostic "gold standard" for acute streptococcal pharyngitis.

Ohio State Faculty: Acute pharyngitis. Columbus, Ohio, Ohio State University Health Plan Clinical Notes, vol 1, no 2, Spring, 1991.
Medical practice guidelines for acute pharyngitis.

Perkins A: An approach to diagnosing the acute sore throat. Am Fam Physician 55:131, 1997.
Discusses guidelines for diagnosing beta-hemolytic streptococci and other causes of acute pharyngitis.

Rapid diagnostic tests for group A streptococcal pharyngitis. Med Lett Drugs Ther 33:40, 1991.
Summarizes available rapid diagnostic test kits and compares their costs.

Roddey OF Jr, Clegg HW, Martin ES, et al: Comparison of throat culture methods for the recovery of group A streptococci in a pediatric office setting. JAMA 274:1863, 1995.
The traditional single-plate method had a sensitivity of 96% and a specificity of 99.5%.

Schlager TA, Hayden GA, Woods WA, et al: Optical immunoassay for rapid detection of group A β-hemolytic streptococci. Arch Pediatr Adolesc Med 150:245, 1996.
The simple blood agar plate is the most reliable test for diagnosing streptococcal pharyngitis.

Schwartz B, Fries S, Fitzgibbon AM, et al: Pediatricians' diagnostic approach to pharyngitis and impact of CLIA 1988 on office diagnostic tests. JAMA 271:234, 1994.
The American Academy of Pediatrics and the American Heart Association recommend culture confirmation of a negative rapid antigen test.

Shulman ST: Streptococcal pharyngitis: Diagnostic considerations. Pediatr Infect Dis J 13:567, 1994.
The presence of typical clinical findings of acute viral infection may dissuade the physician from considering acute streptococcal pharyngitis.

Slawson DC, Baer LJ, Richardson MD: Antibiotic use in the treatment of non-streptococcal pharyngitis. Fam Med 23:198, 1991.
Suggests that antibiotic therapy in patients with non-streptococcal pharyngitis is often inappropriate.

Tenjarla G, Kumar A, Dyke JW: TestPack Strep A kit for the rapid detection of group A streptococci on 11,088 throat swabs in a clinical pathology laboratory. Am J Clin Pathol 96:759, 1991.
Patients with negative rapid antigen tests should be cultured.

Wegner DL, Witte DL, Schrantz RD: Insensitivity of rapid antigen detection methods and single blood agar plate culture for diagnosing streptococcal pharyngitis. JAMA 267:695, 1992.
The single blood agar plate and antigen tests are insensitive.

Williams T: Practice guidelines for management of pharyngitis. (Personal communication, 1997).
   In adult patients, clinical findings can be used to stratify risk and the need for culture and/or antibiotics.

ALLERGIC RHINITIS

Recommendations for allergic rhinitis are from the medical literature.

1. If the diagnosis of allergic rhinitis cannot be made from clinical findings, consider examining a nasal smear for eosinophils, measuring the total serum IgE level, skin testing, and performing radioallergosorbent tests (RASTs) or equivalent in vitro tests. The blood eosinophil count is not helpful.

Allergic rhinitis affects 15 to 20% of the population and accounts for 9% of outpatient visits for the Ohio State University Health Plan.

The differential diagnosis of seasonal allergic rhinitis includes viral infection; abuse of nose drops and sprays; drugs such as ovarian hormones, reserpine, hydralazine, and aspirin and other nonsteroidal anti-inflammatory agents; and premenstrual or pregnancy-related hormonal rhinitis.

The differential diagnosis of perennial allergic rhinitis includes nasal abnormalities such as deviated septum, endocrine abnormalities such as hypothyroidism, nasal mastocytosis, and idiopathic perennial non-allergic rhinitis (vasomotor rhinitis). Symptoms from nasopharyngeal masses can mimic those of allergies.

Nasal secretions should be examined for eosinophilia, even if the blood eosinophil count is normal. The specimen may be collected as follows: having the patient blow the nose onto waxed paper or cellophane, placing a swab in the nose for 2 or 3 minutes, or aspirating the specimen with a small rubber bulb syringe. The specimen is transferred to a slide, dried, and stained with Wright's stain. The blood eosinophil count is not useful because it may be normal or increased in either allergic or nonallergic rhinitis. A positive test for nasal eosinophilia provides the same support for a diagnosis of allergic rhinitis as does an increased total serum IgE level.

Skin tests are of value only in patients with clinical findings and should not be used for screening asymptomatic patients because positive reactions occur in many individuals who have no symptoms. In practice, skin tests are used either to advise patients about avoidance therapy or to help select antigens for use in therapy. Skin tests are the quickest and least expensive way to identify specific allergens.

RAST measures allergen-specific serum IgE antibody titers, and the results correlate well with skin testing. RAST is useful in patients in whom skin testing is inappropriate because of extensive eczema, marked dermatographism, or interfering medications.

2. Evaluate the tests.

A positive nasal smear in a patient with allergic rhinitis shows large numbers of eosinophils (usually more than 25% of all cells present).

A serum total IgE level that is normal practically rules out atopy, whereas one that is high markedly increases the likelihood of this diagnosis.

RAST is usually considered safer, more expensive, less sensitive, but perhaps more specific than skin testing; however, a recent study found that the sensitivity and specificity of RAST and skin tests are almost identical. Although RAST may give false-negative results, it rarely gives false-positive results. Unlike skin tests, it is not affected when the patient is taking antihistamine or sympathomimetic drugs.

Examples of assays that are available at the Ohio State University Medical Center are as follows:

- **Total IgE (reported in IU/mL):** This test may be ordered separately and is performed with both the aeroallergen and food panels described below.
- **Aeroallergen Screening Test:** This test detects IgE antibodies specific for any of the following allergens: mold, dust mite, tree pollen, grass pollen, cat and dog dander, and weed pollen. The screening test is reported as "positive" or "negative."
- **Aeroallergen Panel:** This test, by utilizing separate allergens, is designed to identify allergen-specific IgE. The following individual aeroallergens are included in this panel: birch tree, oak tree, sycamore tree, rye grass, Kentucky blue grass, meadow fescue grass, dog dander, cat dander, ragweed, dust mite, and alternia.
- **Food Allergy Panel:** This test identifies IgE antibodies directed against the following individual food allergens: corn, milk, egg white, wheat, and peanut.

3. If the test results are positive, they support the diagnosis, but the diagnosis must be made by considering the test results together with the clinical features.

A positive nasal smear for eosinophilia and increased serum total IgE support the diagnosis of allergic rhinitis, but they are not diagnostic. Eosinophils can also be found in the syndrome of nonallergic rhinitis with eosinophilia. Large numbers of neutrophils in the nasal smear suggest infection rather than allergic rhinitis. The manifestations of upper respiratory tract infection usually last no longer than a week and include fever, pain, and the presence of neutrophils in secretions.

4. If the test results are negative, do not completely rule out allergic rhinitis.

The tests for allergic rhinitis are not completely sensitive. For example, positive nasal smears for eosinophilia are not found in every patient with proven allergic rhinitis, and the serum total IgE level is not always increased. Achieving relief of symptoms by avoiding the suspected allergen is the best method of diagnosis.

BIBLIOGRAPHY

Eriksson NE: Diagnosis of IgE mediated allergy in clinical practice. Allergol Immunopathol 22:139, 1994.
> *Determination of allergen-specific IgE in the serum could be used when there is suspicion of allergy against only one or a few allergens, whereas skin testing should be used when testing with many allergens is necessary.*

Ferguson BJ: Allergic rhinitis: Recognizing signs, symptoms, and triggering allergens. Postgrad Med 101:110, 1997.
> *Discusses the differentiation of the common cold from allergic rhinitis.*

Georgitis JW, Kaiser HB, Kaliner M: Allergic rhinitis: Taming the troubled nose. Patient Care 31:51, 1997.
> *Reviews the diagnosis and management of allergic rhinitis.*

Kaliner M, Lemanske R: Rhinitis and asthma. JAMA 268:2807, 1992.
> *Discusses the diagnosis and management of allergic rhinitis.*

Nalebuff DJ: In vitro testing methodologies: Evolution and current status. Otolaryngol Clin North Am 25:27, 1992.
> *The American Academy of Otolaryngic Allergy, in its most current position statement, endorses the modified RAST as reproducible, sensitive, and specific. A new organization called the American In Vitro Allergy and Immunology Society has been formed to promote and monitor the use of these tests.*

Ohio State Faculty: Allergic rhinitis. Columbus, OH, Ohio State University Health Plan Clinical Notes, vol 1, no 4, Spring, 1991.
> *Medical practice guidelines for allergic rhinitis.*

Reisman RE: Allergic rhinitis: Update on your therapeutic choices. Consultant 36:1899, 1996.
> *Reviews the diagnosis and treatment.*

Salkie ML: Role of clinical laboratory in allergy testing. Clin Biochem 27:343, 1994.
> *Compares commercially available methods for the screening, diagnosis, and management of patients with allergies.*

Ten RM, Klein JS, Frigas E: Allergy skin testing. Mayo Clin Proc 70:783, 1995.
> *Advocates the use of skin testing.*

VanArsdel PP Jr, Larson EB: Diagnostic tests for patients with suspected allergic disease: Utility and limitations. Ann Intern Med 110:304, 1989.
> *Discusses strategies for the diagnosis of allergic rhinitis.*

ACUTE BACTERIAL SINUSITIS

Recommendations for acute bacterial sinusitis are from the medical literature.

1. In patients with clinical findings of acute bacterial sinusitis, administer antibiotics and appropriate adjunctive therapy (e.g., decongestants, saline sprays, and a room humidifier). Nonspecific symptoms include facial pain, headache, purulent nasal discharge, decreased sense of smell, and fever. Of these, purulent nasal discharge is the most helpful. In one study, preceding common cold, purulent rhinorrhea, pain on bending, unilateral maxillary pain, and pain in the teeth were helpful in improving diagnostic accuracy.

Transillumination, radiographic studies, sinus aspiration, Gram stain, and culture are rarely necessary in uncomplicated infections. Nasal swabs are not recommended for microbiologic studies.

Sinusitis affects up to 12% of adults and complicates approximately 0.5% of viral upper respiratory infections (URIs). If symptoms have lasted less than 7 to 10 days and the patient is improving, a viral URI is the probable cause. Worsening findings that last longer than 7 to 10 days suggest acute bacterial sinusitis. Sinusitis lasting 3 weeks to 3 months is termed subacute; after 3 months it is labeled chronic.

In adults, acute sinusitis is caused by the same bacteria as otitis media: *Streptococcus pneumoniae, Haemophilus influenzae,* and *Moraxella (Branhamella) catarrhalis.* Chronic sinusitis may be caused by anerobic organisms, predominantly by species of *Peptostreptococcus, Fusobacterium,* and *Prevotella* (formerly *Bacteroides*), alone or in combination with *Streptococcus* species or *Staphylococcus* species. In immunocompromised patients, organisms may include gram-negative species and fungi.

2. In patients with complicated acute sinusitis or chronic sinusitis, consider special diagnostic studies, including sinus aspiration.

Sinus aspiration is often reserved for patients with severe symptoms, complicated sinusitis, compromised immunity, and failure to respond to multiple courses of empiric antibiotic therapy. The specimen should be studied with a Gram stain and culture designed to detect unusual infections. Patients with poorly controlled diabetes mellitus or immunosuppression are at risk for unusual infections.

BIBLIOGRAPHY

Grandis JR, Johnson JT: Sinusitis: Tips to direct office diagnosis and effective antibiotic therapy. Consultant 35:789, 1995.
   Base the diagnosis of sinusitis on the history and presenting signs and symptoms.
Hansen JG, Schmidt H, Rosborg J, et al: Predicting acute maxillary sinusitis in a general practice population. BMJ 311:233, 1995.
   Maxillary sinusitis is overdiagnosed, and generally accepted symptoms and signs are not consistently predictive.
Holleman DR Jr, Williams JW Jr, Simel DL: Usual care and outcomes in patients with sinus complaints and normal results of sinus roentgenography. Arch Fam Med 4:246, 1995.
   With usual medical care, the syndrome of sinus symptoms and normal sinus roentgenography persists for at least 14 days in many patients.
Huck W, Reed BD, Nielsen RW, et al: Cefaclor vs amoxicillin in the treatment of acute, recurrent, and chronic sinusitis. Arch Fam Med 2:497, 1993.
   Cefaclor and amoxicillin are equally effective against acute and recurrent sinusitis. Drug susceptibility did not affect clinical outcome.
Lindbaek M: Purulent nasal secretion is strongest clinical predictor of sinusitis. Am Fam Physician 52:2081, 1995.
   A study of 201 patients with a clinical diagnosis of acute sinusitis points to the unreliability of clinical symptoms and signs in the diagnosis of sinusitis. Purulent rhinorrhea was found to be the strongest predictor of acute sinusitis.

Rachelefsky GS, Slavin RG, Wald ER: Sinusitis: Acute, chronic—and manageable. Patient Care 31:105, 1997.
Discusses an algorithm for the diagnosis and management of acute and chronic sinusitis.

Reuler JB, Lucas LM, Kumar KL: Sinusitis: A review for generalists. West J Med 163:40, 1995.
A good review of diagnosis and treatment.

Rosenthal E: A high-tech view of the sinuses offers answer to chronic problems. The New York Times, June 19, 1991, p B7.
Surgery through a fiberoptic scope may become the "gold standard" for chronic sinus problems.

Slavin RG: Sinusitis: Answers to key questions. Consultant 37:745, 1997.
Symptoms for 7 to 10 days after a cold plus purulent discharge are important clues.

van Duijn NP, Brouwer HJ, Lamberts H: Use of symptoms and signs to diagnose maxillary sinusitis in general practice: Comparison with ultrasonography. BMJ 305:684, 1992.
Suggests an algorithm for diagnosing sinusitis based on five weighted symptoms.

Zurlo JJ, Feuerstein IM, Lebovics R, et al: Sinusitis in HIV-1 infection. Am J Med 93:157, 1992.
Godofsky E, Zinreich J, Armstrong M, et al: Sinusitis in HIV-infected patients: A clinical and radiographic review. Am J Med 93:163, 1992.
Sinusitis in HIV-infected patients is common and may be recurrent.

• •

COMMUNITY-ACQUIRED PNEUMONIA

Recommendations for community-acquired pneumonia are from the medical literature.

1. For patients with clinical findings of community-acquired pneumonia (fever, cough, and abnormal breath sounds), decide who can be safely treated as an outpatient and who should be hospitalized. A chest radiograph, complete blood count, electrolyte determinations, and pulse oximetry or arterial blood gases are useful to help assess the severity of the pneumonia.

Depending on the severity of the illness, additional studies to consider include sputum Gram stain and culture, blood and pleural fluid cultures, serologic tests, and fiberoptic bronchoscopy. A recent study predicted the need for hospitalization based on 14 key clinical variables (including age, sex, coexisting illness, vital signs, and mental status) and 7 key laboratory variables (such as arterial oxygen saturation, hematocrit, glucose, urea nitrogen, and pleural effusions on chest radiography).

Although a Gram stain and a culture of sputum are often useful, a Gram stain and a culture of saliva are always useless. The patient should thoroughly rinse his or her mouth with water several times, take some deep breaths and hold them several times, and then attempt to bring up sputum from deep in the bronchial tree. Inhalation of a warmed 3 to 10% saline solution aerosol may be helpful. Sputum can be distinguished from saliva by microscopically evaluating the specimen under low power. More than 25 neutrophils and less than 10 squamous epithelial cells per low-power field indicate an adequate sputum sample. No specimen containing more than 25 squamous epithelial cells per low-power field should be cultured because it is heavily contaminated by oropharyngeal secretions. The Gram stain can be helpful in choosing a good specimen for culture and selecting antibiotics.

Other techniques are available to examine sputum: digestion with 10% potassium hydroxide or fungifluor staining to identify fungi; immunologic techniques for respiratory viruses; and direct fluorescent antibody studies to diagnose *Legionella* species and *Pneumocystis carinii* (induced sputum).

Traditionally, physicians have drawn simultaneous blood cultures from two different sites. Because the increased sensitivity from drawing two blood cultures appears related to the increased volume of blood rather than the two different sites, it does not matter whether the two blood cultures are drawn from the same site or different sites. Blood cultures should be inoculated with the same needle that is used for the venipuncture. An advantage of using two different sites is that chance contamination with skin flora is less likely to occur in two different sites. If a single site is contaminated, all cultures from that site are contaminated.

2. Consider mycoplasmal pneumonia, Legionnaires' disease, influenza, primary tuberculosis, *Chlamydia pneumoniae* (strain TWAR), and other causes of atypical pneumonias in patients with the following clinical findings:

- Occurrence in young adults
- Onset over several days
- Mild fever; patient not severely ill
- No or small amounts of mucopurulent sputum
- Minimal pleurisy; small or no effusion
- Normal to slightly increased leukocyte count
- Patchy "pneumonitis" or nonhomogeneous segmental infiltrate on radiograph

3. Consider pneumococcal pneumonia, *H. influenzae*, staphylococcal pneumonia, gram-negative bacillary pneumonia, and suppurative pulmonary disease in patients with the following clinical findings:

- Patient more often elderly or chronically ill
- Abrupt onset
- High fevers; chills; patient possibly weak, cyanotic, or confused
- Purulent sputum
- Pleurisy and pleural effusion common
- Leukocytosis
- Lobar or segmental consolidation on radiograph

4. In debilitated elderly persons and patients with predisposing conditions, probable causative bacteria are as follows:

- Chronic obstructive pulmonary disease (COPD): *S. pneumoniae*, *M. catarrhalis*, and *H. influenzae*

- Chronic alcoholism: *S. pneumoniae*, anaerobic bacteria (aspiration pneumonia), *H. influenzae, Klebsiella pneumoniae, Staphylococcus aureus*, and *Mycobacterium tuberculosis*
- Postinfluenza bacterial pneumonia: *S. pneumoniae, S. aureus*, and *H. influenzae*
- Elderly nursing home patients: *S. pneumoniae, S. aureus, K. pneumoniae*, and *H. influenzae*
- Patients with mental obtundation, swallowing problems, esophageal disorders, seizure disorders, and poor dental hygiene: usually mixed aerobic and anaerobic bacteria (aspiration pneumonia)
- Cystic fibrosis: *Pseudomonas aeruginosa* and *S. aureus*
- Immunocompromised hosts: multiple causes, including gram-negative bacilli (e.g., *Escherichia coli, K. pneumoniae, P. aeruginosa*), *S. aureus*, and other bacteria, and viral (e.g., cytomegalovirus), fungal (e.g., *Aspergillus*), and protozoal pathogens. The likely spectrum of causative organisms varies, with the cause of the immunodeficiency (e.g., *S. aureus*, aerobic gram-negative bacilli, and *Aspergillus* are likely pathogens in neutropenic patients). Mycobacterial infection is a growing problem, especially in human immunodeficiency virus (HIV)–infected patients. Although any single test must be interpreted with caution, increasing serum lactate dehydrogenase (LD) activity, particularly more than 450 U/L, is suspicious for *P. carinii* in HIV-infected patients with pulmonary disease. Also, the lactate dehydrogenase (LD) activity and APACHE II severity-of-illness score are highly predictive of response to therapy and mortality.

   5. **In patients with mycoplasmal pneumonia, Legionnaires' disease, influenza, primary tuberculosis, and other causes of atypical pneumonias, laboratory test results are as follows.**

Mycoplasmal Pneumonia

Hemolytic anemia caused by cold agglutinins may occur with mycoplasmal pneumonia, but clinically significant hemolysis is rare. A positive direct Coombs' test result occurs in up to 83% of patients. The leukocyte count may be normal to slightly increased, with a minimal left shift and possible mild lymphopenia. The erythrocyte sedimentation rate (ESR) increases to more than 40 mm/hour in at least two thirds of cases. In the sputum, mononuclear cells predominate over neutrophils in a ratio of approximately 60:40 (occasionally neutrophils predominate), and a Gram stain shows no bacteria, although some erythrocytes may be present. The organism can be cultured from the sputum or posterior pharnyx but takes 2 to 3 weeks to grow. A nucleic acid probe for *Mycoplasma pneumoniae* is available but is not always positive in a patient with disease. An enzyme-linked immunosorbent assay (ELISA) for *M. pneumoniae* antibody is also available, but acute and convalescent sera are required. A diagnosis can be made by demonstrating a specific IgM titer of 1:4 or greater or by a single complement-fixing antibody titer of 1:256 or greater. Approximately 50 to 60% of patients show a fourfold or greater rise in the cold agglutinin titer for human type O erythrocytes or a single titer of 1:128 or greater. In more critically ill patients, cold agglutinins are more likely. Titers of 1:32 or lower can occur in patients with infectious mononucleosis and pneumonia caused by adenovirus or influenza.

Legionnaires' Disease

The leukocyte count is normal to moderately increased with a left shift in patients with Legionnaires' disease. A moderate neutrophilia is seen in the sputum, and a Gram stain shows weakly staining gram-negative bacteria. The organism can be cultured from sputum, lung tissue, or pleural fluid and can be directly identified in secretions and tissues using an immunofluorescent technique (for sputum the sensitivity of the immunofluorescent techniques varies from 30 to 70%). A nucleic acid probe detects 50% of infections. Using acute and convalescent sera, 80% of patients have a fourfold rise in titer to 1:128 in 2 to 6 weeks. A single titer of 1:256 or more is also significant. In patients with Legionnaires' disease, an increased aspartate amino-transferase (AST) level occurs in 90% of patients. A *Legionella* urinary antigen test is also available.

Influenza

The diagnosis of influenza depends on the clinical findings. Viral culture requires 7 to 10 days. Secondary bacterial pneumonias can be caused by pneumococci, staphylococci, *H. influenzae*, and gram-negative bacteria, especially *P. aeruginosa*.

Primary Tuberculosis

In 1990, new cases of tuberculosis rose to 26,000 nationwide, and new strains of tuberculosis resistant to multiple drugs have emerged in at least 17 states. The diagnosis of primary tuberculosis depends on clinical findings, radiographs, and results of the tuberculin skin test. Sputum cultures fail to confirm the diagnosis in many adults with mild primary tuberculosis. The diagnosis of tuberculosis in HIV-infected patients is problematic because of undependable skin reactions and non-diagnostic chest radiographs. Watch for the availability of new diagnostic techniques such as (1) specific antigen detection by ELISA or antibody-sensitized latex particles; (2) detection of DNA sequences by probes and polymerase chain reaction; and (3) demonstration of tuberculostearic acid by chromatography and mass spectrometry.

Other Atypical Pneumonias

Many viral agents, particularly adenoviruses, can mimic mycoplasmal pneumonia. Rare causes include Q fever, psittacosis, tularemia, plague, primary histoplasmosis, and primary coccidioidomycosis. *C. pneumoniae* is a relatively common cause of atypical pneumonia.

6. In patients with pneumococcal pneumonia, staphylococcal pneumonia, meningococcal pneumonia, pneumonia caused by *H. influenzae*, *B. catarrhalis*, and gram-negative bacilli, laboratory test results are as follows.

Pneumococcal Pneumonia

Pneumococcal pneumonia accounts for approximately two thirds of the cases of bacterial pneumonia. In patients with pneumococcal pneumonia, the leukocyte count is usually increased to 15 to 30 $\times$ 10^3 cells/μL (15 to 30 $\times$ 10^9 cells/L), with a left shift and often toxic granulation. The white blood cell count may also be normal or low. In the sputum neutrophils are numerous, and the predominant organisms are gram-positive, lancet-shaped diplococci, which can be cultured. The blood culture is positive in 20 to 30% of patients. If anemia is present, it probably represents a pre-existing condition. Hypernatremia may occur, caused by loss of free water secondary to fever and sweating.

Staphylococcal Pneumonia

In patients with staphylococcal pneumonia the leukocyte count is increased, with a left shift, and the sputum smear shows numerous neutrophils and gram-positive cocci in clumps, which may be cultured. Blood cultures may be positive.

Meningococcal Pneumonia

In patients with meningococcal pneumonia, neutrophilic leukocytosis is usual. The sputum smear shows gram-negative diplococci that are often present in the cytoplasm of neutrophils. Blood cultures may be positive.

Pneumonia Caused by *Haemophilus influenzae*

In pneumonia caused by *H. influenzae* there is a neutrophilic leukocytosis, and the sputum smear shows abundant pleomorphic gram-negative organisms, often in neutrophils. Approximately 20% of patients have positive blood cultures.

Moraxella catarrhalis

Formerly regarded as a contaminant, *M. catarrhalis* has emerged as a true pathogen. Patients with COPD are susceptible. The organism can be recovered from respiratory secretions either in pure culture or occasionally in association with other potential pathogens such as *S. pneumoniae*. Many strains of *M. catarrhalis* are β-lactamase positive.

Gram-Negative Bacillary Pneumonias

In patients with gram-negative bacillary pneumonias, neutrophilic leukocytosis is typical, but there may be neutropenia. Numerous gram-negative bacilli are present in the sputum, and they can be cultured. Approximately 20 to 30% of patients have positive blood cultures.

7. In monitoring patients hospitalized for community-acquired pneumonia, follow the respiratory rate, diastolic blood pressure, and serum urea nitrogen level to evaluate prognosis.

A rate of 30 respirations per minute or more, a diastolic blood pressure of 60 mm Hg or less, and a serum urea nitrogen level of more than 42 mg/dL (15 mmol/L) are predictive of mortality. In one study, the presence of any two of these three criteria predicted death with 88% sensitivity and 79% specificity.

8. In patients with viral, mycoplasmal, or other miscellaneous types of pneumonia, the following test results may be increased:

- **Leukocytes**
- Although an **increased ESR** may occur in patients with mycoplasmal pneumonia, increased acute-phase reactants are more characteristic of bacterial pneumonia than viral pneumonia (e.g., an **increased C-reactive protein [CRP]** level is useful to distinguish bacterial from viral pneumonia).
- **AST, lactate dehydrogenase, and alkaline phosphate**

9. In patients with viral, mycoplasmal, or other miscellaneous types of pneumonia, the following test results may be decreased:

- **Hemoglobin and hematocrit**
- **Partial pressure of oxygen (Po$_2$)** caused by pneumonia

10. In patients with bacterial pneumonia, the following test results may be increased:

- **Leukocytes,** characteristically neutrophilic
- **ESR and CRP**

- **Abnormal total carbon dioxide** caused by change in bicarbonate in compensation for abnormal P_{CO_2}
- **AST and LD**
- **Bilirubin**

11. In patients with bacterial pneumonia, the following test results may be decreased:

- **Hemoglobin and hematocrit**
- **Leukocytes** (e.g., in fulminating pneumococcal pneumonia in alcoholics)
- **Albumin**

BIBLIOGRAPHY

American Medical Association Department of Drugs, Division of Drugs and Technology: Drug Evaluations, 6th ed. Chicago, American Medical Association, 1986, p 1238.
Concise approach to the diagnosis of community-acquired pneumonia.

Auwaerter PG, Oldach D, Mundy LM, et al: Hantavirus serologies in patients hospitalized with community-acquired pneumonia. J Infect Dis 173:237, 1996.
Does hantavirus cause community-acquired pneumonia.

Benson CA, Spear J, Hines D, et al: Combined APACHE II score and serum lactate dehydrogenase as predictors of in-hospital mortality caused by first episode *Pneumocystis carinii* pneumonia in patients with acquired immunodeficiency syndrome. Am Rev Respir Dis 144:319, 1991.
Describes an effective way to predict response to therapy and mortality.

Black ER, Mushlin AI, Griner PF, et al: Predicting the need for hospitalization of ambulatory patients with pneumonia. J Gen Intern Med 6:394, 1991.
Identifies factors that predict the need for hospitalization.

Chalasani NP, Valdecanos MAL, Gopal AK, et al: Clinical utility of blood cultures in adult patients with community-acquired pneumonia without defined underlying risks. Chest 108:932, 1995.
Significant cost savings could be incurred by limiting blood cultures to those patients with greatest risk of mortality from bacteremia from pneumonia.

Cunha BA, Ortega AM: Atypical pneumonia: Extrapulmonary clues guide the way to diagnosis. Postgrad Med 99:123, 1996.
Discusses the clinical diagnosis of the most common causative organisms.

Cunha BA, Segreti J, Yamauchi T: Community-acquired pneumonia: New bugs, new drugs. Patient Care 30:142, 1996.
Good update on community-acquired pneumonia.

Curtis JR, Paauw DS, Wenrich MD, et al: Ability of primary care physicians to diagnose and manage *Pneumocystis carinii* pneumonia. J Gen Intern Med 10:395, 1995.
These findings suggest significant delay in diagnosis and treatment had these physicians been treating an actual patient with Pneumocystis carinii *pneumonia.*

Ely JW, Berbaum KS, Bergus GR, et al: Diagnosing left lower lobe pneumonia: Usefulness of the "spine sign" on lateral chest radiographs. J Fam Pract 43:242, 1996.
The lateral chest film was of minimal value in the diagnosis of left lower lobe pneumonia.

Farr BM, Sloman AJ, Fisch MJ: Predicting death in patients hospitalized for community acquired pneumonia. Ann Intern Med 115:428, 1991.
Tachypnea, diastolic hypotension, and an increased serum urea nitrogen level were independently associated with death.

File TM Jr, Tan JS, Plouffe JF: Community-acquired pneumonia: What's needed for accurate diagnosis. Postgrad Med 99:95, 1996.
Discusses the factors that contribute to a reliable diagnosis.

Fine MJ, Auble TE, Yearly DM, et al: A prediction rule to identify low-risk patients with community-acquired pneumonia. N Engl J Med 336:243, 1997.
  Discusses a formula that demonstrated a consistent precision in predicting mortality and, indirectly, need for hospitalization.
Horvath JA, Dummer S: The use of respiratory-tract cultures in the diagnosis of invasive pulmonary aspergillosis. Am J Med 100:171, 1996.
  At least three sputum specimens should be submitted for fungal culture when pulmonary fungal infection is suspected.
Keitz SA, Bastian LA, Bennett CL, et al: AIDS-related *Pneumocystis carinii* pneumonia in older patients. J Gen Intern Med 11:591, 1996.
  Physicians may need to consider HIV-related infections for persons aged 50 years or older at risk of HIV infection.
Leisure MK, Moore DM, Schwartzman JD, et al: Changing the needle when inoculating blood cultures: A no-benefit and high-risk procedure. JAMA 264:2111, 1990.
  There is not much benefit and a lot of risk in changing needles before inoculating blood cultures.
Meeker DP, Matysik GA, Stelmach K, et al: Diagnostic utility of lactate dehydrogenase levels in patients receiving aerosolized pentamidine. Chest 104:386, 1993.
  The percentage elevation from baseline may be more useful than the absolute LD value because of the variability of baseline LD.
Mermel LA, Maki DG: Detection of bacteremia in adults: Consequences of culturing an inadequate volume of blood. Ann Intern Med 119:270, 1993.
  The yield of blood cultures depends on the volume of blood cultured.
Minocha A, Moravec CL Jr: Gram's stain and culture of sputum in the routine management of pulmonary infection. South Med J 86:1225, 1993.
  It may be reasonable to use broad-spectrum antibiotics empirically to routinely manage suspected community-acquired lung infection and use sputum Gram stain and culture more selectively to help patients with poor prognoses.
National action plan to combat multidrug-resistant tuberculosis. MMWR 41:3, 1992.
  Highlights the surge in new cases of tuberculosis, of which many have drug-resistant strains.
Reed WW, Byrd GS, Gates RH Jr, et al: Sputum Gram's stain in community-acquired pneumococcal pneumonia: A meta-analysis. West J Med 165:197, 1996.
  The sputum Gram stain may yield misleading results in community-acquired pneumonia, as its sensitivity and specificity vary substantially in different settings.
Renshaw AA: The frequent sensitivity of special stains and culture in open-lung biopsies. Am J Clin Pathol 102:736, 1994.
  The author concluded that both methenamine silver and acid-fast stains are more sensitive than culture for detecting significant pathogens from open-lung biopsies. Gram stain is as sensitive as bacterial culture but is often misinterpreted.
Roger N, Xaubet A, Agustí C, et al: Role of bronchoalveolar lavage in the diagnosis of fat embolism syndrome. Eur Respir J 8:1275, 1995.
  Positive BAL results (>3% positive macrophages) frequently are found in trauma patients and may be indicative of fat embolism syndrome (FES), but they also may be related to clinically silent fat embolization in trauma patients without clinical evidence of FES.
Smith RL, Yew K, Berkowitz KA, et al: Factors affecting the yield of acid-fast sputum smears in patients with HIV and tuberculosis. Chest 106:684, 1994.
  The acid-fast sputum smear can be expected to be positive in almost all cases of HIV infection with disseminated tuberculosis.
Smith RP, Lipworth BJ: C-reactive protein in simple community-acquired pneumonia. Chest 107:1028, 1995.
  Ninety-five percent of cases of community-acquired pneumonia have an admission CRP of more than 1 mg/dL (100 mg/L).
Smith RP, Lipworth BJ, Cree IA, et al: C-reactive protein: A clinical marker in community-acquired pneumonia. Chest 108:1288, 1995.
  The initial CRP may help diagnose pneumonia when other findings are equivocal, and serial CRP determinations may help determine response to treatment.
Stanley JD, Hanson RR, Hicklin GA, et al: Specificity of bronchoalveolar lavage for the diagnosis of fat embolism syndrome. Am Surg 60:537, 1994.

The resulting low specificity prevents medical personnel from using bronchoalveolar lavage as a diagnostic test for the fat embolism syndrome.

Thamlikitkul V, Chokloikaew S, Tangtrakul T, et al: Blood culture: Comparison of outcomes between switch-needle and no-switch techniques. Am J Infect Control 20:122, 1992.
No need to switch needles in collection of blood cultures.

Williams TW Jr: Community-acquired pneumonia: How to manage this winter's infection. Consultant 35:1621, 1995.
Pneumonia caused by Klebsiella pneumoniae *or* Staphylococcus aureus *is a medical emergency that requires immediate hospitalization and parenteral antibiotic therapy.*

Woodhead MA, Arrowsmith J, Chamberlain-Webber R, et al: The value of routine microbial investigation in community-acquired pneumonia. Respir Med 85:313, 1991.
Mildly ill patients need only an initial blood culture.

PULMONARY EMBOLISM

Recommendations for pulmonary embolism are from the medical literature.

1. In patients with clinical findings (chest pain, dyspnea, tachypnea) of or predisposing factors for pulmonary embolism, request a complete blood count, arterial blood gas analysis, an electrocardiogram (ECG), and a chest radiograph. Consider obtaining a lung scan and pulmonary angiography. Other laboratory studies such as enzymes and fibrin degradation products are generally not useful.

The most sensitive clinical findings are chest pain, dyspnea, and tachypnea, and the most sensitive laboratory test is said to be the arterial P_{O_2}. In the past the triad of high serum bilirubin, high lactate dehydrogenase, and normal transaminase levels has been used, but this triad is only approximately 15% sensitive and thereful not useful. A chest radiograph and an ECG may be helpful, but a lung scan and pulmonary angiography are the definitive studies. The D-dimer test has been recommended for excluding pulmonary embolism in outpatients.

2. Evaluate the tests.

A lung scan can be either a perfusion lung scan (Q lung scan) alone or a combined ventilation-perfusion lung scan (V/Q lung scan). In the Q lung scan, pulmonary blood flow is assessed using intravenous technetium-99m–labeled macroaggregated albumin. In the combined V/Q lung scan, the Q lung scan is coupled with a V lung scan using xenon-133. Although the Q lung scan alone is sensitive for pulmonary embolism, it lacks specificity. The V lung scan increases the specificity of the Q lung scan.

3. If the results of a V/Q lung scan and/or pulmonary angiography are consistent, the diagnosis of pulmonary embolism is confirmed. Decreased arterial P_{O_2} and a compatible Q lung scan are sensitive but not specific for pulmonary embolism.

Pulmonary angiography is the definitive test for the diagnosis of pulmonary embolism, and with some patterns of V/Q lung scans (high-probability lung scans), the diagnosis can be made with virtual certainty. Only rare patients with normal V/Q lung scans have pulmonary embolic disease. A Q lung scan is sensitive for pulmonary embolism (i.e., rarely gives false-negative results) but is not specific (i.e., false-positive results in patients with chronic obstructive pulmonary disease [COPD], asthma, pneumonia, lung cysts, bronchiectasis, and atelectasis).

Decreased arterial P_{O_2} is 87% sensitive for pulmonary embolism but is not specific. The main purpose of the ECG is to exclude acute myocardial infarction. The most common finding in patients with pulmonary embolism is sinus tachycardia. A normal chest radiograph is uncommon in pulmonary embolism, patients, but the changes are nonspecific. Neutral fat droplets in bronchoalveolar lavage fluid are useful for the diagnosis of fat embolism.

4. A normal lung scan reliably excludes pulmonary embolism, but normal blood gas results do not.

Although an unequivocally normal lung scan effectively excludes pulmonary embolism, 29% of patients with pulmonary embolism had a normal alveolar-arterial (A-a) oxygen gradient (20 mm Hg or less), normal Pa_{O_2} (80 mm Hg or more), and normal Pa_{CO_2} (36 mm Hg or more).

5. In patients with pulmonary embolism, the following test results may be increased:

- **Leukocytes** with pulmonary infarction
- **ESR**
- **Bilirubin**
- **LD**

6. In patients with pulmonary embolism, the following blood test results may be decreased:

- **Platelets**
- **P_{CO_2}** less than 35 mm Hg (4.66 kPa) or decreasing P_{CO_2} in patients with known carbon dioxide retention

BIBLIOGRAPHY

Bone RC, Leibovitch E: Pulmonary embolism: An algorithm for diagnosis. Modern Med 59:40, 1991.
Discusses the diagnosis of pulmonary embolism and points out that measurements of enzymes and fibrin degradation products are of no value.
Bounameaux H, Cirafici P, De Moerloose P, et al: Measurement of D-dimer in plasma as diagnostic aid in suspected pulmonary embolism. Lancet 337:196, 1991.
Plasma D-dimer is suggested as a new screening test for pulmonary embolism.
Carson JL, Kelley MA, Duff A, et al: The clinical course of pulmonary embolism. N Engl J Med 326:1240, 1992.
When properly diagnosed and treated, clinically apparent pulmonary embolism was an uncommon cause of death.

Chastre J, Fagon J-Y, Soler P, et al: Bronchoalveolar lavage for rapid diagnosis of the fat embolism syndrome in trauma patients. Ann Intern Med 113:583, 1990.
Increased numbers of cells with neutral fat droplets in bronchoalveolar lavage fluid is a rapid specific test for fat embolism.

Coffman JD: Venous thrombosis and the diagnosis of pulmonary emboli. Hosp Pract 27:99, 1992.
Discusses diagnostic strategy using a case report.

Ginsberg JS: Management of venous thromboembolism. N Engl J Med 335:1816, 1996.
The care of patients with venous thromboembolism is discussed with emphasis on recent advances.

Goldhaber SZ, Simons GR, Elliott CG, et al: Quantitative plasma D-dimer levels among patients undergoing pulmonary angiography for suspected pulmonary embolism. JAMA 270:2819, 1993.
High levels of D-dimer, greater than 500 ng/mL (>500 µg/L), were found in 42 of the 45 patients with angiographically confirmed pulmonary embolism (sensitivity, 93%) and in 96 of the 128 patients without pulmonary embolism (specificity, 25%).

Hull RD, Feldstein W, Stein PD, et al: Cost-effectiveness of pulmonary embolism diagnosis. Arch Intern Med 156:68, 1996.
The strategy that requires pulmonary angiography in the fewest patients is a combination of ventilation-perfusion lung scans and serial impedance plethysmography. This strategy also proved to be the most cost-effective.

Hull RD, Raskob GE, Ginsberg JS, et al: A noninvasive strategy for the treatment of patients with suspected pulmonary embolism. Arch Intern Med 154:289, 1994.
A non-invasive approach to patients with non-diagnostic lung scans appears to have a low probability of adverse outcomes and to be an acceptable alternative to pulmonary angiography.

Hull RD, Raskob GE, Pineo GF, et al: The low-probability lung scan: A need for change in nomenclature. Arch Intern Med 155:1845, 1995.
Authors suggest abandoning the practice of using scan results to categorize pulmonary embolism probabilities as high, intermediate, indeterminant, or low.

Kassirer JP, Kopelman RI: Case 43—Treat: Or keep testing? *In* Learning Clinical Reasoning. Baltimore, Williams & Wilkins, 1991, p 217.
Discusses the clinical reasoning in a patient with pulmonary embolism.

Kerr CP, Yan L: Pulmonary embolism: Clinical decision making to increase diagnostic accuracy. Postgrad Med 91:73, 1992.
Criteria for diagnosing and treating pulmonary embolism.

Monreal M, Lafoz E, Casals A, et al: Platelet count and venous thromboembolism: A useful test for suspected pulmonary embolism. Chest 100:1493, 1991.
Decreased platelet count can be a clue to pulmonary embolism.

Pearson SD, Polak JL, Cartwright S, et al: A critical pathway to evaluate suspected deep vein thrombosis. Arch Intern Med 155:1773, 1995.
Discusses a critical pathway guideline for the emergency department evaluation of patients suspected of having deep vein thrombosis.

Perrier A, Bounameaux H, Morabia A, et al: Diagnosis of pulmonary embolism by a decision analysis–based strategy including clinical probability, D-dimer levels, and ultrasonography: A management study. Arch Intern Med 156:531, 1996.
Discusses the use of D-dimer levels and ultrasonography in patients with non-diagnostic lung scans.

Sherman S: Pulmonary embolism update: Lessons for the '90s. Postgrad Med 89:195, 1991.
Newer concepts in diagnosis, management, and prevention of pulmonary embolism.

Stein PD, Athanasoulis C, Alavi A, et al: Complications and validity of pulmonary angiography in acute pulmonary embolism. Circulation 85:462, 1992.
Confirms the low risk and high accuracy of angiography in most patients.

Stein PD, Goldhaber SZ, Henry JW, et al: Arterial blood gas analysis in the assessment of suspected acute pulmonary embolism. Chest 109:78, 1996.
Pulmonary embolism was present in 29% of all 70 patients with the combination of a normal A-a gradient PaO_2 and $PaCO_2$.

Stein PD, Goldhaber SZ, Henry JW, et al: Alveolar-arterial oxygen gradient in the assessment of acute pulmonary embolism. Chest 107:139, 1995.

A normal alveolar-arterial gradient does not necessarily rule out pulmonary embolism.

Stein PD, Gottschalk A, Saltzman HA, et al: Diagnosis of acute pulmonary embolism in the elderly. J Am Coll Cardiol 18:1452, 1991.
Clinical features of acute pulmonary embolism do not differ with age.

van Beek EJR, Schenk BE, Michel BC, et al: The role of plasma D-dimer concentration in the exclusion of pulmonary embolism. Br J Haematol 92:725, 1996.
The D-dimer test is recommended for excluding pulmonary embolism only in outpatients; it cannot effectively exclude pulmonary embolism in inpatients owing to their higher incidence of both pulmonary embolism and comorbid conditions.

Wirth JA, Matthay RA: Pulmonary embolism: Thirteen questions physicians often ask. Consultant 35:1103, 1995.
Good discussion of the diagnosis and treatment of patients with pulmonary embolism.

• •

CHRONIC OBSTRUCTIVE PULMONARY DISEASE

Recommendations for chronic obstructive pulmonary disease (COPD) are from the medical literature.

1. In patients with clinical findings of COPD (cough, dyspnea, decreased breath sounds, cor pulmonale), perform pulmonary function tests and request a chest radiograph, an ECG, a complete blood count (CBC), and electrolytes. Consider tests for arterial blood gas analysis and the possibility of α_1-antitrypsin deficiency.

Pulmonary function tests are not recommended for the asymptomatic, cigarette-smoking patient. However, the presence of clinical findings (e.g., productive cough in a cigarette smoker, occurring at least 3 months per year for 2 consecutive years) is suggestive of COPD, and pulmonary function tests are appropriate. In individuals with a family history of COPD, test for α_1-antitrypsin deficiency.

Patients with COPD are most commonly seen initially between 55 and 65 years of age. The disease is much more common in males than females (ratio, 9:1), but this may reflect differences in smoking habits. Approximately 75,000 persons per year die of COPD in the United States, which is approximately one half the number of individuals dying annually of lung cancer. Young patients in their twenties and thirties rarely have accumulated enough years of smoking exposure to have COPD. If these young patients have presenting symptoms of severe dyspnea, other diagnoses such as bronchiectasis, asthma, α_1-antitrypsin deficiency, and cystic fibrosis should be considered.

In the average patient with chronic obstructive bronchitis, loss of forced expiratory volume in 1 second (FEV_1) is in the range of 50 to 75 mL per year, two to three times the average rate of decline for nonsmokers. Continued smoking accelerates the deterioration. The best guide to prognosis is the amount of predicted FEV_1 obtained after administration of a bronchodilator.

2. Evaluate the tests.

The FEV_1, forced vital capacity (FVC), FEV_1:FVC ratio, and midmaximal expiratory flow rate (MMEFR) are useful spirometric tests of pulmonary function.

Tests for α_1-antitrypsin deficiency include serum protein electrophoresis, α_1-antitrypsin quantitation by rate nephelometry, and isoelectric focusing for phenotyping.

3. Interpret test results in the context of clinical findings.

In young, minimally symptomatic smokers, the FEV_1, FEV_1:FVC ratio, and MMEFR are not very sensitive for COPD (FEV_1, approximately 10%; MMEFR, approximately 20%); however, in older, more symptomatic patients, the sensitivity increases to 30 to 40%. In both young and old groups the specificity is much higher (80 to 95%).

The chest radiograph is not very useful for diagnosing COPD. Its main value is to exclude other conditions such as infection, malignancy, or bullous disease than can mimic the findings of COPD.

Early in the disease, the ECG usually is normal. Later, there may be changes consistent with pulmonary artery hypertension and cor pulmonale.

The CBC is usually normal except for increased hemoglobin and hematocrit values in some COPD patients with hypoxemia. When eosinophilia is present, consider an asthma-bronchitis component that may be reversible.

Laboratory confirmation of homozygous α_1-antitrypsin deficiency includes almost complete absence of α_1-globulin by serum protein electrophoresis, specifically by a pure Z phenotype. Two M genes (Pi MM phenotype) are present in normal individuals. Individuals homozygous for the disorder (approximately 1 in 4000 persons) have the Pi ZZ phenotype and severely reduced concentrations of α_1-antitrypsin (<50 mg/dL [<0.50 g/L]). Heterozygous individuals (3 to 5% of the population) have reduced antiproteolytic activity but are not at risk for COPD.

4. In patients with COPD, the following blood test results may be increased:

- **Leukocytes** due to pulmonary inflammation or infection
- **Pco_2** with respiratory acidosis
- **Potassium** with acidosis
- **Bicarbonate** with chronic respiratory acidosis

5. In patients with COPD, the following blood test results may be decreased:

- **Hemoglobin and hematocrit** related to high incidence of bleeding peptic ulcer
- **pH** with respiratory acidosis
- **Po_2** with pulmonary insufficiency
- **Chloride** with chronic respiratory acidosis
- **Phosphate,** particularly in those patients receiving mechanical ventilation

6. In patients with α_1-antitrypsin deficiency, the following blood test results may be increased:

- **Liver function tests**

7. In patients with α_1-antitrypsin deficiency, the following blood test results may be decreased:

- **Hemoglobin and hematocrit** with hypersplenism
- **Leukocytes** with hypersplenism
- **Platelets** with hypersplenism

BIBLIOGRAPHY

Boyars MC: COPD: A step-care approach when FEV_1 is deteriorating. Consultant 37:1673, 1997.
Early recognition of COPD is important because treatment of severe disease is often unsatisfactory.

Celli BR, Cosentino A, Fiel S, et al: The challenge of chronic obstructive pulmonary disease: Step by step through the workup. Patient Care 31:21, 1997.
Emphasizes early detection and intervention.

Celli BR, Cosentino A, Fiel S, et al: Managing the special problems of chronic lung disease. Patient Care 31:87, 1997.
Life-threatening infections, acute exacerbations, surgery, impaired sleep, psychosocial problems, and end-of-life decisions are common.

Fitzgerald DJ, Speir WA, Callahan LA: Office evaluation of pulmonary function: Beyond the numbers. Am Fam Physician 54:525, 1996.
Good discussion of pulmonary function tests.

Leighton BM, Kane GC: Chronic obstructive pulmonary disease. *In* Conn RB, Borer WZ, Snyder JW (eds): Current Diagnosis, 9th ed. Philadelphia, WB Saunders, 1997, p 297.
Discusses the differential diagnosis of COPD.

Mayewski RJ: Chronic obstructive lung disease. *In* Panzer RJ, Black ER, Griner PF (eds): Diagnostic Strategies for Common Medical Problems. Philadelphia, American College of Physicians, 1991, p 301.
Suggests strategies for the diagnosis of COPD.

Petty TL: The predictive value of spirometry. Postgrad Med 101:128, 1997.
Spirometry can identify patients with airflow obstruction who are at risk for lung cancer, heart attack, and stroke.

Pina JS, Horan MP: Alpha$_1$-antitrypsin deficiency and asthma. Postgrad Med 101:153, 1997.
Reviews the connection between α_1-antitrypsin deficiency and bronchial asthma.

Schapira RM, Reinke LF: The outpatient diagnosis and management of chronic obstructive pulmonary disease: Pharmacotherapy, administration of supplemental oxygen, and smoking cessation techniques. J Gen Intern Med 10:40, 1995.
Discusses smoking and other unusual causes.

Schapira RM, Schapira MM, Funahashi A, et al: The value of the forced expiratory time in the physical diagnosis of obstructive airways disease. JAMA 270:731, 1993.
The best cutoff for forced expiratory time was 6 seconds, yielding a sensitivity of 74% and a specificity of 75%.

Zaloga GP: Hypophosphatemia in COPD: How serious—And what to do? J Crit Illness 7:364, 1992.
Patients with COPD—particularly those receiving mechanical ventilation—are vulnerable to hypophosphatemia.

PLEURAL FLUID ANALYSIS

Recommendations for pleural fluid analysis are from the medical literature.

1. In patients with a pleural effusion, to diagnose the cause of the effusion, perform a thoracentesis and request pleural fluid total protein and LD determinations, together with serum total protein and LD determinations. Use Light's criteria to distinguish transudates from exudates.

Only 5 to 10 mL of fluid separates the layers of the pleural cavity in normal individuals. Excessive fluid accumulations can be characterized as transudates or exudates. These accumulations may cause pain, dyspnea, and cough; physical and radiologic examination are confirmatory. Common causes of transudates are congestive heart failure, liver disease and ascites, and the nephrotic syndrome. Common causes of exudates are infection, malignancy, and rheumatic disorders.

The appearance of the pleural effusion fluid may be a clue to its cause. For example, transudates are usually clear and straw colored, whereas exudates can be turbid, purulent, or bloody. It takes approximately 10,000 red blood cells/μL to impart a pink color to the fluid. A milky appearance suggests a chylous effusion. Protein and LD measurements are useful to distinguish pleural fluid exudates from transudates.

Collect pleural fluid and venous blood as follows: (1) pleural fluid for chemistry tests—10 mL, heparinized (glucose concentration may decrease if the fluid is not frozen or preserved with fluoride); (2) venous blood for chemistry tests—one clot tube; (3) pleural fluid for cytology—25 to 50 mL, heparinized; (4) pleural fluid for bacterial cultures—10 mL, heparinized; (5) pleural fluid for acid-fast and fungal cultures—10 mL, heparinized (a larger quantity [i.e., 50 mL] increases the sensitivity for culturing acid-fast bacilli); (6) pleural fluid for hematology tests—one ethylenediaminetetra-acetic acid (EDTA) tube; (7) pleural fluid for pH—several milliliters collected anaerobically in a syringe, iced, and quickly sent to the laboratory; and (8) pleural fluid for miscellaneous tests—10 mL, heparinized. These samples should be delivered to the laboratory immediately.

2. Evaluate the tests.

SENSITIVITY AND SPECIFICITY OF TESTS USED FOR CLASSIFICATION OF PLEURAL EFFUSION

Test	Exudate	Sensitivity (%)	Specificity (%)
1. Specific gravity	>1.016	78	89
2. Pleural fluid protein	>3 g/dL (30 g/L)	93	85
3. Pleural fluid/serum protein	>0.5	92	93

Table continued on following page

SENSITIVITY AND SPECIFICITY OF TESTS USED FOR CLASSIFICATION OF PLEURAL EFFUSION *Continued*

Test	Exudate	Sensitivity (%)	Specificity (%)
4. Pleural fluid LD*	>200 U/L	72	100
5. Pleural fluid/serum LD	>0.6	88	96
Test 3 or 5 positive	—	99	89
Tests 3 and 5 positive	—	81	100

*LD method with a reference range >300 U/L. Current LD methods may not be comparable (i.e., pleural fluid LD >two-thirds the upper limit for serum LD).

Light's criteria for an exudate = at least one of 3, 4, or 5 positive.

Source: Skendzel LP: A practical approach to the chemical and microscopic study of pleural and peritoneal fluids. Lab Medica V (1):16, 1988.

A pleural fluid cholesterol greater than 54 mg/dL (>1.40 mmol/L) and a pleural fluid/serum cholesterol ratio greater than 0.32 identifies an exudate with an approximate sensitivity of 96% and specificity of 92%.

3. If the pleural fluid/serum protein ratio, pleural fluid/serum LD ratio, or pleural fluid LD indicate that the fluid is a transudate, then no further testing is usually necessary.

A study of 533 pleural fluid specimens from 340 patients showed that an average of eight to nine tests were performed on each fluid, including white blood cell (WBC), WBC differential, and other specific studies. Although these tests may prove useful when the fluid is an 8xudate, they are of little use when the fluid is a transudate.

4. If the pleural fluid/serum protein ratio, pleural fluid/serum LD ratio, or pleural fluid LD indicate that the fluid is an exudate, perform cytologic studies and cultures. The following additional tests may prove useful.

Test	Diseases
Red blood cell count >100 × 10³/μL (>100 × 10⁹/L)	Trauma, malignancy, pulmonary embolism
WBC count >50–100 × 10³ cells/μL (>50–100 × 10⁹ cells/L)	Empyema (grossly visible pus)
>50% polymorphonuclear leukocytes	Inflammation
>50% lymphocytes	Neoplasm or tuberculosis
Eosinophilia	Previous thoracentesis, pleural air or blood, asbestosis, collagen-vascular disease, drug-induced pleuritis, paragonimiasis, malignancy, tuberculosis

Test	Diseases
pH <7.2	Infection, malignancy, rheumatoid arthritis, esophageal rupture
Glucose <60 mg/dL (<3.33 mmol/L)	Infection, malignancy, rheumatoid arthritis
Amylase increased	Pancreatitis, esophageal rupture, amylase-secreting neoplasm
Triglycerides >100 mg/dL (>1.14 mmol/L)	Chylous effusion seen in trauma, malignancy
Rheumatoid factor, antinuclear antibodies, lupus erythematosus cells, decreased complement	Collagen vascular disease, lupus erythematosus, rheumatoid arthritis

Cytologic studies should include both Wright-Giemsa and Papanicolaou stained preparations. Pleural biopsy may be helpful. Cytologic study has a higher diagnostic yield than pleural biopsy in patients with malignant disease of the pleura but a lower yield than pleural biopsy in patients with tuberculous disease of the pleura. With tuberculous pleuritis, acid-fast smears are 20 to 40% sensitive, a biopsy is 70% sensitive, and a culture is 75% sensitive; all three studies together have a combined sensitivity of 90 to 95%.

BIBLIOGRAPHY

Bassiri AG, Morris W, Kirsch CM: Eosinophilic tuberculous pleural effusion. West J Med 166:277, 1997.
Reports tuberculous pleural effusion with 36% eosinophils.
Brandstetter RD, Velazquez V, Viejo C, et al: Postural changes in pleural fluid constitutents. Chest 105:1458, 1994.
A positional sedimentary effect occurs for pleural fluid exudates but not transudates. This difference generally should not interfere with distinguishing between pleural fluid exudates and transudates.
Burgess LJ, Maritz FJ, Taljaard JJF: Comparative analysis of the biochemical parameters used to distinguish between pleural transudates and exudates. Chest 107:1604, 1995.
The results of this study support the criteria of Light as the diagnostic method of choice for distinguishing between pleural exudates and transudates.
Costa M, Quiroga T, Cruz E: Measurement of pleural fluid cholesterol and lactate dehydrogenase. Chest 108:1260, 1995.
Simultaneous measurement of pleural fluid cholesterol and LD identifies exudates when one or both of these are above the limits of 45 mg/dL (1.17 mmol/L) for cholesterol and 200 U/L for LD, with an accuracy similar to that in the reports using the more complicated criteria of Light and without the need for a blood sample analysis.
Devuyst O, Lambert M, Scheiff JM, et al: High amylase activity in pleural fluid and primary bronchogenic adenocarcinoma. Eur Respir J 3:1217, 1990.
In the absence of pancreatitis and esophageal perforation, high pleural fluid amylase (salivary type) values are consistent with bronchogenic adenocarcinoma.
Ferrer JS, Muñoz XG, Orriols RM, et al: Evolution of idiopathic pleural effusion. Chest 109:1508, 1996.
Idiopathic exudative pleural effusions have a high rate of spontaneous resolution and a low rate of subsequent etiologic diagnosis.

Gottehrer A, Taryle DA, Reed CE, et al: Pleural fluid analysis in malignant mesothelioma. Chest 100:1003, 1991.
Low pleural fluid pH and glucose indicate reduced survival time.

Guarino JR, Guarino JC: Auscultatory percussion: A simple method to detect pleural effusion. J Gen Intern Med 9:71, 1994.
This study shows that auscultatory percussion is a highly sensitive and specific way to detect pleural effusion.

Heffner J, Brown LK, Barbieri C, et al: Pleural fluid chemical analysis in parapneumonic effusions. Am J Respir Crit Care Med 151:1700, 1995.
The available data suggest that pleural fluid pH is the best test for determining whether patients with parapneumonic effusions require chest-tube placement.

Joseph J, Strange C, Sahn SA: Pleural effusions in hospitalized patients with AIDS. Ann Intern Med 118:856, 1993.
Bacterial pneumonia is the most common cause for pleural effusion in AIDS.

Light RW: Pleural Diseases, 3rd ed. Baltimore, Williams & Wilkins, 1995.
Excellent general reference that includes a discussion of Light's indices.

Light RW: Pleural diseases. DM 38(5):1, 1992.
Reviews differential diagnosis of pleural diseases.

Marel M, Stastny B, Melínová L, et al: Diagnosis of pleural effusions. Chest 107:1598, 1995.
Recommends a four-step diagnostic work-up.

Meisel S, Shamiss A, Thaler M, et al: Pleural fluid to serum bilirubin concentration ratio for the separation of transudates from exudates. Chest 98:141, 1990.
Pleural fluid to serum bilirubin ratio can be used to distinguish exudates from transudates.

Menzies R, Charbonneau M: Thoracoscopy for the diagnosis of pleural disease. Ann Intern Med 114:271, 1991.
Thoracoscopy may be helpful in difficult cases.

Peterman TA, Speicher CE: Evaluating pleural effusions: A two-stage laboratory approach. JAMA 252:1051, 1984.
Light's criteria effectively separate transudates from exudates, making further evaluation of transudates unnecessary.

Romero S, Candela A, Martin C, et al: Evaluation of different criteria for the separation of pleural transudates from exudates. Chest 104:399, 1993.
The results show that the criteria of Light provide the greatest accuracy for separating pleural transudates from exudates; misclassifying transudates in patients with congestive heart failure was the greatest error (22.7% misclassified).

Roth BJ, O'Meara TF, Cragun WH: The serum-effusion albumin gradient in the evaluation of pleural effusions. Chest 98:546, 1990.
Gradient between pleural fluid albumin and serum albumin is useful to distinguish exudates from transudates.

Suay VG, Moragón EM, Viedma EC, et al: Pleural cholesterol in differentiating transudates and exudates. Respiration 62:57, 1995.
Both pleural fluid cholesterol and the pleural fluid/serum cholesterol ratio, with respective cutoffs of 54 mg/dL (1.40 mmol/L) and 0.32, are useful in differentiating pleural fluid exudates and transudates.

Vives M, Porcel JM, de Vera MV, et al: A study of Light's criteria and possible modifications for distinguishing exudative from transudative pleural effusions. Chest 109:1503, 1996.
The results of this study support continuously using the unmodified classic criteria of Light to discriminate between pleural transudates and exudates.

5

Gastrointestinal Diseases

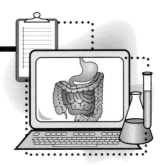

- Acute Abdominal Pain
- Acute Diarrhea
- Intestinal Malabsorption
- Ascites

ACUTE ABDOMINAL PAIN

Recommendations for abdominal pain are from the medical literature.

1. For patients with abdominal pain, assess the clinical findings and obtain appropriate radiographic studies and laboratory tests.

The differential diagnosis of abdominal pain is long, and the reader is referred to other texts for a complete discussion of the various disorders. Although the correct diagnosis of these disorders is primarily a clinical exercise, radiographic studies and laboratory tests may be useful if they are carefully selected and their limitations are understood. Several common disorders are discussed in which laboratory tests may be useful: appendicitis, acute pancreatitis, acute cholecystitis, dyspepsia, and acute intermittent porphyria. Dyspepsia refers to the clinical findings that accompany peptic ulcer disease. These need to be distinguished from gastroesophageal reflux, irritable bowel syndrome, biliary colic, and musculoskeletal pain.

Useful laboratory tests to consider include a complete blood count with differential; determinations of serum glucose, urea nitrogen, creatinine, electrolytes, amylase, lipase, and C-reactive protein; urinalysis; porphyria tests (Watson-Schwartz test and quantitative tests for urine δ-aminolevulinic acid [ALA] and porphobilinogen [PBG]); and dyspepsia tests (gastric acid secretion, serum gastrin, and tests for *Helicobacter pylori*). The use of serial serum human chorionic gonadotropin measurements to diagnose ectopic pregnancy is discussed in Chapter 1, and urinalysis for urinary tract disorders is discussed in Chapter 7.

2. Evaluate the tests.

Recent developments in the methodology for serum lipase and tests for porphyrins and peptic ulcer require comment. For diagnosing acute pancreatitis, the importance of improved lipase methods has been recently elucidated. These newer methods such as the Kodak Ektachem lipase method, which incorporate colipase, result in higher test results and an increased sensitivity for pancreatitis. Appropriate reference ranges should be used.

For diagnosing acute intermittent porphyria, the Watson-Schwartz test for PBG may be used, but it is subject to false-negative and false-positive results; therefore, quantitative methods for determining ALA and PBG are preferable.

For diagnosing dyspepsia, determination of gastric acid secretion is usually unnecessary. *H. pylori* can be detected by the biopsy urease test after endoscopy and noninvasive methods such as serologic antibody measurements and urea breath testing. Serum gastrin can be measured in the fasting state and after secretin or calcium stimulation.

3. Interpret test results in the context of clinical findings.

Appendicitis

The clinical findings of appendicitis include pain (midabdominal, then right lower quadrant); associated with nausea, vomiting, acute loss of appetite; local tenderness; and sometimes local rigidity of muscle.

Consistent laboratory findings include polymorphonuclear leukocytosis with a left shift. Increased hematocrit and serum urea nitrogen values may reflect dehydration, often caused by vomiting and a low fluid intake. Normal results from a urinalysis are important for excluding urinary tract disease; however, 20% of patients with acute appendicitis have a few scattered red blood cells and white blood cells (WBCs) in the urinary sediment. Normal WBC and neutrophil counts are sensitive tests for excluding appendicitis; however, according to a recent report, the addition of a normal C-reactive protein value can increase the negative predictive value to 100%.

Acute Pancreatitis

The clinical findings of acute pancreatitis include pain, shock, vomiting, fever, tenderness, and rigidity.

Serum amylase and lipase tests should be ordered together and then performed two to three times daily during the first 48 hours. Ultrasound and computed tomography studies may be useful. Serum amylase values increase 2 to 3 hours after the onset of acute pancreatitis and return to normal in approximately 4 to 7 days. Serum lipase values increase simultaneously and take longer to return to normal. Slightly increased amylase values are present in many disorders, but values greater than two to three times the upper limit of normal most often indicate acute pancreatitis. High amylase values in the absence of acute pancreatitis occur with renal failure and macroamylasemia. A normal amylase value does not exclude acute pancreatitis. Serum lipase tests (using newer methods) are more sensitive and specific than those for amylase in determining the diagnosis. In asymptomatic alcoholics, lipase values up to three times the upper limit of normal may occur; however, values that exceed five times the upper limit of normal indicate acute pancreatitis. Serum lipase is a better test than serum amylase to diagnose acute alcoholic pancreatitis.

Other consistent test results include leukocytosis, hyperglycemia, hypocalcemia, hyperbilirubinemia, hypertriglyceridemia, and hypoxemia.

Acute Cholecystitis

The clinical findings of acute cholecystitis include pain, nausea, vomiting, loss of appetite; jaundice (with cholestasis); fever; palpable or visibly distended gallbladder; and tenderness and rigidity.

The diagnosis of acute cholecystitis is established by clinical findings and radiographic studies such as ultrasonography, and radionuclide cholescintigraphy. Laboratory tests are ancillary and consist mainly of detecting polymorphonuclear leukocytosis with a left shift and excluding other conditions such as urinary tract disease. Liver function tests, such as serum bilirubin, alkaline phosphatase, and gamma-glutamyl transferase are helpful because they may detect cholestasis secondary to cholelithiasis.

Dyspepsia

Clinical findings of dyspepsia include gnawing epigastic pain relieved by food or antacids. Complications include bleeding, perforation, obstruction, and intractable pain. The symptoms and signs of perforation vary according to the time that has elapsed since the perforation occurred. Within the first 2 hours, great and generalized abdominal pain occurs. The pain leads to lying still rather than walking around.

The definitive diagnosis of dyspepsia depends on visualizing the gastroduodenal mucosa by radiographic or endoscopic studies. Major causes of dyspepsia include nonsteroidal anti-inflammatory drugs (NSAIDs) and *H. pylori*. In the absence of hypergastrinemia, measurement of gastric acid secretion is usually unnecessary. Because the prevalence of the Zollinger-Ellison syndrome is less than 1%, routine measurement of serum gastrin is also usually unnecessary. However, do obtain serum gastrin determinations for patients at increased risk (e.g., family history of peptic ulcer, ulcer associated with hypercalcemia, manifestations of multiple endocrine neoplasia type I, or multiple peptic ulcers).

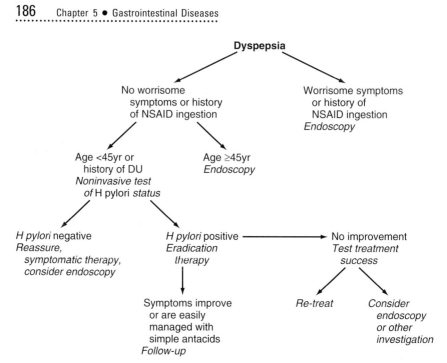

Dyspepsia

Source: Adapted from Goodwin CS, Mendall MM, Northfield NC: *Helicobacter pylori* infection. Lancet 349:265–269, 1997.

In young patients with dyspepsia, without worrisome symptoms or a history of NSAID ingestion, serologic testing for *H. pylori* is an important first step. In *H. pylori*–seropositive patients with dyspepsia, initial anti–*H. pylori* therapy is the most cost-effective management strategy. This recommendation is based on the assumption that serologic testing has a sensitivity and specificity of approximately 90%; therefore, in a population with a 65% prevalence of *H. pylori* infection, serologic testing has a positive predictive value of 95% for active infection.

The following table lists the available methods for diagnosing *H. pylori*, together with their sensitivities, specificities, and relative costs.

Method	Sensitivity (%)	Specificity (%)	Relative Cost
Noninvasive			
Serology	88–99	86–95	$
Urea breath test	90–95	90–100	$$
Invasive			
Biopsy urease test	89–98	95–98	$$$$
Culture	72–92	100	$$$$$
Histology	93–99	95–99	$$$$$

Source: Cave DR, Hoffman JS: Management of *Helicobacter pylori* infection in ulcer disease. Hosp Pract 31:63, 1996. Reproduced with permission. © 1996 McGraw-Hill.

Porphyria

Clinical findings of acute intermittent porphyria include a family history of cramping abdominal pain with episodes precipitated by certain drugs, crash dieting, and infections. In porphyric women the attacks may be menstrually related. A history of repeated attacks of pain, sometimes with surgery and no pathologic findings, may be elicited. During an attack of acute intermittent porphyria, PBG excretion is in the range of 50 to 200 mg/day (220 to 880 μmol/day [reference range, 0 to 2 mg/day]) and ALA excretion is in the range of 20 to 100 mg/day (152 to 763 μmol/day [reference range, 1.5 to 7.5 mg/day]). During an acute attack, the increased concentration of PBG may be detected by a qualitative test, the Watson-Schwartz test.

Porphyrias may be divided into two general categories: cutaneous photosensitivity and neurologic abnormalities. Patients may have cutaneous photosensitivity (e.g., porphyria cutanea tarda), neurologic abnormalities (e.g., intermittent porphyria), or both. Neurologic abnormalities are associated with increased urinary excretion of the porphyria precursors PBG and ALA.

BIBLIOGRAPHY

Albu E, Miller BM, Choi Y, et al: Diagnostic value of C-reactive protein in acute appendicitis. Dis Colon Rectum 37:49, 1994.
  The results show that although a C-reactive protein of 2.5 mg/dL (25 mg/L) is not a definitive indicator of acute appendicitis, a C-reactive protein of less than 2.5 mg/dL (<25 mg/L) 12 hours after onset of symptoms excludes the diagnosis of acute appendicitis.
Altman LK: How tools of medicine get in the way. The New York Times, May 12, 1992, p B6.
  Fascinating account of how medical technology interfered with the diagnosis of acute appendicitis.
Amann ST, DiMagno E, Rubin W: Pancreatitis: Diagnostic and therapeutic interventions. Patient Care 31:200, 1997.
  Recognizing the clinical laboratory and radiologic features of acute and chronic pancreatitis is a critical diagnostic skill.
Andersson R, Hugander A, Thulin A, et al: Indications for operation in suspected appendicitis and incidence of perforation. BMJ 308:197, 1994.
  A strategy of aggressive surgical exploration is unlikely to lower the perforation rate, and the perforation rate probably cannot be used as a measure of quality of care.
Araki T, Ueda M, Taketa K, et al: Pancreatic-type hyperamylasemia in end-stage renal disease. Dig Dis Sci 34:1425, 1989.
  Serum amylase is commonly increased in patients with renal insufficiency.
Berg CL, Wolfe MM: Zollinger-Ellison syndrome. Med Clin North Am 75:903, 1991.
  Reviews the pathophysiology, diagnosis, and management of the Zollinger-Ellison syndrome.
Buchman AL, Ament ME, Moukarzel A: Total serum amylase but not lipase correlates with measured glomerular filtration rate. J Clin Gastroenterol 16:204, 1993.
  In the absence of macroamylasemia or macrolipasemia, even a small elevation of serum amylase or lipase may be clinically significant in a patient with renal insufficiency.
Cave DR, Hoffman JS: Management of *Helicobacter pylori* infection in ulcer disease. Hosp Pract 31:63, 1996.

Well-tolerated drug combinations yield eradication rates exceeding 90% without generating a high frequency of bacterial resistance.

Chi C-H, Shiesh S-C, Chen K-W, et al: C-reactive protein for the evaluation of acute abdominal pain. Am J Emerg Med 14:254, 1996.
The C-reactive protein is a simple, rapid, and relatively inexpensive test to rule in or rule out a serious condition.

Clearfield HR: *Helicobacter pylori*: Aggressor or innocent bystander? Med Clin North Am 75:815, 1991.
Suggests that for most patients the organism is an innocent bystander, but for some patients it facilitates the development and relapse of peptic ulcer disease.

Cooperman AM, Fuhrman SA: Patient with abdominal pain; Shedlofsky SI: Young woman with recurrent abdominal pain; and Henderson AR, Shedlofsky SI: Severe epigastic pain. *In* Tietz NW, Conn RB, Pruden EL (eds): Applied Laboratory Medicine. Philadelphia, WB Saunders, 1992, pp 85, 89, 99.
Discusses three causes of abdominal pain: cholelithiasis, acute intermittent porphyria, and acute pancreatitis.

Corsetti JP, Arvan DA: Acute pancreatitis; and Greene RA, Griner PF: Cholelithiasis and acute cholecystitis. *In* Panzer RJ, Black ER, Griner PF (eds): Diagnostic Strategies for Common Medical Tests. Philadelphia, American College of Physicians, 1991, pp 160, 121.
Recommendations for diagnosing the cause of acute abdominal pain.

Cutler AF, Prasad VM: Long-term follow-up of *Heliobacter pylori* serology after successful eradication. Am J Gastroenterol 91:85, 1996.
During the first year or two after antibiotic treatment for H. pylori, *nearly all successfully treated patients had a decline in IgG by this method, and a minority became seronegative.*

Damianos AJ, McGarrity TJ: Treatment strategies for *Helicobacter pylori* infection. Am Fam Physician 55:2765, 1997.
In patients undergoing endoscopy, the rapid urease test is highly sensitive and specific in diagnosing H. pylori infection. Non-invasive diagnostic methods include serologic antibody measurements and urea breath testing.

Dueholm S, Bagi P, Bud M: Laboratory aid in the diagnosis of acute appendicitis. Dis Colon Rectum 32:855, 1989.
Most efficient test combination for excluding appendicitis consists of a WBC count, a neutrophil count, and a C-reactive protein measurement—negative predictive value of 100%.

Elder GH, Hift RJ, Meissner PN: The acute porphyrias. Lancet 349:1613, 1997.
Discusses three autosomal dominant types: acute intermittent porphyria, variegate porphyria, and hereditary coproporphyria.

Fan S, Lai ECS, Mok FPT, et al: Prediction of the severity of acute pancreatitis. Am J Surg 166:262, 1993.
The admission glucose and urea levels are useful for identifying high-risk pancreatitis patients early so that surveillance or aggressive therapy can be increased.

Frey CF, Gerzof SG, Vennes JA: Progress in acute pancreatitis. Patient Care 26:258, 1992.
Alcohol-related disease or gallstones are common causes. Discusses false-positive and false-negative serum amylase results.

Frucht H, Howard JM, Slaff JI, et al: Secretin and calcium provocative tests in the Zollinger-Ellison syndrome. Ann Intern Med 111:713, 1989.
Calcium provocative test is appropriate for patients with strong clinical suspicion for the Zollinger-Ellison syndrome and a negative secretin test result.

Gullo L: Chronic nonpathological hyperamylasemia of pancreatic origin. Gastroenterology 110:1905, 1996.
Patients who have a persistently elevated serum amylase without clinical, functional, or imaging evidence of pancreatic disease can be assured that they do not have pancreatic disease without undergoing additional costly diagnostic studies.

Gruber PJ, Silverman RA, Gottesfeld S, et al: Presence of fever and leukocytosis in acute cholecystitis. Ann Emerg Med 28:273, 1996.
Singer A, McCracken G, Henry MC, et al: Correlation among clinical, laboratory, and hepatobiliary scanning findings in patients with suspected acute cholecystitis. Ann Emerg Med 28:267, 1996.

These studies suggest that fever and leukocytosis are often absent when patients with acute cholecystitis present initially to the emergency department. But the prevalence of these findings probably rises later during the clinical course.

Gumaste V, Dave P, Sereny G: Serum lipase: A better test to diagnose acute alcoholic pancreatitis. Am J Med 92:239, 1992.
Serum lipase is a better test than amylase for diagnosing acute pancreatitis.

Gumaste VV, Roditis N, Mehta D, et al: Serum lipase levels in nonpancreatic abdominal pain versus acute pancreatitis. J Gastroenterol 88:2051, 1993.
The sensitivity and specificity of serum lipase for diagnosing acute pancreatitis, based on elevated levels of more than three times normal, were 100% and 99%, respectively, compared with only 75% and 99%, respectively, for serum amylase elevated to more than three times normal.

Gurleyik E, Gurleyik G, Unalmiser S: Accuracy of serum C-reactive protein measurements in diagnosis of acute appendicitis compared with surgeon's clinical impression. Colon Rectum 38:1270, 1995.
The C-reactive protein is recommended as a routine laboratory test for patients with suspected acute appendicitis, with use of serial clinical examinations and C-reactive protein tests when the diagnosis is in doubt.

Johnson DA: *Helicobacter pylori* and GI disease: Thirteen questions physicians often ask. Consultant 36:1911, 1996.
At least 90% of duodenal ulcers and most gastric ulcers are thought to be caused by H. pylori *infection.*

Kosunen TU, Seppälä K, Sarna S, et al: Diagnostic value of decreasing IgG, IgA, and IgM antibody titers after eradication of *Helicobacter pylori*. Lancet 339:893, 1992.
Serologic tests may be used to monitor eradication of H. pylori.

Kushner JP: Laboratory diagnosis of the porphyrias. N Engl J Med 324:1432, 1991.
Concise discussion of the porphyrias with strategies for laboratory diagnosis.

Lott JA (ed): Clinical Pathology of Pancreatic Disorders. Totowa, NJ, Humana Press, 1997.
Reviews transplantation of the pancreas as well as inflammatory and neoplastic disorders.

McNamara MJ, Pasquale MD, Evans SRT: Acute appendicitis and the use of intraperitoneal cultures. Surg Gynecol Obstet 177:393, 1993.
The results support abandoning the routine practice of obtaining peritoneal cultures during surgery for acute appendicitis and complicated appendicitis because of their failure to alter patient outcome beyond the use of empiric antibiotic therapy.

Miettinen AK, Heinonen PK, Laippala P, et al: Test performance of erythrocyte sedimentation rate and C-reactive protein in assessing the severity of acute pelvic inflammatory disease. Am J Obstet Gynecol 169:1143, 1993.
The erythrocyte sedimentation rate and C-reactive protein more accurately assess the severity of acute pelvic inflammatory disease than clinical examination alone and also may identify those patients who need antianaerobic antimicrobial therapy.

Ofman JJ, Etchason J, Fullerton S, et al: Management strategies for *H. pylori*–seropositive patients with dyspepsia: Clinical and economic consequences. Ann Intern Med 126:280, 1997.
In H. pylori–*seropositive patients with dyspepsia, initial anti–*H. pylori *therapy is the most cost-effective management strategy.*

Orebaugh SL: Normal amylase levels in the presentation of acute pancreatitis. Am J Emerg Med 12:21, 1994.
The serum amylase is not sensitive enough to be used as the sole laboratory test for diagnosing acute pancreatitis in the emergency department; the serum lipase is much more sensitive.

Puskar D, Vuckovic I, Bedalo G, et al: Urinalysis, ultrasound analysis, and renal dynamic scintigraphy in acute appendicitis. Urology 45:108, 1995.
Abnormal urinalysis, defined as more than four red or white blood cells per high-power field or proteinuria of more than 0.5 g/L, was found in 32 (48%) of the 66 patients with acute appendicitis before appendectomy.

Rabeneck L, Graham DY: *Helicobacter pylori*: When to test, when to treat. Ann Intern Med 126:315, 1997.
Do not test if you are not willing to treat. Whom, then, should we be willing to treat?

On the basis of the available evidence, we should treat all patients who have or have had active peptic ulcer disease.

Ravichandran D, Daltrey I, Uglow M, et al: Urine testing for acute lower abdominal pain in adults. Br J Surg 81:1459, 1994.
Urine dipstick testing is faster, less expensive, and more accurate than microscopy for diagnosing urinary tract infection in patients with acute lower abdominal pain.

Silen W: Cope's Early Diagnosis of the Acute Abdomen, 18th ed. New York, Oxford University Press, 1991.
Classic treatise on the differential diagnosis of acute abdominal pain.

Silver BE, Patterson JW, Kulick M, et al: Effect of CBC results on emergency department management of women with lower abdominal pain. Am J Emerg Med 13:304, 1995.
The complete blood count results very rarely affect patient management or diagnosis in this patient group.

Tham TCK, McLaughlin N, Hughes DF, et al: Possible role of *Helicobacter pylori* serology in reducing endoscopy workload. Postgrad Med J 70:809, 1994.
Thirty-five percent of endoscopies could have been avoided without missing any patient with duodenal ulcer disease if the H. pylori serology had been used as a screening procedure prior to endoscopy for patients up to 45 years old.

Vermeulen B, Morabia A, Unger P-F: Influence of white cell count on surgical decision making in patients with abdominal pain in the right lower quadrant. Eur J Surg 161:483, 1995.
Although the initial WBC count provided clear diagnostic benefit to only 5 of the 221 patients, which may be considered insignificant, the cost of the WBC counts is much less than a single operation or the cost related to a missed diagnosis.

Wagner JM, McKinney P, Carpenter JL: Does this patient have appendicitis? JAMA 276:1589, 1996.
Reviews the literature evaluating the operating characteristics of the most useful elements of the history and physical examination for the diagnosis of appendicitis.

ACUTE DIARRHEA

Recommendations for acute diarrhea are from the medical literature.

1. In patients with acute diarrhea, determine the clinical findings and consider the broad range of causes, infectious and noninfectious. A fecal smear for polymorphonuclear leukocytes may help to distinguish noninflammatory from inflammatory diarrhea, and occult blood testing may be useful.

Acute diarrhea is diarrhea of less than 1 week's duration that is characterized by an increase in daily stool weight of more than 250 g, liquidity, and a frequency of more than three bowel movements per day. It is usually self-limited and requires no treatment; however, it may be prolonged and reflect serious disease, that is, dysentery. Dysentery refers to severe inflammation of the intestine, usually the colon, associated with fever, abdominal pain, and blood, pus, and mucus in the stool.

Acute diarrhea is divided into two types, noninflammatory and inflammatory, on the basis of whether or not polymorphonuclear leukocytes are present in the feces. This is a clinically relevant classification because in the United States noninflammatory disease usually is self-limited and is associated with cramping, bloating, periumbilical pain, and large-volume, watery stools. Fever, leukocytosis, and constitutional symptoms are absent. In contrast, inflammatory diarrhea or dysentery is associated with mucosal invasion and commonly is accompanied by fever, constitutional symptoms, lower abdominal pain, and tenesmus. Stools may be small in volume and often are bloody or mucoid.

To look for fecal leukocytes, apply a thin layer of feces or mucus to a slide, mix with one drop of Löffler's methylene blue stain, seal with a coverslip, and examine for polymorphonuclear leukocytes (Wright's stain of dried fecal smears may also be used). More than five leukocytes per high-power field in five or more fields is considered positive for inflammatory diarrhea. The presence of erythrocytes or occult blood suggests an inflammatory cause, but there are exceptions such as ischemia.

In the United States, Norwalk virus and other viral agents are common causes of noninflammatory diarrhea in adults; the diarrhea is explosive and lasts approximately 24 to 48 hours. Rotavirus infection predominates in infants and young children and produces watery diarrhea of 5 to 8 days' duration. Other causes of noninflammatory diarrhea include enterotoxigenic *Escherichia coli, Vibrio cholerae, Bacillus cereus, Cryptosporidum, Giardia lamblia*, and bacterial toxins associated with food poisoning *(Staphylococcus* and *Clostridium perfringens)*. These organisms or toxins do not invade the mucosa but induce a secretory, watery diarrhea; thus, fecal leukocytes are typically absent.

Noninflammatory diarrhea has a number of non-infectious causes. Drugs that can cause diarrhea include laxatives, warfarin, thyroid hormones, magnesium-containing antacids, quinidine, colchicine, cholestyramine, digoxin, and antimetabolites. Diarrhea can occur with toxins such as heavy metals (lead, zinc, cadmium, copper), poisonous fish (ciguatoxin, scombrotoxin, puffer fish, shellfish), monosodium glutamate, botulism, and mushroom poisoning. Fecal impaction is an additional cause. Some patients with an irritable bowel or an inflamed rectum pass several loose bowel movements each day that do not exceed a total of 250 g. Diabetic diarrhea is common in patients with diabetic peripheral and autonomic neuropathy, and bacterial overgrowth may play a role. A watery diarrhea can also occur with other chronic conditions: irritable bowel syndrome, inflammatory bowel disease, villous adenoma, ischemic colitis, and mesenteric thrombosis.

It may be useful to distinguish osmotic diarrhea from secretory diarrhea. Osmotic diarrhea is caused by the accumulation in the gut lumen of nonabsorbable solutes (e.g., divalent or trivalent ions [Mg^{2+}, PO^{2-}, SO^{2-}]) from saline solution laxatives and of lactose secondary to disaccharidase deficiency. In contrast, secretory diarrhea (usually >1000 mL/day) is caused by a net luminal gain of secretions, that is, electrolytes and water. Examples of secretory diarrhea include enterotoxin-induced diarrhea, pancreatic cholera syndrome, carcinoid syndrome, glucagonoma, Zollinger-Ellison syndrome, and surreptitious ingestion of cathartic agents such as phenolphthalein (pink color of alkalinized stool). Osmotic diarrhea can be distinguished from secretory diarrhea by calculating the stool osmotic gap as follows:

Stool osmotic gap = Measured stool osmolality − $2[(Na^+) + (K^+)]$

A high stool osmotic gap (commonly >160 mOsm/kg), indicates osmotic diarrhea. A gap that is approximately zero or negative (may be negative because of multivalent anions), indicates secretory diarrhea. The stool sample must be fresh or stored at 39.2°F (4°C). Measured osmolality of diarrheal stool is normally 285 to 330 mOsm/kg. Osmotic diarrhea typically stops after a 24-hour fast, whereas secretory diarrhea persists.

2. In patients with findings suggestive of infectious diarrhea, request a stool culture and stool examination for ova and parasites.

A single stool submission for bacterial culture and/or ova and parasite analysis provides high diagnostic sensitivity. In general, no more than two stool specimens should be submitted for bacteriology and no more than three stool specimens for parasitology. Repeat specimens should be submitted on separate days.

Consider stool culture for viruses in immunocompromised patients and testing for *Clostridium difficile* toxin in patients with antibiotic exposure and no other recognized cause for diarrhea.

3. In patients with specific clinical findings suggestive of infections that cannot be detected by routine stool cultures and ova and parasite analyses, request specific stool studies depending on the clinical and epidemiologic findings.

Specific agents that fall in this category include: *E. coli* 0157:H7, *Vibrio* species, *Yersinia enterocolitica, Cryptosporidium, Cyclospora*, and microsporidia.

4. In patients with diarrhea noted 3 or more days after hospitalization, stool cultures and ova and parasite analyses are not indicated; consider testing for *C. difficile* toxin.

In this group of patients, routine stool studies are not productive. However, these patients have often been on antibiotics, and *C. difficile* toxin may be the causative agent. No more than two studies for *C. difficile* toxin should be requested. Wait for the result of the first study before requesting the second study.

5. Perform proctosigmoidoscopy in patients with toxicity, bloody diarrhea, antibiotic-associated diarrhea, or prolonged diarrhea.

Sigmoidoscopy can reveal the yellow-gray plaques of antibiotic-associated colitis, and the diagnosis can be confirmed by rectal biopsy, measuring *C. difficile* toxin, or anaerobic culture of *C. difficile*. In a patient with antibiotic-associated diarrhea and negative studies for *C. difficile*, consider *Candida*. A patient with amebiasis has colonic ulcerations containing amebas, and serologic tests using gel diffusion precipitin or indirect hemagglutination tests are positive in 85 to 95% of patients. In patients with ulcerative colitis, the rectal and colonic mucosa are diffusely red and friable, and cultures are negative. Consider ischemic colitis in older patients with atherosclerotic vascular disease and diarrhea. A barium enema examination may be useful to diagnose ischemic colitis, even though it is ordinarily not part of the evaluation of acute diarrhea.

6. In patients with acute diarrhea, the following test results may be increased:

- **Hemoglobin and hematocrit** caused by loss of salt and water with contraction of the extracellular compartment and hemoconcentration
- **Leukocytes** with inflammatory diarrhea
- **Urea and creatinine** associated with prerenal azotemia
- **Sodium and chloride** with dehydration related to water loss. (With diarrhea, **decreased electrolytes** may occur if water is replaced and not electrolytes.)
- **Albumin and calcium** (bound to albumin) with dehydration
- **Alkaline phosphatase** (intestinal type) in ulcerative lesions of the intestine such as with ulcerative colitis

BIBLIOGRAPHY

Chitkara YK, McCasland KA, Kenefic L: Development and implementation of cost-effective guidelines in the laboratory investigation of diarrhea in a community hospital. Arch Intern Med 156:1445, 1996.
Neither the fecal leukocyte test nor multiple cultures are particularly useful.
Community outbreaks of shigellosis—United States. MMWR 39:509, 1990.
Incidence of shigellosis is increasing. Physicians should suspect shigellosis in community outbreaks of diarrheal illness that involve young children especially.
Danna PL, Urban C, Bellin E, et al: Role of candida in pathogenesis of antibiotic-associated diarrhea in elderly inpatients. Lancet 337:511, 1991.
In antibiotic-associated diarrhea with negative assays for C. difficile, *consider* Candida.
Greenwald DA, Brandt LJ: Recognizing *E. coli* 0157:H7 infection. Hosp Pract 32:123, 1997.
Discusses the various clinical presentations and their diagnosis and management.
Guerrant RL, Bobak DA: Bacterial and protozoal gastroenteritis. N Engl J Med 325:327, 1991.
Excellent review with an algorithm for patient management.
Juckett G: Intestinal protozoa. Am Fam Physician 53:2507, 1996.
Reviews the diagnosis and treatment of giardiasis and other intestinal protozoa.
Lee LA, Taylor J, Carter GP, et al: *Yersinia enterocolitica* 0:3: An emerging cause of pediatric gastroenteritis in the United States. J Infect Dis 163:660, 1991.
Y. enterocolitica *infections are increasing. Eating raw chitterlings (pork intestines) can cause the disease.*
Massey BT, Suchman AL: Acute diarrhea. *In* Panzer RJ, Black ER, Griner PF (eds): Diagnostic Strategies for Common Medical Problems. Philadelphia, American College of Physicians, 1991, p 113.
Recommends strategies for the diagnosis of acute diarrhea.
Neal KR, Scott HM, Slack RCB, et al: Omeprazole as a risk factor for *Campylobacter gastroenteritis*: Case-control study. BMJ 312:414, 1996.
Results showed a powerful relation between omeprazole use and Campylobacter *infection.*
Novak RW: Identifying leukocytes in fecal specimens. Lab Med 27:433, 1996.
Discusses tests for fecal leukocytes and occult blood to diagnose inflammatory diarrhea.

Outbreaks of *Cyclospora cayetanesis* infection—United States, 1996. MMWR 45:549, 1996.
Update: Outbreaks of *Cyclospora cayetanensis* infection—United States and Canada, 1996. MMWR 45:611, 1996.
Cyclospora can be diagnosed by identifying oocytes in stool, but the procedures (wet-mount phase microscopy, acid-fast staining, and epifluorescence microscopy) are not routine in most clinical laboratories.

Senay H, MacPherson D: Parasitology: Diagnostic yield of stool examination. Can Med Assoc J 140:1329, 1989.
At least 90% of enteric parasites are detected in the first stool sample. Obtaining up to two additional samples is appropriate if the first sample is negative.

Shiau Y-F, Feldman GM, Resnick MA, et al: Stool electrolyte and osmolality measurements in the evaluation of diarrheal disorders. Ann Intern Med 102:773, 1985.
Stool osmotic gap in patients with osmotic diarrhea is substantially higher than previously reported—commonly greater than 160 mOsm/kg.

Siegel DL, Edelstein PH, Nachamkin I: Inappropriate testing for diarrheal diseases in the hospital. JAMA 263:979, 1990.
With rare exceptions, routine stool culture and examination for ova and parasites are not appropriate for inpatients who develop diarrhea more than 3 days after admission.

Smith PD, Quinn TC, Strober W, et al: Gastrointestinal infections in AIDS. Ann Intern Med 116:63, 1992.
National Institutes of Health conference on the gastrointestinal pathogens in human immunodeficiency virus–infected patients.

Topazian M, Binder HJ: Brief report: Factitious diarrhea detected by stool osmolality. N Engl J Med 330:1418, 1994.
It is appropriate to search for factitious disease to exclude laxative use or abuse when the cause of chronic diarrhea is elusive. Measuring the stool osmolality can identify those cases of factitious diarrhea caused by adding water to stool specimens.

Update: *Salmonella enteritidis* infections and Grade A shell eggs—United States, 1989. MMWR 38:877, 1990.
Salmonellosis is increasing. Consumers should be advised to avoid eating raw or undercooked eggs.

INTESTINAL MALABSORPTION

Recommendations for intestinal malabsorption are from the medical literature.

1. In patients with clinical findings of steatorrhea, obtain a 72-hour stool collection for quantitative fecal fat analysis. To perform a 72-hour fecal fat analysis, start the individual on an 80 to 100 g/day fat diet and continue this diet during the collection period. Microscopic examination of a random stool sample may be used as a qualitative screening test. Serum carotene and vitamin A concentrations may be helpful.

Intestinal malabsorption, or steatorrhea, is a type of chronic diarrhea that must be distinguished from other causes of chronic diarrhea such as irritable bowel and inflammatory bowel disease (Crohn's disease and ulcerative colitis). *Malabsorption* is a term used to indicate defective absorption of nutrients by the small intestine.

A key feature is the marked difficulty the patient describes in flushing stool down the toilet because of increased stool volume and fat content (when fecal fat is approximately 20 g/day, at least two flushings are required to clear the toilet water).

Although microscopic examination of a random stool sample may be used as a screening test, quantitative documentation of increased fecal fat over a 3-day period is the best method for diagnosing intestinal malabsorption. Serum carotene and vitamin A concentrations may be decreased, but these tests are not reliable enough to use as diagnostic tests.

For a 72-hour quantitative fecal fat study, the individual should be instructed as follows: avoid castor, mineral, or nut oils and the use of suppositories. After 3 to 5 days of the diet, begin a 72-hour stool collection for quantitative fecal fat analysis. Collect the specimens in glass or plastic containers (clean paint cans work well). Wax-coated containers should not be used. During the collection period the fecal specimens should be refrigerated, and contamination of feces with urine should be avoided. Any obvious foreign matter should be removed before proceeding with the analysis.

2. To perform a microscopic examination for increased fecal fat, obtain a random stool sample and proceed in the following manner.

When done properly, the Sudan stain has an 80 to 90% sensitivity for detecting clinically significant steatorrhea. If it is positive, it should be confirmed with a 72-hour quantitative fecal fat study.

> **a. Place a small amount of stool (size of one half of a split pea) on a glass slide. If stool is not liquid, add several drops of water or saline solution and make a homogenate by using an applicator stick as a pestle.**
> **b. Add 2 or 3 drops of glacial acetic acid and 4 or 5 drops of alcoholic solution of Sudan stain, mix, and add coverslip.**
> **c. Heat with alcohol lamp or burner to boiling to facilitate hydrolysis of soaps to free fatty acids and to facilitate staining.**
> **d. Examine under a microscope while the slide is warm, using low power to locate stained fat droplets and high power to examine droplets.**
>
> > **Normal:** A few small droplets should be noticeable and represent normal fat excretion; they reassure the examiner that the slide has been prepared properly.
> > **Abnormal:** A much larger number and size of reddish colored round droplets indicate steatorrhea.
>
> **e. Pitfalls: The skillful examiner gains experience by comparing stool from patients with steatorrhea with that from healthy individuals. False-positive results can occur in patients receiving castor oil, mineral oil, and oil-based suppositories. False-negative results can result from dilution of the stool with barium. Failure to examine the slide while warm can result in conversion of the stained melted fat droplets to unstained needle-like crystals. If this occurs, the slide should be reheated and re-examined.**

3. Evaluate the tests.

In addition to fecal fat and serum beta-carotene and vitamin A concentrations, the ^{14}C-triolein breath test also screens for steatorrhea.

REFERENCE RANGES

Test	Specimen	Conventional Units	International Units
Fat, fecal	Feces (72 hr)	<6 g/day	<6 g/day
Betacarotene	Serum	60–200 μg/dL	1.12–3.72 μmol/L
Vitamin A	Serum	30–65 μg/dL	1.05–2.27 μmol/L

Test	Normal Fat Excreters (<6 g/24 hr)	Abnormal Fat Excreters (>6 g/24 hr)
Number of microscopic fat droplets per high-lower field	2.5 ± 0.8	26.6 ⊥ 4

Compared with the quantitative fecal fat test, the ^{14}C-triolein breath test has a sensitivity of 85 to 100% and a specificity of 93 to 96%. False-positive results with the breath test can occur in patients with obesity, gastric retention, and chronic liver disease.

4. If fecal fat is increased, the patient has malabsorption. Perform a xylose absorption test to differentiate maldigestion (pancreatic disease) from malassimilation (intestinal disease). A small bowel series is appropriate.

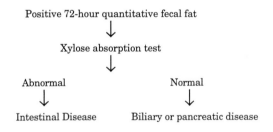

The degree of increase of fecal fat is not useful in differentiating between pancreatic and intestinal disease. To perform the xylose absorption test, the patient ingests 25 grams of xylose and collects urine for the next 5 hours. The patient must drink 500 mL of water during the first 3 hours of the collection period to ensure adequate urinary filtration of the xylose. A normal xylose absorption test shows 10 to 20 mg/dL/1.73 m^2 (0.67 to 1.33 mmol/L/1.73 m^2) of body surface area increase of the serum concentration within 60 to 75 minutes after ingestion of xylose or 4 grams or more of xylose in the urine within 5 hours. False-positive xylose absorption tests occasionally occur in the following situations:

a. Decreased renal function in patients more than 60 years of age or patients of any age with renal disease (false-positive urine test, but serum test is valid).
b. Patients with increased extracellular fluid, particularly with ascites or massive edema.
c. Patients with delayed gastric emptying (can be overcome by instilling the test dose through a tube directly into the proximal intestine).

In patients with decreased renal function, only serum values should be used in the interpretation of xylose absorption.

A small bowel series may be used to detect the presence of malabsorption and may help to differentiate intraluminal maldigestion from malassimilation.

5. If fecal fat is increased and the xylose absorption test result is abnormal, consider intestinal disease.

In this circumstance a small bowel biopsy may diagnose such intestinal diseases as celiac sprue, Whipple's disease, hypogammaglobulinemia (IgA), lymphangiectasia, and lymphoma. A recent study suggests that the xylose absorption test is not useful to diagnose adult celiac disease or to monitor the effect of dietary treatment. A normal biopsy result suggests bacterial overgrowth. The most common disorders of the small bowel that lead to malabsorption (other than bowel resection) are celiac disease, tropical sprue, and bacterial overgrowth.

6. If fecal fat is increased and the xylose absorption test result is normal, consider biliary or pancreatic disease. Evaluate the patient for diabetes mellitus and perform appropriate radiographic and endoscopic studies.

Pancreatic diabetes occurs in one third of all patients with chronic pancreatitis and in approximately twice this number of patients with calcific pancreatitis. Radiographic and sometimes endoscopic studies are necessary to evaluate the patient adequately. The secretin test is a sensitive test of impaired pancreatic function, but it requires intubation and is complex to perform. The bentiromide assay is a noninvasive test for detecting advanced chronic pancreatitis or cancer of the pancreatic head with ductal obstruction. When 500 mg of bentiromide is ingested, patients with normal amounts of trypsin excrete at least 50% of the bentiromide as para-aminobenzoic acid (PABA) in the urine within 6 hours. Patients with pancreatic disease excrete less. Determination of serum trypsin-like immunoreactivity level is another test to detect chronic pancreatitis or cancer of the pancreatic head causing ductal obstruction. It is decreased in patients with these disorders. Also, decreased values of other serum analytes such as pancreatic isoamylase, lipase, and pancreatic polypeptide may be used to detect chronic pancreatitis. Unfortunately, the noninvasive tests of pancreatic function usually are positive only in patients with severe pancreatic insufficiency but not with milder forms of the disease.

7. If the fecal fat excretion is normal, intestinal malabsorption is ruled out; however, fecal fat excretion may be normal in patients with specific absorption defects such as disaccharidase deficiency.

Disaccharidase deficiency, which can be caused by giardiasis, can be diagnosed by an assay of tissue from the small intestine by peroral biopsy. Usually this is not necessary because the clinical findings can be produced by ingestion of 50 grams of the sugar and because dramatic improvement results when milk products are eliminated from the diet. In the oral lactose tolerance test, a fasting healthy individual shows a 20 to 30 mg/dL (1.11 to 1.67 mmol/L) increase in serum glucose in the first 2 hours after ingesting 50 grams of lactose. A lactose breath test is also available.

8. In patients with intestinal malabsorption, the following test results may be increased:

- **Hematocrit** suggests dehydration.
- **Sodium and urea nitrogen** suggest dehydration.
- **Eosinophils** suggest parasites or eosinophilic gastroenteritis.
- **Platelets** suggest ulcerative colitis, Whipple's disease, and celiac sprue.
- **Prothrombin time** may be caused by impaired absorption of vitamin K.*
- Chronic diarrhea can cause metabolic acidosis or metabolic alkalosis with **decreased or increased bicarbonate,** with reciprocal changes in chloride.
- **Glucose** from pancreatic diabetes
- **Lactate dehydrogenase and aspartate aminotransferase** from **decreased vitamin B_{12}** absorption with megaloblastic anemia and intramedullary death of megaloblasts
- **Alkaline phosphatase** caused by vitamin D deficiency with **decreased calcium** absorption causing osteomalacia

9. In patients with intestinal malabsorption, the following test results may be decreased:

- **Hematocrit** suggests blood loss of anemia caused by malabsorption (e.g., iron, folate, vitamin B_{12}).*
- **Lymphocytes** may indicate excessive leakage of lymph into the gut.
- **Potassium and sodium** may be caused by diarrhea.
- **Calcium** related to hypoalbuminemia and/or vitamin D deficiency

---

*Because the absorption of carotene, vitamin K, vitamin D, folate, and iron is independent of pancreatic enzyme digestion, the presence of a low serum carotene value, hypocalcemia, hypoprothrombinemia, or anemia suggests a small bowel disorder rather than a pancreatic disorder.

with decreased calcium absorption; rare in pancreatic insuffi-
ciency.*
- **Glucose and urea nitrogen** may be caused by malabsorption of
  glucose and protein.
- **Magnesium;** rare in pancreatic insufficiency
- **Albumin**
- **Bilirubin** related to hypoalbuminemia
- **Cholesterol**
- **Iron**

BIBLIOGRAPHY

Aberger FL: Chronic diarrhea and malabsorption. *In* Conn RB, Borer WZ, Snyder JW
(eds): Current Diagnosis, 9th ed. Philadelphia, WB Saunders, 1997, p 596.
  *Discusses the diagnosis of chronic diarrhea, emphasizing clinical findings and patho-
  physiologic principles.*
Bardella MT, Fraquelli M, Quatrini M, et al: Prevalence of hypertransaminasemia in adult
celiac patients and effect of gluten-free diet. Hepatology 22:833, 1995.
  *Increased aspartate aminotransferase or alanine aminotransferase commonly occurs
  in a large proportion of untreated adult celiac patients and usually normalizes on a
  gluten-free diet.*
Gambino SR: Fecal fat. Lab Report Physicians 3:57, 1981.
  *Compares microscopic stool examination for fecal fat with quantification of fecal fat
  for 24 hours.*
Simko V: Fecal fat microscopy: Acceptable predictive value in screening for steatorrhea.
Am J Gastroenterol 75:204, 1981.
  Found that microscopic stool examination for fecal fat is useful.
Trier JS: Celiac sprue. N Engl J Med 325:1709, 1991.
  Reviews pathogenesis, diagnosis, and management of celiac sprue.
Trier JS: Intestinal malabsorption: Differentiation of cause. Hosp Pract 23:195, 1988.
  Discusses the differential diagnosis of intestinal malabsorption.

ASCITES

Recommendations for ascites are from the medical literature.

**1. In patients with ascites, perform paracentesis and measure serum
and ascites-fluid albumin to determine the serum-ascites albumin
gradient. Also, perform an ascites fluid cell count and differential,
total protein, Gram stain, and culture. Optional tests include amylase
(pancreatic ascites), triglyceride (chylous ascites), lactate dehydrogenase (LD) and glucose (secondary peritonitis), cytology (malignant
ascites), and acid-fast bacillus studies (tuberculous ascites).**

Clinical findings for ruling out ascites include a negative history
of ankle swelling or increased abdominal girth plus lack of bulging

---

*Because the absorption of carotene, vitamin K, vitamin D, folate, and iron is
independent of pancreatic enzyme digestion, the presence of a low serum carotene
value, hypocalcemia, hypoprothrombinemia, or anemia suggests a small bowel disorder
rather than a pancreatic disorder.

flanks, flank dullness, or shifting dullness. The presence of a positive fluid wave, shifting dullness, or peripheral edema supports the diagnosis of ascites. The term *pseudoascites* denotes the clinical impression of ascites when, in fact, free fluid is not present within the peritoneal cavity.

The gradient (difference) between the serum albumin and ascitic fluid albumin levels accurately reflects the oncotic pressure of ascitic fluid and has real pathophysiologic significance. It provides a new way to categorize patients with ascites.

2. Evaluate the tests.

The reference ranges and the sensitivity and specificity of the tests are important.

REFERENCE RANGES FOR GRADIENT OF SERUM ALBUMIN MINUS ASCITIC FLUID ALBUMIN

Ascites	Conventional Units	International Units
With portal hypertension	$\geq$1.1 g/dL	$\geq$11 g/L
Without portal hypertension	<1.1 g/dL	<11 g/L

SENSITIVITY AND SPECIFICITY OF TESTS FOR DIFFERENTIATING BETWEEN TRANSUDATIVE AND EXUDATIVE ASCITIC EFFUSIONS

Test	Exudate Criteria	Sensitivity (%)	Specificity (%)
1. Total protein	>3 g/dL (>30 g/L)	86	83
2. Ascitic fluid/serum protein ratio	>0.5	93	85
3. Ascitic fluid/serum LD ratio	>0.6	79	92
4. LD	>400 Sigma units (SU) (normal serum range, 200–500 SU)	57	100
5. WBC	>500/mm3	—	90
6. Serum albumin minus ascitic fluid albumin	<1.1 g/dL (<11 g/L)	87	78
2, 3, and 4 positive		57	100

LD, lactate dehydrogenase; WBC, white blood cells.
Source: Skendzel LP: A practical approach to the chemical and microscopic study of pleural and peritoneal fluids. Lab Medica V(1):19, 1988.

3. The gradient of serum albumin minus ascitic fluid albumin can be used to classify the types of ascites.

The following table gives the causes of high-gradient and low-gradient ascites. A gradient equal to or greater than 1.1 g/dL (≥11 g/L) indicates the pressure of portal hypertension.

Transudative Ascites High Gradient (≥1.1 g/dL [≥11 g/L])	Exudative Ascites Low Gradient (<1.1 g/dL [<11 g/L])
Cirrhosis	Peritoneal carcinomatosis
Alcoholic hepatitis	Peritoneal tuberculosis
Cardiac failure	Pancreatic ascites
Massive liver metastases	Biliary ascites
Fulminant hepatic failure	Nephrotic syndrome
Budd-Chiari syndrome	Serositis
Portal vein thrombosis	Bowel obstruction or infarction
Veno-occlusive disease	
Fatty liver of pregnancy	
Myxedema	
"Mixed" ascites*	

*Found in patients with portal hypertension and another cause of ascites formation, such as cirrhosis plus peritoneal tuberculosis. The portal pressure remains elevated in such patients, and the serum-ascites albumin gradient is high.

Source: Runyon BA: Care of patients with ascites. N Engl J Med 330:337–342, 1994. Copyright 1994, Massachusetts Medical Society. All rights reserved.

BIBLIOGRAPHY

Albillos A, Cuervas-Mons V, Millán I, et al: Ascitic fluid polymorphonuclear cell count and serum to ascites albumin gradient in the diagnosis of bacterial peritonitis. Gastroenterology 98:134, 1990.
Suggests a polymorphonuclear cell count greater than 0.5 × 10³ cells/L (>0.5 × 10⁹ cells/L) for diagnosing spontaneous bacterial peritonitis and a serum ascites albumin gradient less than 1.1 g/dL (<11 g/L) for diagnosing malignancy.
Antillon MR, Runyon BA: Effect of marked peripheral leukocytosis on the leukocyte count in ascites. Arch Intern Med 151:509, 1991.
Increased ascites fluid neutrophil count indicates a peritoneal inflammation regardless of the peripheral blood leukocyte count.
Candocia SA, Locker GY: Elevated serum CA 125 secondary to tuberculous peritonitis. Cancer 72:2016, 1993.
CA 125 has only limited specificity for any one disease, but its high sensitivity makes it useful in monitoring various intra-abdominal processes in which ascites and marked peritoneal inflammation are present.
Chen S-J, Wang S-S, Lu C-W, et al: Clinical value of tumor markers and serum-ascites albumin gradient in the diagnosis of malignancy-related ascites. J Gastroenterol Hepatol 9:396, 1994.
The serum-ascites albumin gradient provides the highest diagnostic accuracy in differentiating malignancy-related ascites at values of less than 1.1 g/dL (<11 g/L), but it is not a sufficiently sensitive indicator for this diagnosis.
D'Amelio LF, Rhodes M: A reassessment of the peritoneal lavage leukocyte count in blunt abdominal trauma. J Trauma 30:1291, 1990.
Grossly clear peritoneal lavage fluid after blunt abdominal trauma indicates that serious intraperitoneal injury is extremely unlikely.
DeLaurier GA, Ivey RK, Johnson RH: Peritoneal fluid lactic acid and diagnostic dilemmas in acute abdominal disease. Am J Surg 167:302, 1994.
Determining the difference between the lactic acid level in peritoneal fluid and plasma

may be useful in patients with possible intra-abdominal catastrophe, particularly when neurologic status hampers clinical evaluation, and in critically ill patients for whom negative exploration may be catastrophic.

Fiedorek SC, Casteel HB, Reddy G, et al: The etiology and clinical significance of pseudoascites. J Gen Intern Med 6:77, 1991.
Discusses the differential diagnosis of pseudoascites.

Gerbes AL, Hoermann R, Mann K, et al: Human chorionic gonadotropin-beta in the differentiation of malignancy-related and nonmalignant ascites. Digestion 57:113, 1996.
Elevated ascitic fluid β-hCG (>10 mIu/mL; >10 IU/L) was found in 18 of 27 patients with peritoneal carcinomatosis and 4 of 9 patients with miscellaneous malignancy-related ascites without peritoneal carcinomatosis.

Gupta R, Misra SP, Dwivedi M, et al: Diagnosing ascites: Value of ascitic fluid total protein, albumin, cholesterol, their ratios, serum-ascites albumin and cholesterol gradient. J Gastroenterol Hepatol 10:295, 1995.
The measurement of ascitic fluid cholesterol provides for a simple and cost-effective method to differentiate cirrhotic from malignant and tuberculous ascites at the cut-off of less than 55 mg/dL (<1.42 mmol/L) for cirrhosis, with sensitivity, specificity, positive and negative predictive values, and overall diagnostic accuracy of 94%.

Habeeb KS, Herrera JL: Management of ascites: Paracentesis as a guide. Postgrad Med 101:191, 1997.
Recommends mandatory and optimal studies for the diagnosis of ascites.

Ho H, Zuckerman MJ, Ho TK, et al: Prevalence of associated infections in community-acquired spontaneous bacterial peritonitis. Am J Gastroenterol 91:735, 1996.
In this study, spontaneous bacterial peritonitis was associated with a surprisingly high prevalence of bacteriuria.

Runyon BA: Care of patients with ascites. N Engl J Med 330:337, 1994.
Reviews the diagnosis and management of patients with ascites.

Sartori M, Andorno S, Gambaro M, et al: Diagnostic paracentesis: A two-step approach. Ital J Gastroenterol 28:81, 1996.
Culture and cytology would be carried out for those with albumin gradient of less than 1.1 g/dL (<11 g/L) or white blood cell count of 0.5 × 10³/μL (0.5 × 10⁹/L) or more, or both.

Shakil AO, Korula J, Kanel GC, et al: Diagnostic features of tuberculous peritonitis in the absence and presence of chronic liver disease: A case control study. Am J Med 100:179, 1996.
Ascitic fluid analysis is recommended as the initial study for patients with suspected tuberculous peritonitis, with high sensitivity provided by total protein greater than 2.5 g/dL (>25 g/L), LD greater than 90 U/L (>90 U/L), and serum–ascitic fluid albumin gradient less than 1.1 g/dL (<11 g/L).

Simmen HP, Battaglia H, Giovanoli P, et al: Biochemical analysis of peritoneal fluid in patients with and without bacterial infection. Eur J Surg 161:23, 1995.
Although total white cell count is a criterion for diagnosing infection in peritoneal fluid, biochemical analysis can be of diagnostic help in immunocompromised patients without the classic signs of infection and in patients with accumulation of peritoneal fluid of unknown cause.

Wang S-S, Lu C-W, Chao Y, et al: Malignancy-related ascites: A diagnostic pitfall of spontaneous bacterial peritonitis by ascitic fluid polymorphonuclear cell count. J Hepatol 20:79, 1994.
The diagnosis of peritoneal carcinomatosis or massive liver metastases was indicated by serum to ascites albumin difference of 1.1 g/dL (11 g/L) or less and ratio of ascitic fluid polymorphonuclear to total leukocyte count of up to 75%.

6

Liver Diseases

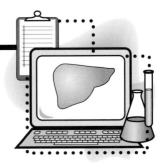

- Jaundice, Abnormal Liver Function Tests, and Liver Failure
- Acute Viral Hepatitis
- Fatty Liver and Alcoholic Hepatitis
- Acute Nonviral, Nonalcoholic Hepatitis
- Chronic Hepatitis
- Cirrhosis
- Cholestasis and Obstructive Liver Disease

JAUNDICE, ABNORMAL LIVER FUNCTION TESTS, AND LIVER FAILURE

Recommendations for jaundice, abnormal liver function tests, and liver failure are from the American Gastroenterological Association and the medical literature.

1. In patients with jaundice, use clinical findings, liver function tests, and other procedures to diagnose liver disease and to help decide whether it is due to hepatocellular disease, infiltrative disease, or extrahepatic obstruction.

The Patient Care Committee of the American Gastroenterological Association recommends the following work-up of patients with jaundice.

In patients with probable hepatocellular disease or infiltrative disease, categorize the disease as either probably benign or possibly malignant. Observe patients with probably benign disease and consider performing liver biopsy and ultrasonography. Study patients with possibly malignant tumors, using ultrasonography or computed tomography (CT).

In patients with possible extrahepatic obstruction, consider using ultrasonography or CT with or without biopsy. If the results are equivocal or negative, consider using endoscopic retrograde cholangiopancreatography (ERCP) or percutaneous transhepatic cholangiography.

In patients with probable extrahepatic obstruction, consider using ERCP or percutaneous transhepatic cholangiography.

2. Interpret liver function tests in the context of clinical findings.

The composition of liver function tests (often referred to as LFTs) varies from one health care facility to another. One useful combination of serum tests for acute liver disease follows:

- Aspartate aminotransferase (AST)
- Alanine aminotransferase (ALT)
- Alkaline phosphatase (ALP)
- Bilirubin, total and conjugated
- Gamma-glutamyl transferase (GGT)

For chronic or severe liver disease, consider using two additional tests: (1) prothrombin time (PT) and (2) albumin and globulin determinations.

Serum GGT is a sensitive test for liver disease of any variety. The sensitivity of routine liver function tests for excluding liver disease can be increased by measuring serum GGT; however, the increased sensitivity is accompanied by decreased specificity.

In addition to clinical findings and abnormal serum test results, increased urinary bilirubin and urobilinogen determinations may serve as clues to the presence of liver disease. Negative test results may not be reliable because these analytes are destroyed in urine that is not promptly analyzed.

Liver function tests are easier to understand and interpret if they are viewed according to the pathophysiologic derangements that cause the test results to become abnormal. Thus, five pathophysiologic questions are useful to ask.

a. Is liver disease present or not? Measure all liver functions.

If all test results are normal, significant liver disease is unlikely.

b. Is there liver cell injury, and what is its severity? Measure serum transaminase levels—AST and ALT.

Both AST and ALT are liver cell enzymes that are released into the blood after injury to the liver cell membranes, and significantly increased values are characteristic of acute hepatitis. Increased serum transaminase values correlate poorly with abnormal liver cell morphology by light microscopy. Remember that ALT usually is higher than AST in patients with viral hepatitis and that the reverse is true in patients with alcoholic hepatitis. ALT has been used as a surrogate test for viral hepatitis.

In patients with AST levels of 3000 U/L or higher, acute hypotension was the most common cause and severe toxic hepatic injury (e.g., acetaminophen poisoning) was second. Other causes included liver trauma, viral hepatitis, heart failure, metastatic liver cancer, and rhabdomyolysis. The major diseases associated with low serum AST and ALT levels were alcoholic liver disease, uremia, malnutrition, and diabetes.

c. Is there cholestasis? Measure serum ALP and total and conjugated bilirubin.

Serum ALP and bilirubin are good tests to detect cholestasis. Cholestasis occurs with either biliary obstruction or infiltrative disease, which may be due to either malignancy or inflammation, especially granulomatous inflammation. ALP usually is more sensitive than bilirubin. Serum GGT is another good test for cholestasis. GGT is particularly useful when the patient has an increased serum ALP value and it is unclear whether the increased ALP is originating in liver or bone. GGT is high in liver disease but not in bone disease. GGT values can be useful in diagnosing liver disease in adolescents and pregnant women when the ALP cannot be used to assess the liver because it is high as a result of bone growth and the placenta, respectively. Also, GGT is useful to screen for alcohol abuse and can be used along with AST and ALT to monitor a return to abstinence (see Alcohol Abuse in Chapter 1). Serum bile acid values are always increased in patients with cholestasis, but they are normal in patients with hereditary hyperbilirubinemias such as Gilbert's disease. Cholesterol is also increased in patients with cholestasis.

d. Are the metabolic functions of the liver compromised? Measure plasma PT and serum albumin.

Determination of decreased synthesis of proteins, especially serum albumin and the plasma coagulation factors (i.e., PT), is a sensitive test for metabolic derangement of the liver. A low serum albumin is a useful indicator of the severity of hepatocellular disease in patients with chronic liver disease. Because of the short half-life of Factor VII (about 4 hours), PT is affected more quickly than serum albumin in acute liver disease.

e. Is the disease process acute or chronic? Measure serum globulins.

Most acute liver diseases do not cause a significant increase of serum globulins, but chronic liver diseases commonly show an increase of gamma globulins (>3 g/dL [>30 g/L]). Measurement of gamma globulins by protein electrophoresis is useful to assess whether the liver disease is acute or chronic. For example, with chronic hepatitis and cirrhosis, hypergammaglobulinemia is a common finding.

3. If one or more test results are abnormal, liver disease may be present. Analyze the pattern of abnormalities for clues about the type of liver disease and consider drug-related liver disease.

The best method for diagnosing liver disease is microscopic examination of a liver biopsy. Serum tests provide indirect information about hepatic pathophysiology. Although there is a great deal of overlap, four major patterns of liver function test results can occur:

- Acute hepatitis pattern: significantly increased serum transaminase values with varying abnormalities of other liver function tests
- Cirrhosis pattern: decreased albumin, hypergammaglobulinemia,

often with beta-gamma bridging, and prolonged PT with varying abnormalities of other liver function tests
- Chronic hepatitis pattern: combinations of the first two patterns
- Obstructive liver disease pattern: increased ALP and bilirubin, with varying abnormalities of other liver function test results

Drug-related liver disease can take the form of acute hepatitis, chronic hepatitis, cirrhosis, and obstructive liver disease and therefore can show any of the above patterns. Drugs that can cause liver disease follow:

Hepatocellular Injury	Cholestatic Injury	Both Hepatocellular and Cholestatic Injury
Acetaminophen	Aminosalicylic acid	Allopurinol
Acetohexamide	Amitriptyline (Elavil,	(Zyloprim)
(Dymelor)	Endep)	Cimetidine
Bleomycin	Androgens	(Tagamet)
(Blenoxane)	Azathioprine (Imuran)	Dantrolene
Carbenicillin	Benzodiazepines	(Dantrium)
(Geocillin)	Busulfan (Myleran)	Dapsone
Chlorambucil	Captopril (Capoten)	Gold sodium
(Leukeran)	Carbamazepine (Tegretol)	thiomalate
Clindamycin	Carisoprodol (Soma)	(Myochrysine)
(Cleocin)	Chloramphenicol	Haloperidol
Colchicine	(Chloromycetin)	(Haldol)
Cyclophosphamide	Chlordiazepoxide	Hydralazine
(Cytoxan)	(Librium)	(Apresoline)
Emetine	Chlorpropamide	Inhalation
Ketoconazole	(Diabinese)	anesthetics
(Nizoral)	Chlorthalidone	Isoniazid (INH,
Methimazole	(Hygroton)	Laniazid,
(Tapazole)	Diazepam (Valium)	Nydrazid)
Methotrexate	Disopyramide (Norpace)	Nitrofurantoin
(Folex,	Disulfiram (Antabuse)	(Furadantin,
Rheumatrex)	Erythromycin estolate	Macrodantin)
Methyldopa	(Ilosone)	Nonsteroidal anti-
(Aldomet)	Erythromycin	inflammatory
Mithramcyin	ethylsuccinate (E.E.S.)	drugs
(Mithracin)	Estrogens	Phenytoin (Dilantin)
Monoamine	Ethambutol (Myambutol)	Rifampin (Rifadin,
oxidase	Flurazepam (Dalmane)	Rimactane)
inhibitors	Griseofulvin (Fulvicin,	Sulfonamides
Niacin (Nicobid)	Grifulvin, Grisactin)	Tetracyclines
Phenazopyridine	Mercaptopurine	Tricyclic
(Pyridium)	(Purinethol)	antidepressants
Propylthiouracil	Nifedipine (Adalat,	
Pyrazinamide	Procardia)	
Quinidine	Oral contraceptives	
(Quinaglute,	Oxacillin (Bactocill,	
Quinidex)	Prostaphlin)	

Hepatocellular Injury	Cholestatic Injury	Both Hepatocellular and Cholestatic Injury
Salicylates	Penicillamine (Cuprimine,	
Sulfasalazine	Depen)	
(Azulfidine)	Phenobarbital	
Tamoxifen	Phenothiazines	
(Nolvadex)	Progestins	
	Propoxyphene (Darvon)	
	Thiabendazole (Mintezol)	
	Thiazides	
	Tolazamide (Tolinase)	
	Tolbutamide (Orinase)	
	Trimethoprim	
	Troleandomycin (Tao)	
	Verapamil (Calan, Isoptin)	
	Warfarin (Coumadin,	
	Panwarfin)	

Source: McKnight JT, Jones JE: Jaundice. Am Fam Physician 45:1139–1148, 1992. Republished with permission from the American Academy of Family Physicians.

Remember that tissues other than the liver can be the source for increased serum transaminase and ALP values. If the serum ALP is elevated and you are uncertain about the cause, request ALP fractionation (isoenzymes). High transaminase values can originate in heart, pancreas, and skeletal muscle, and high ALP values can originate in bone, intestines, and placenta.

4. If the liver function test results are all normal, the liver is probably normal—the level of confidence is higher if serum GGT values are also normal.

Normal results for liver function tests are good evidence against liver disease, and if serum GGT values are also normal, the probability of liver disease is very low indeed, perhaps only 1 to 2%. Still, a liver disorder occasionally is present with normal liver function test results—a common example is fatty liver.

5. In patients with persistently increased liver enzyme values who are otherwise well (discovered during blood donation or routine health checks), perform a thorough evaluation and consider a liver biopsy.

In studies of this clinical situation, the most common abnormality was fatty liver. Other disorders in decreasing order of frequency included non-cirrhotic alcoholic liver disease; chronic active (viral) hepatitis; chronic persistent hepatitis; cirrhosis; hemochromatosis; granulomatous liver disease; and autoimmune liver disease. Drug-related hepatitis was rare. Several hematologic, biochemical, and serologic tests may further aid the diagnosis: mean red cell volume; serum iron, transferrin, ferritin, ceruloplasmin, and α_1-antitrypsin levels; smooth muscle, antimitochondrial, and antinuclear antibodies; immunoglobulins; and markers for hepatitis A, B, and C. Ultrasonography should be done to exclude infiltrative liver disease and extrahepatic abnormalities. Ultrasound and isotope scans, CT, or magnetic resonance imaging techniques are of little value in differentiating the major forms of parenchymal liver disease. Liver biopsy is essential for the evaluation of a patient with persistently (>6 months) increased enzymes. Asymptomatic individuals with three- to eight-fold increased transaminase values frequently have chronic active hepatitis and often cirrhosis.

6. If you intend to perform a percutaneous liver biopsy (mortality rate, 0.01%), remember to exclude a bleeding disorder and other contraindications.

A negative history of unusual bleeding after surgery, previous biopsies, or dental work plus normal or only mildly abnormal tests for coagulation excludes a significant bleeding disorder. Minimal acceptable guidelines include a PT no more than 4 seconds greater than midrange normal, an activated partial thromboplastin time no more than 9 seconds greater than midrange normal, a platelet count greater than $50 \times 10^3/\mu L$ ($50 \times 10^9/L$), and a normal bleeding time. Aspirin and other non-steroidal anti-inflammatory agents can prolong the bleeding time and, ideally, should be omitted for approximately 1 to 2 weeks before the test. Correction of any coagulation abnormality should be undertaken before biopsy. Other relative contraindications to biopsy include lack of patient cooperation, ascites, and right lower lobe pneumonia.

7. In patients with liver disease with clinical findings of hepatic failure (hepatorenal syndrome, hepatic encephalopathy), request determinations of serum urea nitrogen, creatinine, and urine sodium together with arterial blood ammonia.

Ordinary liver function tests may not be useful to monitor hepatic failure (e.g., the serum transaminase level may be low in a patient with massive hepatic necrosis because the hepatic cell transaminase content has been exhausted). Rising serum urea nitrogen and creatinine values and falling urinary volume and sodium excretion characterize the renal failure of the hepatorenal syndrome as intrarenal shunting deprives the renal cortex of blood. Because these findings do not differentiate the hepatorenal syndrome from prerenal azotemia, patients should be initially treated as though they had prerenal azotemia. Although blood ammonia, short-chain fatty acids, false neurotransmitters, and amino acids have been implicated as the cause of hepatic encephalopathy, determination of arterial blood ammonia is the only widely available test to diagnose this syndrome.

Fulminant hepatic failure may be caused by viruses, drugs and toxins, vascular disorders, and miscellaneous causes as follows:

Viruses
   Hepatitis B (especially with hepatitis D virus)
   Occasionally hepatitis A through hepatitis E
   Probably not hepatitis C
Drugs and toxins
   Acetaminophen (common cause)
   Carbon tetrachloride
   Certain mushrooms
   Medicinal herbs
   Hypersensitivity reactions (e.g., halothane,
      isoniazid, phenytoin)
Vascular disorders
   Cardiogenic shock
   Occlusion of vessels
Miscellaneous
   Fatty liver of pregnancy
   Heatstroke
   Wilson's disease
   Reye's syndrome

BIBLIOGRAPHY

Brooks GS, Zimbler AG, Bodenheimer HC Jr, et al: Patterns of liver test abnormalities in patients with surgical sepsis. Am Surg 57:656, 1991.
   Surgical sepsis may be associated with two patterns of test abnormalities: a rapid rise in bilirubin and a normal alkaline phosphatase in severe sepsis; and a rapid rise in alkaline phosphatase with a slow rise in bilirubin in moderate sepsis.
Cassidy WM, Reynolds TB: Serum lactic dehydrogenase in the differential diagnosis of acute hepatocellular injury. J Clin Gastroenterol 19:118, 1994.
   Within 24 hours of admission, an aminotransferase:lactic dehydrogenase ratio of 1.5 or more favors viral hepatitis over ischemic and acetaminophen hepatitis.
Frank BB, Members of the Patient Care Committee of the American Gastroenterological Association: Clinical evaluation of jaundice: A guideline of the Patient Care Committee of the American Gastroenterological Association. JAMA 262:3031, 1989.
   Recommendations for the work-up of patients with jaundice.
Garcia-Tsao G, Boyer JL: Outpatient liver biopsy: How safe is it? Ann Intern Med 118:150, 1993.
   Discusses pros and cons of outpatient liver biopsy.
Ginsberg AL: Liver enzyme abnormalities: How to interpret the diagnostic implications. Consultant 36:575, 1996.
   Case histories of patients with similar liver enzyme abnormalities which illustrate the importance of clinical findings in the interpretation of test results.
Hay JE, Czaja AJ, Rakela J, et al: The nature of unexplained chronic aminotransferase elevations of a mild to moderate degree in asymptomatic patients. Hepatology 9:193, 1989.
   Asymptomatic patients with mildly to moderately increased aminotransferase values frequently have chronic active hepatitis and often cirrhosis.

Jacobs J, Von Behren J, Kreutzer R: Serious mushroom poisonings in California requiring hospital admission, 1990 through 1994. West J Med 165:283, 1996.
If amatoxin poisoning is suspected, institute prompt and aggressive treatment and consider early referral to a liver transplant unit.

Janes CH, Lindor KD: Outcome of patients hospitalized for complications after outpatient liver biopsy. Ann Intern Med 118:96, 1993.
In selected patients, outpatient liver biopsy is safe. Any serious complications are likely to be evident in several hours.

Janssen HLA, Brouwer JT, Nevens F, et al: Fatal hepatic decompensation associated with interferon alfa. BMJ 306:107, 1993.
Fatal liver decompensation is a rare complication of interferon-alpha therapy.

Johnson RD, O'Connor ML, Kerr RM: Extreme serum elevations of aspartate aminotransferase. Am J Gastroenterol 90:1244, 1995.
Acute hypotension and severe toxic hepatic injury were the most common causes of very high serum AST levels.

Kamath PS: Concise review for primary-care physicians: Clinical approach to the patient with abnormal liver test results. Mayo Clin Proc 71:1089, 1996.
Discusses the interpretation of liver function tests.

Kassirer JP, Kopelman RI: Case 13—A picture is worth a thousand words. *In* Learning Clinical Reasoning. Baltimore, Williams & Wilkins, 1991, p 97.
Discusses clinical reasoning in a patient with alcoholic liver disease and the hepatorenal syndrome.

Koff RS: Herbal hepatotoxicity: Revisiting a dangerous alternative. JAMA 273:502, 1995. Gordon DW, Rosenthal G, Hart J, et al: Chaparral ingestion: The broadening spectrum of liver injury caused by herbal medications. JAMA 273:489, 1995.
Consider herbal hepatotoxicity in patients with hepatic injury of unknown origin.

Kothur R, Marsh F Jr, Posner G: Liver function tests in nonparenteral cocaine users. Arch Intern Med 151:1126, 1991.
Minimally increased liver enzymes are common in non-parenteral cocaine users without evidence of severe hepatotoxicity.

Kumar S, Rex DK: Failure of physicians to recognize acetaminophen hepatotoxicity in chronic alcoholics. Arch Intern Med 151:1189, 1991.
High index of suspicion is necessary to detect acetaminophen-related hepatitis in alcoholics.

Kundrotas LW, Clement DJ: Serum alanine aminotransferase elevation in asymptomatic U.S. Air Force basic trainee blood donors. Digest Dis Sci 38:2145, 1993.
Extensive investigation, including serologic investigation for viral disease, should be limited in asymptomatic healthy subjects to those with two ALT elevations separated by an undefined period of time.

Lee WM: Acute liver failure. N Engl J Med 329:1862, 1993.
Reviews acute liver failure and its causes—viruses, drugs, toxins, vascular events, and miscellaneous factors.

Lum G: Low activities of aspartate and alanine aminotransferase. Lab Med 26:273, 1995.
Alcoholic liver disease, uremia, malnutrition, and diabetes were the main diseases associated with low levels of AST and ALT.

Mas A, Rodés J: Fulminant hepatic failure. Lancet 349:1081, 1997.
Discusses the diagnosis and management of liver failure.

Mason A, Sallie R: What causes fulminant hepatic failure of unknown etiology? Am J Clin Pathol 104:491, 1995.
Over 40% of patients with fulminant hepatic failure have no known cause.

McKnight JT, Jones JE: Jaundice. Am Fam Physicians 45:1139, 1992.
Good discussion of the differential diagnosis and management of jaundice.

McVay PA, Toy P: Lack of increased bleeding after liver biopsy in patients with mild hemostatic abnormalities. Am J Clin Pathol 94:747, 1990.
Mildly abnormal platelet count, PT, and activated partial thromboplastin time do not increase the risk of bleeding after liver biopsy.

Neuschwander-Tetri BA: Common blood tests for liver disease: Which ones are most useful? Postgrad Med 98:49, 1995.
A good discussion of serum tests and liver biopsy in the differential diagnosis of liver disease.

O'Grady JG: Paracetamol hepatotoxicity: How to prevent. J R Soc Med 90:368, 1997.
Acetaminophen (paracetamol) is the main cause of acute liver failure in the United Kingdom.

Riordan SM, Williams R: Treatment of hepatic encephalopathy. N Engl J Med 337:473, 1997.
Reviews the pathophysiology, diagnosis, and management of hepatic encephalopathy.

Rockey DC: Utility of "liver function tests" in alcoholic patients. West J Med 156:319, 1992.
Good discussion of the laboratory test abnormalities that may be encountered in alcoholic patients.

Sherman KE: Alanine aminotransferase in clinical practice. Arch Intern Med 151:260, 1991.
Reviews the biochemistry and clinical relevance of alanine aminotransferase in patient care.

Singer AJ, Carracio TR, Mofenson HC: The temporal profile of increased transaminase levels in patients with acetaminophen-induced liver dysfunction. Ann Emerg Med 26:49, 1995.
When encountering an overdose patient with an early rise in the serum AST, clinicians should not rule out the possibility of acetaminophen overdose within the previous 24 hours.

Speicher CE, Widish JR, Gaudot FJ, et al: An evaluation of the overestimation of serum albumin by bromcresol green. Am J Clin Pathol 69:347, 1978.
Bromcresol green reacts with alpha and beta globulins. This can cause overestimation of albumin when these globulins are high (e.g., with nephrotic syndrome).

Theal RM, Scott K: Evaluating asymptomatic patients with abnormal liver function test results. Am Fam Physician 53:2111, 1996.
Good discussion of the differential diagnosis of asymptomatic patients with persistently abnormal liver function test results.

Van Ness MN, Diehl AM: Is liver biopsy useful in the evaluation of patients with chronically elevated liver enzymes? Ann Intern Med 111:473, 1989.
The higher the liver enzyme values (AST, ALT, GGT), the more accurate is the noninvasive diagnosis, but liver biopsy ensures maximal diagnostic accuracy.

What's up with the enzymes? [editorial] Lancet 335:140, 1990.
Outlines the most common diagnoses in patients with increased liver enzymes and encourages performance of a liver biopsy.

Yasuda K, Okuka K, Endo N, et al: Hypoaminotransferasemia in patients undergoing long-term hemodialysis: Clinical and biochemical appraisal. Gastroenterology 109:1295, 1995.
Discusses low transaminase values in patients undergoing hemodialysis.

Yoshida EM, Steinbrecher UP: Interpreting liver function tests: A practical guide for clinical use. Consultant 37:569, 1997.
Groups liver function tests into hepatocellular enzymes, markers of cholestasis, tests of liver excretion, and tests of liver synthetic function.

ACUTE VIRAL HEPATITIS

Recommendations for acute hepatitis are from the medical literature.

1. For patients at risk for acute hepatitis or with clinical findings and liver function test results of acute viral hepatitis, request serologic tests for hepatitis A, B, and C; namely, anti-hepatitis A IgM antibody; hepatitis B surface antigen, anti-hepatitis B core IgM antibody; and anti-hepatitis C antibody. In patients with hepatitis B, request anti-hepatitis D antibody to detect hepatitis D. Other causes of viral hepatitis, for which there are no readily available tests, are hepatitis E, hepatitis G, and other unknown hepatitis viruses.

Clinical findings of viral hepatitis include malaise, nausea, fatigue, jaundice, and a tender enlarged liver. Vaccination is now available for hepatitis A and B. In the United States, about 3% of acute hepatitis cases and 17% of chronic hepatitis cases are caused by viruses other than A through E. About 10% of patients with transfusion-associated hepatitis have negative test results.

The following clues about different varieties of viral hepatitis are helpful. Hepatitis A has fecal and oral transmission, a 15- to 60-day incubation period, and up to a 75% prevalence in some groups in the United States; whereas hepatitis B has percutaneous or venereal transmission, a 35- to 150-day incubation period, and up to a 5 to 15% prevalence in some groups in the United States. The transmission of hepatitis C and G resembles that of hepatitis B, whereas the transmission of hepatitis E resembles that of hepatitis A. Hepatitis C causes many cases of post-transfusion hepatitis. Hepatitis E should be considered in individuals who have travelled to Africa, central Asia, the Far East, the Indian subcontinent, and the Middle East. Recently, hepatitis G was identified; it may cause 20% of post-transfusion hepatitis and 15% of community-acquired hepatitis not caused by hepatitis A through E.

The clinical features of acute hepatitis C infection are milder than those of acute hepatitis B infection: lower peak transaminase and bilirubin levels, jaundice in only 20% of patients. Fulminant hepatitis due to hepatitis C is rare in Western countries.

The serum aspartate aminotransferase (AST) and alanine aminotransferase (ALT) values are usually increased from 600 to 5000 U/L or more, but may be less than 500 U/L in mild illness. Asymptomatic blood donors with positive serologic tests for hepatitis B or C may have normal transaminase values. Usually the ALT exceeds the AST. The magnitude of the transaminase increase is not well correlated with the severity of liver damage. Serum bilirubin is commonly increased from 5 to 20 mg/dL (85 to 342 μmol/L); values greater than 30 mg/dL (>513 μmol/L) suggest severe disease or hemolysis. Alkaline phosphatase is slightly increased but may be markedly increased in the presence of severe cholestasis. Serum gamma globulins may be slightly increased: concentrations greater than 3 g/dL (>30 g/L) suggest chronic disease. Decreased serum albumin and a prolonged plasma prothrombin time (PT) reflect impairment of liver protein synthesis and parallel the severity of the disease. A PT greater than 20 seconds suggests the development of acute hepatic insufficiency.

2. If anti-hepatitis A IgM antibody is present, diagnose hepatitis A. If hepatitis B surface antigen and/or anti-hepatitis B core IgM antibody is present, diagnose acute hepatitis B, and if anti-hepatitis C antibody is present, diagnose hepatitis C (confirm diagnosis of hepatitis C with recombinant immunoblot assay or polymerase chain reaction).

Diagnosis of hepatitis A is confirmed by the presence of anti-hepatitis A IgM antibody. After several months, the IgM antibody titer decreases and anti-hepatitis A IgG antibody rises and persists indefinitely.

The serologic profile for acute hepatitis B follows:

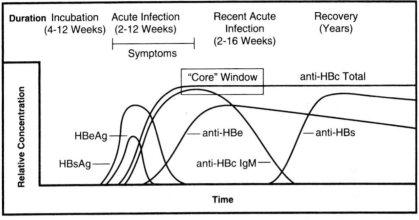

Serodiagnostic assessment of acute viral hepatitis. HBsAg = hepatitis B surface antigen; HBeAg = hepatitis B e antigen; anti-HBe = antibody to hepatitis B e antigen; anti-HBc IgM = antibody (IgM) to core antigen; anti-HBc total = total antibody (IgG and IgM) to core antigen; anti-HBs = antibody to hepatitis B surface antigen. Source: Abbott Diagnostics Educational Services, Abbott Laboratories, Abbott Park, IL, January, 1990.

As one can see, the presence of hepatitis B surface antigen and/or anti-hepatitis B core IgM antibody confirms the diagnosis of hepatitis B. Hepatitis B vaccination causes a positive test for hepatitis B surface antibody but does not cause a positive test for hepatitis B surface antigen or hepatitis B core antibody. Only patients with hepatitis B can acquire hepatitis D. Hepatitis D is diagnosed by the presence of a positive serologic test for anti-hepatitis D antibody.

Anti-hepatitis C is not completely sensitive or specific for hepatitis C; that is, both false positives and false negatives may occur. Use the latest generation enzyme immunoassay for the greatest sensitivity and specificity, and confirm positive test results with the latest generation recombinant immunoblot assay and/or a qualitative polymerase chain reaction test for hepatitis C virus RNA.

3. If diagnostic test results for hepatitis A, hepatitis B, and hepatitis C are negative, consider other causes of an acute viral hepatitis–like syndrome.

Hepatitis E
Hepatitis E may occur sporadically but is probably rare in the United States. Because no serologic tests for hepatitis E are readily available,

the diagnosis relies on clinical findings and surrogate test results such as increased ALT. Like hepatitis A, hepatitis E does not progress to chronic disease.

Hepatitis G
Approximately 3% of cases of acute hepatitis are not explained by hepatitis A through E. Other hepatitis viruses, such as G, are under active investigation.

Epstein-Barr Hepatitis
Consider Epstein-Barr hepatitis (often part of the infectious mononucleosis syndrome) with these findings: nausea and vomiting, jaundice, and increased serum transaminase values. The presence of heterophil antibodies (positive Monospot test) or a rise in titer of specific antibodies to Epstein-Barr virus confirms the diagnosis, that is, viral capsid antigen antibody IgM (VCA-IgM).

Cytomegalovirus Hepatitis
Consider cytomegalovirus hepatitis (sometimes as part of an infectious mononucleosis syndrome without adenopathy or tonsillopharyngeal involvement) in patients with clinical and laboratory findings of mild acute hepatitis. Infection can be demonstrated by culture or serology.

4. After diagnosing acute viral hepatitis, begin therapy and monitor the patient's progress, using chemical and serologic (immunologic) test results.

For acute hepatitis A and E there is no carrier state or possibility of chronic hepatitis, so serologic monitoring of these patients is not necessary.

For acute hepatitis B, serologic monitoring is mandatory. Anti-hepatitis B core antibody appears before hepatitis B surface antibody and persists throughout life. Anti-hepatitis B core IgG antibody is the best single marker of exposure to hepatitis B virus. To determine when the infection has resolved, test for hepatitis B surface antibody monthly. If by 6 months after the acute episode the patient is no longer hepatitis B surface antigen positive and is anti-hepatitis B surface IgG antibody positive, the patient has eliminated the virus, and a full and complete recovery has occurred. Such a patient has no chronic sequelae and can no longer infect others. After 1 to 23 months anti-hepatitis B surface antibody may be lost, but anti-hepatitis B core IgG antibody always persists. In patients who do not develop anti-hepatitis B surface IgG antibody, the finding of two positive hepatitis B surface antigen results 6 months or more apart indicates chronic hepatitis.

For acute hepatitis C, continue monitoring because the majority of these patients are at risk for chronic hepatitis.

5. In patients with acute viral hepatitis, in addition to abnormal liver function tests, the following blood test results may be increased:

- **Platelets** in fulminant disease
- **Lactate dehydrogenase** from hepatocellular damage
- **Lymphocytes** and atypical lymphocytes; mild leukocytosis may occur.
- **Uric acid** related to hepatocellular damage
- **Amylase** with concurrent pancreatitis

6. In patients with acute viral hepatitis, in addition to abnormal liver function tests, the following blood test results may be decreased:

- **Hemoglobin and hematocrit,** mild and transient; rarely, aplastic anemia
- **Glucose,** often mild and insignificant; profound hypoglycemia can occur in fulminant hepatitis.
- **Cholesterol** from decreased liver synthesis; degree parallels severity of hepatitis.

BIBLIOGRAPHY

Altman LK: Newly found viruses may cause hepatitis. The New York Times, April 11, 1995, p B6.
In the United States, 3% of acute hepatitis and 17% of chronic hepatitis are not caused by hepatitis A through E.

Becherer PR: Viral hepatitis: What have we learned about risk factors and transmission? Postgrad Med 98:65, 1995.
Reviews the current information on viral hepatitis A, B, C, D, and E.

Brodell RT, Helms SE, Devine M: Office dermatologic testing: The Tzanck preparation. Am Fam Physician 44:857, 1991.
Describes how to do a Tzanck preparation.

Bryan JP: Viral hepatitis: Update on preventing hepatitis A. Consultant 35:1027, 1995.
Hepatitis A virus is the most common cause of viral hepatitis in the United States.

Bryan JP: Viral hepatitis: Update on hepatitis D and E. Consultant 35:1846, 1995.
Hepatitis D usually occurs in injectable drug users and to a lesser extent in persons who receive multiple blood products. Hepatitis E is transmitted enterically.

de Franchis R, Meucci G, Vecchi M, et al: The natural history of asymptomatic hepatitis B surface antigen carriers. Ann Intern Med 118:191, 1993.
Blood donors who were positive for hepatitis B surface antigen had normal alkaline phosphatase and transaminase levels.

Dubois F, Francois M, Mariotte N, et al: Serum alanine aminotransferase measurement as a guide to selective testing for hepatitis C during medical check-up. J Hepatol 21:837, 1994.
Serum alanine aminotransferase is an effective screening test for hepatitis C.

Eng TR, Borges ML, Harlin VK, et al: Screening for hepatitis B during pregnancy: Awareness of current recommendations among Washington hospitals. West J Med 155:613, 1991.
The Centers for Disease Control recommend prenatal hepatitis B surface antigen screening of all women or, for women who do not have a history of prenatal care, screening at the time of delivery.

Harpaz R, von Seidlein L, Averhoff FM, et al: Transmission of hepatitis B virus to multiple patients from a surgeon without evidence of inadequate infection control. N Engl J Med 334:549, 1996.
Emphasizes need to develop safer surgical techniques and equipment.

Healey CJ, Chapman RWG, Fleming KA: Liver histology in hepatitis C infection: A comparison between patients with persistently normal or abnormal transaminases. Gut 37:374, 1995.

Rossini A, Gazzola GB, Ravaggi A, et al: Long-term follow-up of and infectivity in blood donors with hepatitis C antibodies and persistently normal alanine amino-transferase levels. Transfusion 35:108, 1995.

Patients with chronic hepatitis C may have persistently normal serum ALT levels.

Hepatitis E among U.S. travelers: 1989–1992. MMWR 42:1, 1993.

Transmission of hepatitis E has not been confirmed in the United States.

Kao J-H, Hwang Y-T, Chen P-J, et al: Transmission of hepatitis C virus between spouses: The important role of exposure duration. Am J Gastroenterol 91:2087, 1996.

Transmission between spouses is not rare. Other routes may be involved.

Katkov WN Ault MJ, Dubin SB: Absence of hepatitis B surface antigenemia after vaccina-tion. Arch Pathol Lab Med 113:1290, 1989.

Positive hepatitis B surface antigen should not be attributed to vaccination.

Kelen GD, Green GB, Purcell RH, et al: Hepatitis B and hepatitis C in emergency depart-ment patients. N Engl J Med 326:1399, 1992.

There is a high incidence of markers for hepatitis B, hepatitis C, and human immunode-ficiency virus in the sera of emergency department patients.

Linnen J, Wages J Jr, Zhang-Keck Z-Y, et al: Molecular cloning and disease association of hepatitis G virus: A transfusion-transmissible agent. Science 271:505, 1996.

Hepatitis G virus is distantly related to the hepatitis C virus.

Marsano LS, Greenberg RN, Kirkpatrick BB, et al: Comparison of a rapid hepatitis B immunization schedule to the standard schedule for adults. Am J Gastroenterol 91:111, 1996.

Hepatitis G may cause 20% of post-transfusion hepatitis and 15% of community-acquired hepatitis not caused by hepatitis A through E.

Nalpas B, Romeo R, Pol S, et al: Serum hepatitis C virus (HCV) RNA: A reliable tool for evaluating HCV-related liver disease in anti-HCV–positive blood donors with persistently normal alanine aminotransferase values. Transfusion 35:750, 1995.

Discusses the evaluation of "healthy" anti-hepatitis C–positive blood donors with persis-tently normal transaminase values.

Olynyk JK, Bacon BR: Hepatitis C: Recent advances in understanding and management. Postgrad Med 98:79, 1995.

Good discussion of the diagnosis and treatment of patients with hepatitis C.

Osmond DH, Padian NS, Sheppard HW, et al: Risk factors for hepatitis C virus seropositiv-ity in heterosexual couples. JAMA 269:361, 1993.

Weinstock HS, Bolan G, Reingold AL, et al: Hepatitis C virus infection among patients attending a clinic for sexually transmitted diseases. JAMA 269:392, 1993.

Sexually transmitted hepatitis C is uncommon.

Scharschmidt BF: Hepatitis E: A virus in waiting. Lancet 346:519, 1995.

Hepatitis E is a serious global health menace.

Schifman RB, Rivers SL, Samplinger RE, et al: Significance of isolated hepatitis B core antibody in blood donors. Arch Intern Med 153:2261, 1993.

Presence of an isolated anti-hepatitis B in blood donors may be a false positive.

Schwartz JG, Stellato KM: A lesson in the ABCs of hepatitis. Med Lab Observer 29:30, 1997.

A clear discussion of the use of serologic tests to diagnose hepatitis A, B, and C.

Scotiniotis I, Brass CA, Malet PF: Hepatitis C: Diagnosis and treatment. J Gen Intern Med 10:273, 1995.

Reviews the clinical features, laboratory diagnosis, and treatment of patients with hepatitis C.

Serfaty L, Nousbaum JB, Elghouzzi MH, et al: Prevalence, severity, and risk factors of liver disease in blood donors positive in a second-generation anti-hepatitis C virus screening test. Hepatology 21:725, 1995.

Assesses the clinical significance of antibody to hepatitis C virus in asymptomatic blood donors.

Tedeschi V, Seeff LB: Diagnostic tests for hepatitis C: Where are we now? Ann Intern Med 123:383, 1995.

Outlines the latest information on hepatitis C testing.

Werzberger A, Mensch B, Kuter B, et al: A controlled trial of a formalin-inactivated hepatitis A vaccine in healthy children. N Engl J Med 327:453, 1992.

Hepatitis A vaccine is highly effective.
Zuckerman AJ: Alphabet of hepatitis virus. Lancet 347:558, 1996.
  The list of hepatitis viruses continues to grow; namely hepatitis A, B, C, D, E, GGV, and HGV.

FATTY LIVER AND ALCOHOLIC HEPATITIS

Recommendations for fatty liver and alcoholic hepatitis are from the medical literature.

1. In patients with clinical findings and liver function test results of fatty liver or alcoholic hepatitis, to accurately diagnose the lesion, consider a needle biopsy of the liver. To screen for alcoholism, see alcohol abuse in Chapter 1.

Clinical findings of fatty liver and alcoholic hepatitis may include hepatomegaly, fever, anorexia, and jaundice.

In fatty liver, the aspartate aminotransferase (AST) value may be normal to modestly increased, up to 400 U/L (ratio of AST to alanine aminotransferase [ALT] is often ≥2:1). Increased serum bilirubin values to 5 mg/dL (85 μmol/L) may occur with mildly increased ALP. Occasionally, intense cholestasis develops. Serum albumin and globulin values are abnormal in approximately 25% of patients, and serum gamma glutamyltransferase (GGT) is usually increased. Mild anemia and leukocytosis may occur. An increased GGT level by itself may not warrant a liver biopsy. Occasionally, severe fatty liver may be the only significant finding in sudden unexpected death.

Patients with alcoholic hepatitis have fever, and leukocytosis may exceed 30 to 40 × 10^3 cells/μL (30 to 40 × 10^9 cells/L). The AST may be increased to 600 U/L, and AST is usually higher than ALT. Frequently, the AST is more than twice as high as ALT. A high AST:ALT ratio may also occur in nonhepatic diseases such as acute myocardial infarction, skeletal muscle necrosis, hemolysis, renal necrosis, and cerebral necrosis. Serum bilirubin and ALP levels may increase moderately, and a small percentage of patients develops a cholestatic picture, with high bilirubin (up to 30 mg/dL [513 μmol/L]) and high ALP levels as the predominant abnormalities. Prolongation of the prothrombin time (PT), hypoalbuminemia, and hyperglobulinemia may be present.

Very high (>10 times normal) AST levels are quite unusual in alcoholic liver disease, and their presence should make one think of other causes of liver injury, particularly those in which hepatocellular injury is prominent.

2. Evaluate the tests.

The best method for the diagnosis of fatty liver and alcoholic hepatitis is microscopic examination of a liver biopsy sample.

3. A liver biopsy finding of fatty changes of the large droplet variety is consistent with the fatty liver of alcohol abuse.

Large-droplet fatty change is not specific for alcohol abuse but may be seen in other conditions such as obesity, protein-calorie malnutrition (e.g., kwashiorkor, jejunoileal bypass), hyperlipidemia, and/or diabetes mellitus. The lesion may also be caused by corticosteroids, methotrexate, and perhexilene. Alcoholic fatty liver is reversible if the patient stops drinking.

4. A liver biopsy finding of hepatocellular necrosis with infiltration by polymorphonuclear leukocytes is consistent with alcoholic hepatitis.

The essential feature of alcoholic hepatitis is hepatocellular necrosis and infiltration by polymorphonuclear leukocytes. Alcoholic hyalin may be present or absent. Fibrosis may be present within the lobule and around the central vein, where it can cause obstruction of blood flow and portal hypertension. Patients with alcoholic hepatitis may develop the hepatorenal syndrome—rising serum urea nitrogen and creatinine levels indicate a poor prognosis, and these patients may develop cirrhosis. Amiodarone toxicity can simulate alcoholic hepatitis.

5. To monitor an alcoholic who is abstaining from alcohol, see alcohol abuse in Chapter 1.

In a study of the prognostic value of various laboratory test results on mortality, a prolonged plasma PT was the best test. The AST, ALT, and GGT had no prognostic significance.

BIBLIOGRAPHY

Blake J, Orrego H: Monitoring treatment of alcoholic liver disease: Evaluation of various severity indices. Clin Chem 37:5, 1991.
   Discusses monitoring of the effectiveness of treatment for alcoholic liver disease.
Christiansen M, Andersen JR, Torning J, et al: Serum alpha-fetoprotein and alcohol consumption. Scand J Clin Lab Invest 54:215, 1994.
   Discusses the significance of elevated serum alpha-fetoprotein in chronic alcoholic outpatients.
Gupta S, Slaughter S, Akriviadis EA, et al: Serial measurement of serum C-reactive protein facilitates evaluation in alcoholic hepatitis. Hepatogastroenterology 42:516, 1995.
   C-reactive protein is useful in assessing clinical activity.
Ireland A, Hartley L, Ryley N, et al: Raised gamma-glutamyltransferase activity and the need for liver biopsy. BMJ 302:388, 1991.
   Isolated increase in GGT may not by itself be enough to warrant a liver biopsy.
Lieber CS: Alcoholic liver disease: A public health issue in need of a public health approach. Semin Liver Dis, vol 13, no 2, 1993. Foreword.
   Reviews all aspects of alcoholic liver disease.
Lieber CS, Guadagnini KS: The spectrum of alcoholic liver disease. Hosp Pract 25:51, 1990.
   Good discussion of the pathophysiology of alcoholic liver disease, including fatty liver, early fibrosis, alcoholic hepatitis, and cirrhosis.
Rockey DC: Utility of "liver function tests" in alcoholic patients. West J Med 156:319, 1992.
   Good discussion of the laboratory test abnormalities that may be encountered in

alcoholic patients. *Discusses the use of PT and serum bilirubin to assess prognosis by a discriminant function analysis.*

Sherlock S: Alcoholic liver disease. Lancet 345:227, 1995.
Reviews the pathogenesis, clinical recognition, and management of alcoholic liver disease.

Sheth SG, Gordon FD, Chopra S: Nonalcoholic steatohepatitis. Ann Intern Med 126:137, 1997.
Non-alcoholic steatohepatitis is an important differential diagnosis for asymptomatic patients with chronically elevated plasma liver enzyme levels, especially if obesity, diabetes, or hyperlipidemia is present.

Teli MR, Day CP, Burt AD, et al: Determinants of progression to cirrhosis or fibrosis in pure alcoholic fatty liver. Lancet 346:987, 1995.
Fatty liver can no longer be regarded as benign.

Thomson AD: Alcoholic hepatitis. Lancet 343:810, 1994.
Mortality from severe, acute alcoholic hepatitis is about 60% after hospitalization.

Zakim D, Boyer TD: Hepatology: A Textbook of Liver Disease, 2nd ed. Philadelphia, WB Saunders, 1990.
Good discussion of fatty liver and alcoholic hepatitis.

ACUTE NONVIRAL, NONALCOHOLIC HEPATITIS

Recommendations for acute nonviral, nonalcoholic hepatitis are from the medical literature.

In patients with clinical findings and liver function test results of acute hepatitis in whom acute viral hepatitis and alcoholic hepatitis have been excluded, consider hepatitis caused by drugs, toxins, heart failure, hepatic vein occlusion, and Reye's syndrome.

All of these kinds of hepatitis may be confused with acute viral hepatitis because of similar clinical and laboratory findings such as an increased serum transaminase level. Because few specific tests are available, diagnosis often depends on a careful analysis of the history, physical examination, laboratory findings, and results of other studies.

Drug-related Hepatitis

Consider drug-related hepatitis in patients with these findings: clinical and chemical evidence of acute hepatitis and onset of hepatitis 2 to 6 weeks after starting drug therapy (but may occur as early as the first day or not until 6 months later). The hepatitis may progress even after drug withdrawal, and failure to withdraw the offending drug can cause death. Almost any drug can occasionally cause unpredictable hepatitis. Older patients and women appear more susceptible. Acetaminophen can cause hepatitis, especially in alcoholics; acetylcysteine treatment is safe and effective even in later stages of poisoning. Isoniazid administration can rarely result in serious hepatotoxicity and death.

See the discussion of jaundice, abnormal liver function tests, and liver failure in this chapter for drugs that can cause jaundice.

Examples of different types of tissue reactions related to drugs follow:

Tissue Reaction	Examples
Microvesicular fat	Tetracycline, salicylates
Cholestasis (with or without hepatocellular injury)	Chlorpromazine, sex steroids, including oral contraceptives
Hepatitis, acute or chronic	Isoniazid, oxyphenisatin, alpha-methyldopa, nitrofurantoin, phenytoin, cinchophen
Macrovesicular fat	Methotrexate, perhexiline, ethanol
Centrilobular necrosis	Acetaminophen, halothane
Massive necrosis	Halothane, acetaminophen, alpha-methyldopa
Fibrosis-cirrhosis	Methotrexate, cinchophen, amiodarone
Veno-occlusive disease	Cytotoxic drugs
Granuloma formation	Sulfonamides, alpha-methyldopa, quinidine, phenylbutazone, hydralazine, allopurinol
Adenoma	Oral contraceptives
Hepatocellular carcinoma	?Anabolic steroids, oral contraceptives
Hepatic or portal vein thrombosis	Estrogens, including oral contraceptives
Focal nodular hyperplasia	?C-17 alkylated steroids, including oral contraceptives

Source: Cotran RS, Kumar V, Robbins SL: The liver and biliary tract. *In* Robbins Pathologic Basis of Disease, 4th ed. Philadelphia, WB Saunders 1989, p 963.

Toxic Hepatitis

Consider toxic hepatitis in patients with severe acute hepatitis who were exposed to poisoning such as carbon tetrachloride or the wild mushroom *Amanita phalloides*. The mortality rate is high. Also, inquire about herbal medications, which may be toxic to the liver. Recently, fulminant liver failure was described in association with the emetic toxin of *Bacillus cereus*.

Heart-failure Hepatitis

Consider heart-failure hepatitis in patients with increased serum trans-aminase values up to thousands of units per liter and sometimes jaundice. These patients may have marked hypotension, shock, or severe acute congestive heart failure.

Hepatic Vein Occlusion Hepatitis

Consider hepatic vein occlusion hepatitis (Budd-Chiari syndrome) in patients with these findings: acute abdominal pain, tender hepatomeg-aly, ascites, and liver function test results consistent with acute hepati-tis. Causes include polycythemia vera, pregnancy, the postpartum state, the use of oral contraceptives, paroxysmal nocturnal hemoglobinuria, and intra-abdominal cancers, particularly hepatocellular carcinoma.

Reye's Syndrome

Consider Reye's syndrome in children with these findings: sudden onset of intractable vomiting a few days after a viral illness, history of aspirin ingestion, cloudy sensorium, seizures, coma, enlarged liver, hypoglycemia, and abnormal liver function tests. Liver biopsy reveals fatty change of the small-droplet variety, with little or no inflammation. Small-droplet fatty change may also occur in patients with acute fatty liver of pregnancy, Jamaican vomiting sickness, drug (tetracycline and valproic acid) hepatotoxicity, and occasionally ethanol ingestion.

BIBLIOGRAPHY

Abramowicz M (ed): Acetaminophen, NSAID, and alcohol. Med Lett 38:55, 1996.
  Severe liver damage has been reported in alcoholics who took less than 4 grams of acetaminophen per day.
Cassidy WM, Reynolds TB: Serum lactic dehydrogenase in the differential diagnosis of acute hepatocellular injury. J Clin Gastroenterol 19:118, 1994.
  An alanine aminotransaminase/lactate dehydrogenase ratio of 1.5 or more within 24 hours of admission favors viral over ischemic and acetaminophen hepatitis.
Cohen JA, Kaplan MM: Left-sided heart failure presenting as hepatitis. Gastroenterology 74:583, 1978.
  Discusses several cases of heart-failure hepatitis that presented as a viral hepatitis–like syndrome.
Feinfeld DA, Mofenson HC, Caraccio T, et al: Poisoning by amatoxin-containing mushrooms in suburban New York: Report of four cases. J Toxicol Clin Toxicol 32:715, 1994.
  Discusses four cases in suburban Long Island—one dead.
Hench PK, Weart CW, Whitcomb DC: Acetaminophen toxicity: When to worry, what to do. Patient Care 30:87, 1996.
  Excellent review of the diagnosis and treatment of acetaminophen toxicity.
Janssen HLA, Brouwer JT, Nevens F, et al: Fatal hepatic decompensation associated with interferon alfa. BMJ 306:107, 1993.
  Fatal liver decompensation is a rare complication of interferon-alpha therapy.
Keays R, Harrison PM, Wendon JA, et al: Intravenous acetylcysteine in paracetamol induced fulminant hepatic failure: A prospective controlled trial. BMJ 303:1026, 1991.
  Acetylcysteine therapy is effective even in late stages of poisoning.
Koff RS: Herbal hepatotoxicity: Revisiting a dangerous alternative. JAMA 273:502, 1995.
  Gordon DW, Rosenthal G, Hart J, et al: Chaparral ingestion: The broadening spectrum of liver injury caused by herbal medications. JAMA 273:489, 1995.
  Consider herbal hepatotoxicity in patients with hepatic injury of unknown origin.
Kothur R, Marsh F Jr, Posner G: Liver function tests in nonparenteral cocaine users. Arch Intern Med 151:1126, 1991.
  Minimally increased liver enzymes are common in non-parenteral cocaine users without evidence of severe hepatotoxicity.
Kumar S, Rex DK: Failure of physicians to recognize acetaminophen hepatotoxicity in chronic alcoholics. Arch Intern Med 151:1189, 1991.
  High index of suspicion is necessary to detect acetaminophen-related hepatitis in alcoholics.
Larsen LC, Fuller SH: Management of acetaminophen toxicity. Am Fam Physician 53:185, 1996.

Vale JA, Proudfoot AT: Paracetamol (acetaminophen) poisoning. Lancet 346:547, 1995.
  Treatment of acetaminophen poisoning consists of preventing gastrointestinal absorption, administration of N-acetylcysteine, and supportive care.
Lee WM: Drug-induced hepatotoxicity. N Engl J Med 333:1118, 1995.
  Reviews the kinds of toxic reactions occurring in the liver secondary to drugs.
Mahler H, Pasi A, Kramer JM, et al: Fulminant liver failure in association with the emetic toxin of *Bacillus cereus*. N Engl J Med 336:1142, 1997.
  Schafer DF, Sorrell MF: Power failure, liver failure. N Engl J Med 336:1173, 1997.
  Food poisoning with B. cereus can cause liver failure.
Millard PS, Wilcosky TC, Reade-Christopher SJ, et al: Isoniazid-related fatal hepatitis. West J Med 164:486, 1996.
  Fatal isoniazid-related hepatitis was no greater than 4.2 per 100,000 persons beginning therapy and no greater than 7 per 100,000 completing therapy.
Severe isoniazid-associated hepatitis—New York, 1991–1993. MMWR 42:545, 1993.
  When prescribing isoniazid, follow guidelines and monitor patients monthly for hepatitis.
Singer AJ, Carracio TR, Mofenson HC: The temporal profile of increased transaminase levels in patients with acetaminophen-induced liver dysfunction. Ann Emerg Med 26:49, 1995.
  Serum ALT and AST levels may increase within 24 hours and peak within 48 to 72 hours after toxic acetaminophen ingestion.
Whitcomb DC, Block GD: Association of acetaminophen hepatotoxicity with fasting and ethanol use. JAMA 272:1845, 1994.
  Moderate doses of acetaminophen can cause hepatotoxicity after fasting and recent alcohol use.
Zakim D, Boyer TD: Hepatology: A Textbook of Liver Disease, 2nd ed. Philadelphia, WB Saunders, 1990.
  Good discussion of non-viral, non-alcoholic liver disease.

CHRONIC HEPATITIS

Recommendations for chronic hepatitis are from the National Institutes of Health (NIH) and the medical literature.

1. For patients at risk for chronic hepatitis or with clinical findings and liver function test results of chronic hepatitis, request serologic tests for viral hepatitis (namely, hepatitis B surface antigen, anti-hepatitis B core antibody, and anti-hepatitis C antibody) and consider the possibility of autoimmune hepatitis, drug-induced hepatitis, and other less common disorders. Request anti-hepatitis D antibody to detect hepatitis D. To diagnose the lesion accurately, consider a needle biopsy of the liver. According to NIH, persons with the following risk factors should be tested for hepatitis C:

- History of transfusions of blood or blood products before 1990
- Long-term hemodialysis
- History of parenteral drug use
- Multiple sexual partners
- Spouse or close household contact of patient with hepatitis C
- Sharing of instruments for intranasal cocaine use

Chronic hepatitis is a smoldering inflammation of the liver that lasts 6 months or longer. Clinical findings include fatigue, malaise, and mild abdominal pain. Causes range from viruses, autoimmunity, and drugs to a variety of miscellaneous disorders such as α_1-antitrypsin deficiency, Wilson's disease, primary biliary cirrhosis, sclerosing cholangitis, and other agents.

When chronic hepatitis follows acute hepatitis, persistence longer than 6 months can be used to make the diagnosis. Sometimes the disease begins insidiously, or the problem may arise when an apparently healthy person is found to have a high serum transaminase value by laboratory screening, or a positive serologic test for hepatitis is discovered when an individual attempts to donate blood. In these latter instances, hypergammaglobulinemia on serum protein electrophoresis may be a clue that the patient has chronic hepatitis.

In patients with chronic hepatitis, serum transaminase values may be increased up to 400 U/L or more. The values may fluctuate. Serum alkaline phosphatase, bilirubin, albumin, and plasma prothrombin time may be normal or abnormal, depending on the stage of the disease. Increased serum gamma globulins up to the 3 to 7 g/dL (30 to 70 g/L) range are characteristic of autoimmune hepatitis but not viral hepatitis.

2. Evaluate the tests.

Although identification of the cause of chronic hepatitis may generally be accomplished by routine laboratory tests plus immunologic and serologic testing, liver biopsy may be required to confirm the diagnosis and stage the disease (e.g., periodic acid-Schiff reaction–positive material in hepatocytes after diastase treatment is characteristic of α_1-antitrypsin deficiency and increased copper stains of Wilson's disease).

3. If the diagnosis is chronic hepatitis, determine the cause so that appropriate therapy may be chosen.

Viral Hepatitis

In chronic hepatitis, the results of viral serologic tests are as follows:

Type of Hepatitis*	Diagnostic Serologic Test Results
B	Hepatitis B surface antigen *positive*; anti-hepatitis core antibody *positive*
C	Anti-hepatitis C antibody *positive* (confirm with supplemental assay)
D	Hepatitis B surface antigen *positive*; anti-hepatitis D antibody *positive*

*See the discussion of testing for acute hepatitis.

If anti-hepatitis C antibody is present, confirm the diagnosis with the latest generation recombinant immunoblot assay and/or a qualitative polymerase chain reaction test for hepatitis C virus RNA. Hepatitis A and E do not cause chronic hepatitis.

Autoimmune Hepatitis

In Western countries, about 20% of patients with chronic hepatitis have autoimmune hepatitis; most patients are women, but up to one-third are men. Almost all patients have autoantibodies, but only about two-thirds have one of the classic autoimmune markers: antinuclear or anti-smooth-muscle antibodies. Tests for additional autoantibodies can identify most other cases. Hypergammaglobulinemia, mostly IgG, is a characteristic finding.

Drug-induced Hepatitis

A number of drugs have been associated with chronic hepatitis: acetaminophen, amiodarone, aspirin, dantrolene, ethanol, isoniazid, methyldopa, nitrofurantoin, oxyphenisatin, perhexilene maleate, phenytoin, propylthiouracil, and sulfonamides.

Other Causes

Consider α_1-antitrypsin deficiency, Wilson's disease, primary biliary cirrhosis, sclerosing cholangitis, and other possible causes (cryptogenic chronic hepatitis).

4. **In patients with chronic hepatitis, in addition to abnormal liver function tests, the following blood test results may be increased:**

- Ferritin
- Iron

5. **In patients with chronic hepatitis, in addition to abnormal liver function tests, the following blood test result may be decreased:**

- HDL cholesterol

BIBLIOGRAPHY

Adachi H, Kaneko S, Matsushita E, et al: Clearance of HBsAg in seven patients with chronic hepatitis B. Hepatology 16:1334, 1992.
  Regardless of the clearance of hepatitis B surface antigen, patients with chronic hepatitis B should be monitored for the development of liver cancer.
Alter HJ, Purcell RH, Shih JW, et al: Detection of antibody to hepatitis C virus in prospectively followed transfusion recipients with acute and chronic non-A, non-B hepatitis. N Engl J Med 321:1494, 1989.
  Hepatitis C is the predominant agent of transfusion-associated non-A, non-B hepatitis.

Babb RR: Chronic liver disease: The scope of causes and treatments. Postgrad Med 91:89, 1992.
Discusses the differential diagnosis of chronic liver disease.

Batts KP, Ludwig J: Chronic hepatitis: An update on terminology and reporting. Am J Surg Pathol 19:1409, 1995.
The terms chronic active hepatitis, chronic persistent hepatitis, and chronic lobular hepatitis have become obsolete, and one should not use them without further specifications.

Bell H, Skinningsrud A, Raknerud N, et al: Serum ferritin and transferrin saturation in patients with chronic alcoholic and nonalcoholic liver diseases. J Intern Med 236:315, 1994.
Although serum ferritin is often increased in alcoholic liver disease, during abstinence it falls and then transferrin saturation is normal.

Büschenfelde K-H, Lohse AW: Autoimmune hepatitis. N Engl J Med 333:1004, 1995.
Reviews the diagnosis and management of autoimmune hepatitis.

Cahen DL, van Leeuwen DJ, ten Kate FJW, et al: Do serum ALT values reflect the inflammatory activity in the liver of patients with chronic viral hepatitis? Liver 16:105, 1996.
The results suggest that the serum ALT is useful as an indicator of inflammatory activity in chronic viral hepatitis and may play a role in reducing the number of liver biopsies for follow-up therapy.

Di Bisceglie AM: Chronic hepatitis B: Hope for decreasing its impact. Postgrad Med 98:99, 1995.
Reviews the prevention, diagnosis, and management of chronic hepatitis B.

Dove L, Wright TL: Hepatitis C virus: A pathogen for all people. West J Med 164:532, 1996.
Hepatitis C infects 3.5 million people in the United States and is acquired largely by parenteral or sexual modes of transmission.

Dubois F, Francois M, Mariotte N, et al: Serum alanine aminotransferase measurement as a guide to selective testing for hepatitis C during medical check-up. J Hepatol 21:837, 1994.
Serum ALT is an effective screening test for hepatitis C.

Fattovich G, Giustina G, Degos F, et al: Morbidity and mortality in compensated cirrhosis type C: A retrospective follow-up study of 384 patients. Gastroenterology 112:463, 1997.
A substantial minority of patients develop complications during the 10 years following the diagnosis of hepatitis C–related cirrhosis.

Haber MM, West AB, Haber AD, et al: Relationship of aminotransferases to liver histological status in chronic hepatitis C. Am J Gastroenterol 90:1250, 1995.
The lack of enzyme correlation indicates that liver biopsy is still necessary to determine disease grade and stage in patients with chronic hepatitis C.

Harrison PM, Lau JYN, Williams R: Hepatology. Postgrad Med J 67:719, 1991.
Reviews the diagnosis and management of viral hepatitis.

Healey CJ, Chapman RWG, Fleming KA: Liver histology in hepatitis C infection: A comparison between patients with persistently normal or abnormal transaminases. Gut 37:274, 1995.
The results show that significant liver disease can occur with hepatitis C virus (HCV) infection, despite persistently normal transaminase. Liver biopsy is the only means of accurately determining the degree of histologic disease in HCV infection.

Hoofnagle JH, Di Bisceglie AM: Serologic diagnosis of acute and chronic hepatitis. Semin Liver Dis 11:73, 1991.
Reviews the serologic diagnosis of viral hepatitis.

Irving WL, Neal KR, Underwood JCE, et al: Chronic hepatitis in United Kingdom blood donors infected with hepatitis C virus. BMJ 308:695, 1994.
Bruno S, Rossi S, Petroni ML, et al: Normal aminotransferase concentrations in patients with antibodies to hepatitis C virus. BMJ 308:697, 1994.
Serum alanine aminotransferase values may not be increased in patients with hepatitis C.

Lunel F, Musset L, Cacoub P, et al: Cryoglobulinemia in chronic liver disease: Role of hepatitis C and liver damage. Gastroenterology 106:1291, 1994.

The incidence was 54% in chronic hepatitis C, 15% in chronic hepatitis B, and 32% in other types of chronic hepatitis.

McCormick SE, Goodman ZD, Maydonovitch CL, et al: Evaluation of liver histology, ALT elevation and HCV RNA titer in patients with chronic hepatitis C. Am J Gastroenterol 91:1516, 1996.
Liver biopsy continues to be the "gold standard" for determining liver abnormalities and making therapeutic decisions for these patients.

Primary Care Update: Hepatitis C: Latest management guidelines from the NIH. Consultant 137:1864, 1997.
Gives NIH recommendations for testing of patients at risk for hepatitis C.

Rossini A, Gazzola GB, Ravaggi A, et al: Long-term follow-up of and infectivity in blood donors with hepatitis C antibodies and persistently normal alanine aminotransferase levels. Transfusion 35:108, 1995.
Persistently normal or slightly elevated ALT does not exclude HCV chronic hepatitis and supports the need for long-term follow-up and evaluation of liver histology.

Sánchez-Tapias JM, Barrera JM, Costa J, et al: Hepatitis C virus infection in patients with nonalcoholic chronic liver disease. Ann Intern Med 112:921, 1990.
Testing for anti–hepatitis C antibody may be helpful in the differential diagnosis between viral and autoimmune chronic liver disease.

Sato Y, Nakata K, Kato Y, et al: Early recognition of hepatocellular carcinoma based on altered profiles of alpha-fetoprotein. N Engl J Med 328:1802, 1993.
New alpha-fetoprotein tests aid liver cancer diagnosis.

Scotiniotis I, Brass CA, Malet PF: Hepatitis C: Diagnosis and treatment. J Gen Intern Med 10:273, 1995.
Reviews the diagnosis and management of hepatitis C.

Summary of a workshop on screening for hepatocellular carcinoma. MMWR 39:619, 1990.
Suggests serum alpha-fetoprotein and ultrasonography to detect hepatocellular carcinoma.

Tong MJ, El-Farra NS: Clinical sequelae of hepatitis C acquired from injection drug use. West J Med 164:399, 1996.
Hepatitis C from injection drug use is a serious disease that can lead to chronic hepatitis and hepatocellular carcinoma.

Tong MJ, El-Farra NS, Reikes AR, et al: Clinical outcomes after transfusion-associated hepatitis C. N Engl J Med 332:1463, 1995.
Chronic post-transfusion hepatitis C may cause progressive disease and, in some patients, lead to death from either liver failure or hepatocellular carcinoma.

Tsukuma H, Hiyama T, Tanaka S, et al: Risk factors for hepatocellular carcinoma among patients with chronic liver disease. N Engl J Med 328:1797, 1993.
Chronic hepatitis C, like chronic hepatitis B, greatly increases the risk of liver cancer.

Vail BA: Management of chronic viral hepatitis. Am Fam Physician 55:2749, 1997.
Discusses the diagnosis and management of chronic viral hepatitis.

Van Thiel DH, Friedlander L, Malloy P, et al: Gamma-glutamyl transpeptidase as a response predictor when using α-interferon to treat hepatitis C. Hepatogastroenterology 42:888, 1995.
An increase in GGT level during interferon therapy identifies patients with chronic hepatitis C disease who are unlikely to respond to interferon therapy.

Williams ALB, Hoofnagle JH: Ratio of serum aspartate to alanine aminotransferase in chronic hepatitis. Gastroenterology 95:734, 1988.
An AST:ALT ratio greater than 1 in patients with nonalcoholic chronic liver disease suggests that cirrhosis is present or developing.

Yarze JC, Martin P, Muñoz SJ, et al: Wilson's disease: Current status. Am J Med 92:643, 1992.
Discusses pathophysiology, diagnosis, and management of Wilson's disease.

CIRRHOSIS

Recommendations for cirrhosis are from the medical literature.

1. In patients with clinical findings and liver function test results of

cirrhosis, consider a needle biopsy of the liver to accurately diagnose the lesion.

In patients with cirrhosis, the liver function test results vary according to the rate of hepatocellular destruction and the amount of tissue replaced by fibrosis. Thus, aspartate aminotransferase (AST) and alanine aminotransferase (ALT) activities may be normal or increased. In patients with alcoholic cirrhosis, AST values can increase to 200 to 300 U/L. The increase of ALT is typically less. Alkaline phosphatase may be normal to increased up to three times the upper limit, and the bilirubin is normal to increased up to 20 to 40 mg/dL (342 to 684 μmol/L). Albumin is typically decreased, the globulins increased, and the plasma prothrombin time prolonged.

2. Evaluate the tests.

Percutaneous liver biopsy is the procedure of choice to accurately diagnose cirrhosis. In 10 to 20% of cases of presumed alcoholic cirrhosis, another disease is found on biopsy. Whereas a needle biopsy is usually diagnostic for micronodular cirrhosis, a single needle biopsy can miss the morphologic diagnosis of macronodular cirrhosis, and three separate biopsies may be necessary to exclude macronodular cirrhosis because the needle can puncture the center of a large macronodule in which the histology does not show cirrhosis.

3. If the liver biopsy shows cirrhosis, determine its cause so that appropriate therapy can be chosen.

The most common types of cirrhosis in the Western world are alcoholic cirrhosis, cryptogenic cirrhosis, postnecrotic cirrhosis, biliary cirrhosis (primary and secondary), and pigment cirrhosis (in hemochromatosis). Cirrhosis associated with Wilson's disease and α_1-antitrypsin deficiency is rare.

4. In patients with cirrhosis, in addition to abnormal liver function tests, the following blood test results may be increased:

- **Erythrocyte sedimentation rate**
- **Creatinine** caused by the hepatorenal syndrome
- **Uric acid**
- **Urea nitrogen** due to gastrointestinal hemorrhage or the hepatorenal syndrome
- **Amylase**, which correlates with high incidence of patients with pancreatic disease
- **α-Fetoprotein** as a marker for hepatoma: greater than 200 ng/mL (>200 μg/L), sensitive but not specific; greater than 1000 ng/mL (>1000 μg/L), highly suggestive

5. In patients with cirrhosis, in addition to abnormal liver function tests, the following blood test results may be decreased:

- **Hemoglobin and hematocrit** related to chronic disease, gastrointestinal bleeding, and/or hypersplenism

- **Glucose**
- **Uric acid**
- **Potassium** frequently in patients with ascites and edema
- **Phosphorous**, particularly after glucose administration
- **Leukocytes** related to hypersplenism
- **Platelets** related to hypersplenism and/or disseminated intravascular coagulation
- **Urea nitrogen** caused by decreased synthesis of urea
- **Sodium**, especially in patients with ascites
- **Calcium**
- **Magnesium**

BIBLIOGRAPHY

Adachi H, Kaneko S, Matsushita E, et al: Clearance of HBsAg in seven patients with chronic hepatitis B. Hepatology 16:1334, 1992.
In patients with chronic hepatitis B, clearance of hepatitis B surface antigen does not rule out development of hepatocellular carcinoma.

Castilla A, Prieto J, Fausto N: Transforming growth factors beta-1 and alpha in chronic liver disease: Effects of interferon alfa therapy. N Engl J Med 324:933, 1991.
Schiff ER: Hepatic fibrosis: New therapeutic approaches. N Engl J Med 324:987, 1991.
New information on the pathogenesis of cirrhosis.

Colombo M, DeFranchis R, Del Ninno E, et al: Hepatocellular carcinoma in Italian patients with cirrhosis. N Engl J Med 325:675, 1991.
Cirrhotic patients should be carefully followed for the development of hepatoma.

Czaja AJ, Wolf AM, Baggenstoss AH: Clinical assessment of cirrhosis in severe chronic active liver disease: Specificity and sensitivity of physical and laboratory findings. Mayo Clin Proc 55:360, 1980.
Three separate needle biopsies may be required to exclude macronodular cirrhosis.

Imaeda T, Doi H: A retrospective study on the patterns of sequential fluctuation of serum alpha-fetoprotein level during progression from liver cirrhosis to hepatocellular carcinoma. J Gastroenterol Hepatol 7:132, 1992.
In cirrhotic patients, suspect hepatocellular carcinoma when serum α-fetoprotein increases to more than three times the level found the previous month.

Kuwahara T, Sakai T, Majima Y, et al: Serial changes in serum alpha-fetoprotein prior to detection of hepatocellular carcinoma in liver cirrhosis. Hepatogastroenterology 40:347, 1993.
Suspect carcinoma when the serum alpha-fetoprotein elevation shows a spiky or high plateau pattern, despite negative diagnostic imaging studies.

Little DR: Hemochromatosis: Diagnosis and management. Am Fam Physician 53:2623, 1996.
Liver biopsy can confirm the diagnosis and document the presence of cirrhosis.

Melato M, Laurino L, Mucli E, et al: Relationship between cirrhosis, liver cancer, and hepatic metastases: An autopsy study. Cancer 64:455, 1989.
Most neoplasms in cirrhotic livers are primary.

Oka H, Tamori A, Kuroki T, et al: Prospective study of alpha-fetoprotein in cirrhotic patients monitored for development of hepatocellular carcinoma. Hepatology 19:61, 1994.
Cirrhotic patients should be screened more often for hepatocellular carcinoma when the alpha-fetoprotein levels are greater than 20 ng/mL (>20 μg/L).

Plevris JN, Dhariwal A, Elton RA, et al: The platelet count as a predictor of variceal hemorrhage in primary biliary cirrhosis. Am J Gastroenterol 90:959, 1995.
Platelet count below $200 \times 10^3/\mu L$ ($200 \times 10^9/L$) is a good predictor of variceal bleeding.

Violi F, Leo R, Vezza F., et al: Bleeding time in patients with cirrhosis: Relation with degree of liver failure and clotting abnormalities. J Hepatol 20:531, 1994.
About 40% of cirrhotic patients have prolonged bleeding time secondary to a low platelet count and/or low fibrinogen.

CHOLESTASIS AND OBSTRUCTIVE LIVER DISEASE

Recommendations for cholestasis and obstructive liver disease are from the medical literature.

1. For patients with clinical findings and liver function test results of obstructive liver disease, consider appropriate radiographic and other studies and liver biopsy. See the discussion of jaundice, abnormal liver function tests, and liver failure in this chapter for the work-up of patients with jaundice.

Cholestasis refers to disorders that impair bile formation or bile flow. It is sometimes referred to as *obstructive liver disease*, which may be either intrahepatic or extrahepatic. Intrahepatic obstructive processes may be due to hepatocellular disease (e.g., acute viral hepatitis, drug-induced hepatitis); hepatocellular and cholestatic disease (e.g., acute cholestatic viral hepatitis, chronic active hepatitis, cirrhosis, drug-related cholestatic hepatitis); and cholestatic disease (drug-related cholestasis [e.g., chlorpromazine, sex steroids], infiltrative neoplastic or granulomatous hepatic disease, and primary biliary cirrhosis). Extrahepatic obstruction is usually due to mechanical obstruction (e.g., common duct stone and periampullary carcinoma). Some additional causes of cholestatic jaundice follow:

Alcoholic hepatitis	Postoperative cholestasis
Amyloidosis	Sarcoidosis
Benign recurrent cholestasis	Sclerosing cholangitis
Biliary cirrhosis	Shock
Cholestasis of pregnancy	Sickle cell disease
Chronic active hepatitis	Total parenteral nutrition
Congestive heart failure	Toxic chemicals (e.g., paraquat)
Drugs*	Transplant rejection
Hepatic cirrhosis	Viral hepatitis
Mechanical obstruction	

*See the discussion of jaundice, abnormal liver function tests, and liver failure in this chapter for drugs that can cause jaundice.

Source: McKnight JT, Jones JE: Jaundice. Am Fam Physician 45:1139–1148, 1992. Republished with permission from the American Academy of Family Physicians.

By strict definition, cholestasis does not include prehepatic jaundice (hemolysis) or the hereditary hyperbilirubinemias such as Gilbert's disease, the Crigler-Najjar syndrome, the Dubin-Johnson syndrome, and Rotor's syndrome. Cholestasis is characterized by increased serum bile acids. In all the hereditary hyperbilirubinemias, bile acids are typically normal.

Increased alkaline phosphatase, bilirubin, and gamma-glutamyltransferase levels are valuable in identifying cholestasic disorders but are not very useful in determining the cause of the cholestasis and whether the obstruction is intrahepatic or hepatic. Moreover, in this regard even liver biopsy has limitations. Radiographic and endoscopic studies are often necessary to diagnose the nature and location of the obstruction.

Appropriate procedures to consider include ultrasonography, computed tomography, endoscopic retrograde cholangiopancreatography, and percutaneous transhepatic cholangiography. See the recommendations for the work-up of patients with jaundice at the beginning of this chapter.

2. Interpret test results in the context of clinical findings.

If the liver function test results show a cholestatic pattern, determine whether the biliary obstruction is intrahepatic or extrahepatic (i.e., medical versus surgical obstruction). Serum bile acid values may be helpful in excluding prehepatic jaundice. Determine the exact cause of either medical or surgical obstruction so that appropriate therapy can be chosen.

BIBLIOGRAPHY

Arvan DA: Obstructive jaundice. In Panzer RJ, Black ER, Griner PF (eds): Diagnostic Strategies for Common Medical Problems. Philadelphia, American College of Physicians, 1991, p 131.
    Recommends strategies for the differential diagnosis of obstructive jaundice.

Gershwin ME, Mackay IR: New knowledge in primary biliary cirrhosis. Hosp Pract 30:29, 1995.
    Reviews pathogenesis, diagnosis, and therapy of primary biliary cirrhosis.

Hadjis NS, Blenkharn JI, Hatzis G, et al: Patterns of serum alkaline phosphatase activity in unilateral hepatic duct obstruction: A clinical and experimental study. Surgery 107:193, 1990.
    Increased serum alkaline phosphatase may be the only abnormality in patients with unilateral hepatic duct obstruction.

Halevy A, Gold-Deutch R, Negri M, et al: Are elevated liver enzymes and bilirubin levels significant after laparoscopic cholecystectomy in the absence of bile duct injury? Ann Surg 219:362, 1994.
    Transient increase of liver enzymes after laparoscopic cholecystectomy is not clinically significant.

Kurzweil SM, Shapiro MJ, Andrus CH, et al: Hyperbilirubinemia without common duct abnormalities and hyperamylasemia without pancreatitis in patients with gallbladder disease. Arch Surg 129:829, 1994.
    The cause of hyperbilirubinemia without common bile duct stones may be cholestasis

secondary to sepsis. There is no explanation for hyperamylasemia in gallbladder disease without pancreatitis.

Lacerda MA, Ludwig J, Dickson ER, et al: Antimitochondrial antibody–negative primary biliary cirrhosis. Am J Gastroenterol 90:247, 1995.

About 5% of patients with clinical, biochemical, and histologic features of primary biliary cirrhosis do not have antimitochondrial antibody.

Lee Y-M, Kaplan MM: Primary sclerosing cholangitis. N Engl J Med 332:924, 1995.

Reviews the diagnosis and management of primary sclerosing cholangitis.

Monaghan G, Ryan M, Seddon R, et al: Genetic variation in bilirubin UDP-glucuronosyl-transferase gene promoter and Gilbert's syndrome. Lancet 347:578, 1996.

Sato H, Adachi Y, Koiwai O: The genetic basis of Gilbert's syndrome. Lancet 347:557, 1996.

There may be two genetic varieties of Gilbert's syndrome, one with a high bilirubin concentration and the other with a low bilirubin concentration.

Panzer RJ: Hepatic metastases. *In* Panzer RJ, Black ER, Griner PF (eds): Diagnostic Strategies for Common Medical Problems. Philadelphia, American College of Physicians, 1991, p 152.

Recommends strategies for the diagnosis of hepatic metastases.

Rocklin MS, Senagore AJ, Talbott TM: Role of carcinoembryonic antigen and liver function tests in the detection of recurrent colorectal carcinoma. Dis Colon Rectum 34:794, 1991.

Carcinoembryonic antigen measurements are sufficient to monitor patients for metastatic colorectal cancer. Liver function tests are unnecessary.

Sartin JS, Walker RC: Granulomatous hepatitis: A retrospective review of 88 cases at the Mayo Clinic. Mayo Clinic Proc 66:914, 1991.

Discusses differential diagnosis of granulomatous hepatitis.

Schmid R: Gilbert's syndrome: A legitimate genetic anomaly? N Engl J Med 333:1217, 1995.

Bosma PJ, Chowdhury JR, Bakker C, et al: The genetic basis of the reduced expression of bilirubin UDP-glucuronosyltransferase 1 in Gilbert's syndrome. N Engl J Med 333:1171, 1995.

Gilbert's syndrome is a genetically determined, benign, and clinically inconsequential entity that requires neither treatment nor follow-up.

Tai D-I, Shen F-H, Liaw Y-F: Abnormal predrainage serum creatinine as a prognostic indicator in acute cholangitis. Hepatogastroenterology 39:47, 1992.

Elevated predrainage creatinine is not unusual in acute cholangitis and indicates an increased mortality in those patients presenting with more than mild symptoms.

Wang M-J, Chao A, Huang C-H, et al: Hyperbilirubinemia after cardiac operation: Incidence, risk factors, and clinical significance. J Thorac Cardiovasc Surg 108:429, 1994.

The overall incidence of hyperbilirubinemia after cardiac surgery is 35.1% and is largely tied to unconjugated bilirubin due to hemolysis caused by blood trauma by the roller pump, the cardiotomy suction, or the replacement mechanical prostheses.

7

Urinary Tract Diseases

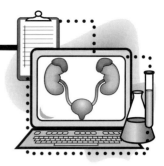

- The Urinalysis
- Glucosuria
- Proteinuria
- Hematuria and Colored Urine
- Urinary Tract Infection in Women
- Acute Renal Failure

THE URINALYSIS

Recommendations for urinalysis are from the medical literature. The United States Preventive Services Task Force (USPST) does not recommend screening for asymptomatic bacteriuria in the general population but does recommend this screening by urine culture in all pregnant women. The American Academy of Family Physicians recommends urine dipstick testing to detect bacteriuria in preschool children, morbidly obese persons, persons older than 65, and persons with diabetes or history of gestational diabetes.

1. Screen asymptomatic persons at risk for urinary tract disease using a reagent strip (dipstick) that includes the nitrite test and leukocyte esterase test. Pregnant women require special surveillance for asymptomatic bacteriuria. In asymptomatic individuals, if all urine dipstick test results are negative, omit microscopic examination of the sediment.

Performance of a urinalysis for wellness screening is controversial. Because a urine dipstick test is such an economical and effective way to detect urinary tract disease and because urinary tract disorders are so prevalent, many physicians perform dipstick screening. Use of dipstick testing is particularly well suited for screening asymptomatic high-risk populations (e.g., diabetics, pregnant women, preschool children, persons older than age 65). Pregnant women should have regular urinalyses with urine cultures if pyuria is noted. The USPST recommends urine culture for pregnant women at 12 to 16 weeks of gestation and periodically at the discretion of the attending physician because evidence is strong that treatment is efficacious in improving outcome. General screening may be useful in other groups, such as infants, toddlers, preschool children, school children, adolescents, adults, and institutionalized elderly persons.

In the routine health care setting, urinalysis may be compromised by a poorly collected specimen, delays in testing, lack of standardization of procedures, and lack of proficiency by the examiner. Microscopic examination of the sediment is particularly vulnerable to these poor practices. To obtain medically reliable information, emphasis must be placed on proper collection of a fresh specimen, which is quickly tested by a competent examiner, using standardized and controlled techniques.

The traditional macroscopic examination consists of a description of the urine, including its color and specific gravity. The usual dipstick provides a semiquantitative estimation of pH, glucose, protein, hemoglobin, ketones, bilirubin, and urobilinogen. Newer dipsticks have two additional tests: the nitrite test and the leukocyte esterase test. Each of these new tests is designed to detect the presence of urinary tract infections (UTIs). Many gram-negative bacteria reduce nitrates to nitrites, and polymorphonuclear leukocytes in urine release leukocyte esterase.

The microscopic examination is done by centrifuging 10 mL of urine at 2000 rpm for 5 minutes at approximately 450 g and resuspending the sediment in 1 mL of urine. Under high power, red blood cells (RBCs), white blood cells (WBCs), and renal epithelial cells are counted in 10 representative fields. Bacteria and yeast are noted. Crystals are reported if their number is unusually large or they are abnormal. If casts are present, they are identified, and the number of casts per low-power field in 10 fields is reported. With the introduction of the nitrite and leukocyte esterase tests to detect bacteria and WBCs in the urine, a number of studies have been done to determine whether it is necessary to perform a labor-intensive microscopic examination of the urinary sediment if all reagent strip tests are completely negative.

A study of the results of a nine-parameter dipstick examination of 1385 urine specimens gave the following results: all positive protein tests confirmed by the sulfosalicylic acid test; 81.9% sensitivity for pyuria (five WBCs per high-power field); 94.5% sensitivity for blood; 25.9% sensitivity for bacteria; and 82.2% for one or more elements of any kind. Only 3.8% of the 730 specimens with negative reagent strip tests had positive microscopic findings. The reagent strip had a 98.1% sensitivity for bacteria in specimens that had positive cultures.

A practical approach seems advisable—a urine dipstick test is an effective test to detect covert pyuria, hematuria, and proteinuria as a part of a routine physical examination. The test is inexpensive and can detect diseases that cause serious morbidity. A negative result is useful as baseline information. A urine dipstick test may also be useful to detect sexually transmitted disease in men. Clearly, the microscopic examination is the most time-consuming and costly part of the urinalysis, and it can be omitted in the context of screening for urinary tract disorders if all the dipstick test results are negative.

2. In patients with clinical findings of urinary tract disease, obtain a complete urinalysis—dipstick test and microscopic examination of the sediment—regardless of the dipstick test results. Consider obtaining a culture.

Because a dipstick test is not 100% sensitive for abnormal findings in the microscopic sediment and because the results of both a dipstick test and microscopic examination are clinically useful, it is prudent to perform both a dipstick test and microscopic examination of the sediment in patients who are symptomatic. If there are clinical findings of UTI, a urine culture may be appropriate.

3. Collect urine samples for culture without contamination.

Verbally instructing the patient on proper collection technique is a very important aspect in obtaining a contamination-free urine sample. Instruct the patients to clean themselves well with the materials provided in the collection kit (for females, spread themselves with one hand and wipe, rinse, and dry the vaginal area with the other hand; for males, retract the foreskin [if uncircumcised] and wipe, rinse, and dry the glans). Tell the patients not to touch the inside of the collection container. The clean-catch technique is preferred—pass a small amount of urine into the toilet, then pass enough urine into the sterile container to fill it half full, and place the lid on the container.

4. Interpret urinalysis test results in the context of clinical findings.

Positive test results, either macroscopic or microscopic, should always be explored. The presence of glucose, protein, or hemoglobin in the urine may be a clue to serious disease or may represent a benign finding that, once explained, can be disregarded. RBCs, WBCs, epithelial cells, bacteria, casts, and other findings in the urinary sediment may constitute key information in diagnosing a urinary tract disorder. The problems that follow discuss the work-up of glucosuria, proteinuria, and hemoglobinuria and the use of urinalysis in the diagnosis of UTI in women.

BIBLIOGRAPHY

Abyad A: Screening for asymptomatic bacteriuria in pregnancy: Urinalysis vs urine culture. J Fam Pract 33:471, 1991.
  Suggests complete urinalysis at first prenatal visit with cultures if five or more leukocytes per high-power field are present.
Akin BV, Hubbell FA, Frye EB, et al: Efficacy of routine admission urinalysis. Am J Med 82:719, 1987.
  Concludes that routine hospital admission urinalysis is not very useful.
Bachman JW, Heise RH, Naessens JM, et al: A study of various tests to detect asymptomatic urinary tract infections in an obstetric population. JAMA 270:1971, 1993.
  Recommends low-cost urine dipstick screening of asymptomatic pregnant women to detect urinary tract infection as well as glycosuria and proteinuria.
Belsey R, Baer DM: Specimen collection for diagnosing UTI. Med Lab Observer 28:29, 1996.
  The most important factor affecting the identification of urinary pathogens is the quality of the specimen.
Cramer AD, Chogyoji M, Saxena S, et al: Macroscopic screening urinalysis. Lab Med 20:623, 1989.
  A study of 1385 urine specimens that supports omission of the microscopic sediment examination if all urine dipstick results are negative.

Is routine urinalysis worthwhile? [editorial] Lancet 1:747, 1988.
Concludes that the high prevalence of urinary abnormalities justifies routine urinalysis in both the ambulatory care and hospital settings.

Kawamura T, Ohta T, Ohno Y, et al: Significance of urinalysis for subsequent kidney and urinary tract disorders in mass screening of adults. Intern Med 34:475, 1995.
Urine dipstick analysis is required for all students, workers, and residents in Japan for detecting renal and urinary tract disorders in the early stages. Proteinuria and hematuria were the best markers for urinary tract disorders.

Kiel DP, Moskowitz MA: The urinalysis: A critical appraisal. Med Clin North Am 71:607, 1987.
Good review of the technical and medical aspects of urinalysis.

Lachs MS, Nachamkin I, Edelstein PH, et al: Spectrum bias in the evaluation of diagnostic tests: Lessons from the rapid dipstick test for urinary tract infection. Ann Intern Med 117:135, 1992.
Sensitivity and specificity of the leukocyte esterase and nitrite urine dipstick tests for UTI may differ among different patient groups.

Monane M, Gurwitz JH, Lipsitz LA, et al: Epidemiologic and diagnostic aspects of bacteriuria: A longitudinal study in older women. J Am Geriatr Soc 43:618, 1995.
Transient bacteriuria is a common event in elderly women and can be excluded by inexpensive routine urinalysis.

Mortier E, Pouchot J, Girard L, et al: Assessment of urine analysis for the diagnosis of tuberculosis. BMJ 312:27, 1996.
Urine cultures for tuberculosis are not appropriate in cases of suspected pulmonary tuberculosis and may be limited to those patients with suspected genitourinary tuberculosis.

Mimoz O, Bouchet E, Edouard A, et al: Limited usefulness of urinary dipsticks to screen out catheter-associated bacteriuria in ICU patients. Anaesth Intensive Care 23:706, 1995.
Use of the urine dipstick as a screen for significant bacteriuria cannot be recommended for determining the need for quantitative urine culture in ICU patients with prolonged urethral catheterization.

Nunns D, Smith ARB, Hosker G: Reagent strip testing urine for significant bacteriuria in a urodynamic clinic. Br J Urol 76:87, 1995.
It is unnecessary to culture urine samples for asymptomatic bacteriuria if the urine dipstick test is negative for leukocytes and nitrite.

Pappas PG: Laboratory in the diagnosis and management of urinary tract infections. Med Clin North Am 75:313, 1991.
Good discussions of urinalysis, urine culture, non-invasive methods of UTI localization, and office diagnosis of UTIs.

Rouse DJ, Andrews WW, Goldenberg RL, et al: Screening and treatment of asymptomatic bacteriuria of pregnancy to prevent pyelonephritis: A cost-effectiveness and cost-benefit analysis. Obstet Gynecol 86:119, 1995.
Either dipstick urinalysis or urine culture is cost-beneficial compared with no screening, but screening with culture becomes cost-beneficial compared with dipstick urinalysis only at high asymptomatic bacteriuria prevalence rates.

Sadof MD, Woods ER, Emans J: Dipstick leukocyte esterase activity in first-catch urine specimens: A useful screening test for detecting sexually transmitted disease in the adolescent male. JAMA 258:1932, 1987.
Shafer MA, Schachter J, Moscicki AB, et al: Urinary leukocyte esterase screening test for asymptomatic chlamydial and gonococcal infections in males. JAMA 262:2562, 1989.
Urine dipstick leukocyte esterase testing can detect sexually transmitted disease in the male.

Screening for asymptomatic bacteriuria. *In* Guide to Clinical Preventive Services: Report of the U.S. Preventive Services Task Force, 2nd ed. Baltimore, Williams & Wilkins, 1996, p 347.
The American Academy of Family Physicians recommends periodic screening by dipstick combining leukocyte esterase and nitrite tests to detect bacteriuria in preschool children, those who are morbidly obese, persons with diabetes or a history of gestational diabetes, and persons aged 65 years and older.

GLUCOSURIA

Recommendations for glucosuria are from the medical literature. Although the presence of glucosuria may indicate diabetes mellitus, urine dipstick testing for glucose is not an adequate test to screen for diabetes.

1. In patients with glucosuria, assess the clinical findings, perform a complete urinalysis, including microscopic examination of the urinary sediment, and measure serum glucose, creatinine, and urea nitrogen.

Glucosuria usually occurs when the serum glucose concentration is greater than 180 to 200 mg/dL (9.99 to 11.10 mmol/L), but glucose may appear in the urine at lower serum glucose values, varying in individuals. The serum glucose concentration at which glucose appears in the urine is termed the *renal threshold* for glucose. Glucosuria should be distinguished from other conditions involving sugars in the urine such as lactosuria and galactosuria. In addition to the serum glucose concentration, other factors that affect the appearance of glucose in the urine include glomerular blood flow, tubular reabsorption rate, and the urine flow rate. Follow-up studies are necessary to determine whether the glucosuria is caused by hyperglycemia or renal tubular dysfunction. Glucosuria in the absence of hyperglycemia is called *renal glucosuria*.

Glucosuria may occur as an isolated finding, or it may be accompanied by other abnormal findings. A complete urinalysis can provide clues to a variety of disorders such as diabetic nephropathy. A serum glucose measurement can help determine whether glucosuria is an overflow phenomenon or related to a renal disorder, and serum urea nitrogen and creatinine measurements are useful to assess renal function.

2. Evaluate the tests.

Reduction methods (copper reduction test) for measuring urinary glucose are too cumbersome for routine use. A dipstick test using glucose oxidase currently is the most commonly used technique, and it is specific for glucose. Large doses of ascorbic acid (vitamin C) can cause a false-negative urinary glucose test result using the glucose oxidase method. Ascorbic acid does not affect reduction methods, but other drugs can give false-positive results or unusual colors with the copper reduction test, especially the cephalosporins (e.g., cephalexin [Keflex]) and radiocontrast agents. Reduction methods are useful to detect nonglucose meliturias, which can occur in infants. In the presence of other sugars such as lactose and galactose, the reduction test is positive and the glucose oxidase test is negative.

3. If the serum glucose concentration is increased in a patient with glucosuria, conclude that the urinary glucose is an overflow phenomenon, and determine whether the increased serum glucose is due to diabetes mellitus or hyperglycemia secondary to some other cause.

Serum glucose may be increased in diabetes mellitus, during stress, and with a variety of diseases such as acute pancreatitis, central nervous system lesions, and disorders secondary to drugs (e.g., corticosteroids).

4. If the serum glucose concentration is normal in a patient with glucosuria, consider renal tubular dysfunction (i.e., renal glucosuria).

Glucosuria without hyperglycemia is usually caused by renal tubular dysfunction, which may be inherited (uncommon) or acquired. In patients with renal tubular dysfunction, glucose is not the only substance with impaired tubular reabsorption. For example, in patients with Fanconi's syndrome, the reabsorption of water, amino acids, sodium, bicarbonate, and phosphate is also impaired. Other examples of conditions associated with renal tubular dysfunction include galactosemia, cystinosis, lead poisoning, and myeloma. Glucosuria secondary to renal tubular dysfunction is less common than glucosuria due to hyperglycemia.

BIBLIOGRAPHY

Freeman JA, Beeler MF: Laboratory Medicine: Urinalysis and Medical Microscopy, 2nd ed. Philadelphia, Lea & Febiger, 1983.
  Good general reference on urinalysis and glucosuria.
Grady D: Newer guidelines redefine diabetes in broader terms. The New York Times, June 24, 1997, p A1.
  The urine dipstick test for glucose is not an adequate test to screen for diabetes mellitus.
Kiel DP, Moskowitz MA: The urinalysis: A critical appraisal. Med Clin North Am 71:607, 1987.
  Discusses differential diagnosis of glucosuria.
Lenhard MJ, DeCherney GS, Maser RE, et al: A comparison between alternative and trade name glucose test strips. Diabetes Care 18:686, 1995.
  Physicians should use caution when advising use of the less expensive alternative test strips to avoid introducing further error in diabetic patient blood glucose monitoring.

PROTEINURIA

Recommendations for proteinuria and microalbuminuria are from the medical literature.

1. In patients with proteinuria, assess the clinical findings, request a complete urinalysis, including microscopic examination of the urinary sediment, and measure serum creatinine and urea nitrogen. Consider testing diabetic and hypertensive patients for microalbuminuria.

Proteinuria is a common and easily detected sign of urinary tract disease, especially renal disease. In the past normal urine was believed free of protein. It now is known that healthy individuals excrete a small amount of protein, which is undetectable by routine methods. Normally the composition of urinary protein is approximately 40% albumin, 40% tissue proteins from renal and other urogenital tissues, 15% immunoglobulins, and 5% other plasma proteins. Proteinuria may be caused by (1) an overflow of increased plasma proteins, (2) increased glomerular permeability, (3) tubular proteinuria, and (4) altered renal hemodynamics.

Proteinuria may occur as an isolated finding during a urinalysis or together with other abnormal findings. A urinalysis can provide clues to a variety of disorders such as fatty casts, oval fat bodies, and doubly refractile fat globules for the nephrotic syndrome; erythrocyte casts for glomerulonephritis; and glucosuria for diabetes mellitus. When these other findings are present, they corroborate the significance of the proteinuria. Serum creatinine and urea nitrogen measurements are useful to evaluate renal function.

Many diabetologists and nephrologists believe that the early detection and reversal of microalbuminuria in diabetics may delay or prevent frank diabetic nephropathy. Thus, there is a growing interest in detecting and reversing microalbuminuria not only in diabetics but also in hypertensive patients. The usual urine dipstick test is not sensitive enough to screen for microalbuminuria; a special method is required. To measure urine microalbuminuria, submit a random or 24-hour urine collection to the laboratory.

2. Evaluate the tests.

Urine protein can be measured by a urine dipstick test as well as by turbidimetric, chemical, and immunologic methods. With the urine dipstick test, false-positive results can occur with highly concentrated urine, highly alkaline (pH >7) urine, and contamination of the urine with bacteria, blood, quaternary ammonium compounds, and chlorhexidine. False-negative results can occur with urinary immunoglobulin light chains (Bence Jones protein) and highly dilute urine. With turbidimetric methods, false-positive results can occur if the urine contains tolbutamide, radiocontrast agents, or high levels of cephalosporin, penicillin, or sulfonamide derivatives.

The usual urine dipstick test can detect 5 to 20 mg/dL (50 to 200 mg/L) of albumin (depending on the method) and is less sensitive to globulins, Bence Jones protein, and mucoprotein. To quantify microalbuminuria, a special method is necessary: a detection limit of at least 0.5 mg/dL (5 mg/L) and a range of 0.5 to 200 mg/dL (5 to 2000 mg/L) are preferred. Normal values are less than about 2 mg/dL (20 mg/L) (depending on the method).

3. If proteinuria is present, documented, and confirmed, measure serum creatinine, urea nitrogen, and a 24-hour protein excretion (alternatively, measure urinary protein and creatinine in a random urine specimen and calculate the protein:creatinine ratio to estimate protein excretion). Consider the possibility of transient and orthostatic proteinuria.

Spot urinary measurements of protein and creatinine reliably detect significant proteinuria. This method avoids the cumbersome, inconvenient, and often unreliable collection of a 24-hour urine sample. The protein:creatinine ratio can distinguish healthy individuals from those with renal disease and can differentiate nephrotic-range proteinuria from that seen with other renal diseases. The protein:creatinine ratio in healthy individuals seldom exceeds 0.2 mg of protein per mg of creatinine. For patients with nephrotic range proteinuria, the ratio exceeds 3.5 mg/mg.

Transient proteinuria may be associated with strenuous exercise, emotional stress, extreme cold, epinephrine administration, congestive heart failure, and seizures. Transient proteinuria can be documented by several protein-free urinalyses after the precipitating cause has passed. The mechanism of proteinuria is believed to be related to hemodynamic changes. The patient should be reassured, and no further work-up is indicated.

Orthostatic proteinuria is characterized by the presence of proteinuria with the patient in the erect position and the absence of proteinuria as shown by a negative reagent strip test result or one less than 50 mg/L with the patient in the recumbent position. The true mechanism is unknown but probably is increased glomerular permeability. The proteinuria usually does not exceed 2 g/day. Long-term follow-up studies over several decades have shown excellent prognosis, with normal renal function.

4. If proteinuria is persistent and nonorthostatic, perform a more extensive evaluation. Other useful laboratory tests include blood glucose, antinuclear antibody, complement, VDRL, HIV, hepatitis B and C, as well as renal biopsy.

The spectrum of lesions in isolated proteinuria is wide, and it is important to perform a thorough evaluation. Nephrotoxic agents such as nonsteroidal anti-inflammatories, gold compounds, penicillamine, ACE inhibitors, and lithium are an important cause of proteinuria to consider.

BIBLIOGRAPHY

Ali H: Proteinuria: How much evaluation is appropriate? Postgrad Med 101:173, 1997.
  Reviews the types of proteinuria and outlines diagnostic and management options.
Cembrowski GS: Testing for microalbuminuria: Promises and pitfalls. Lab Med 21:491, 1990.
  Suggests strategies for monitoring microalbuminuria in diabetic patients.
Ginsberg JM, Chang BS, Matarese RA, et al: Use of single voided urine samples to estimate quantitative proteinuria. N Engl J Med 309:1543, 1983.
  In the presence of stable renal function, a protein:creatinine ratio greater than 3.5 mg/mg can be taken to represent "nephrotic-range" proteinuria, and a ratio of less than 0.2 mg/mg is within normal limits.
Kaplan NM: Microalbuminuria: A risk factor for vascular and renal complications of hypertension. Am J Med 92(Suppl 4B):8S, 1992.
  In hypertensive patients, testing for microalbuminuria should be routinely performed.

Krolewski AS, Laffel LMB, Krolewski M, et al: Glycosylated hemoglobin and the risk of microalbuminuria in patients with insulin-dependent diabetes mellitus. N Engl J Med 332:1251, 1995.
To decrease risk for microalbuminuria, strive to maintain the hemoglobin A_{1C} below 10% in patients with insulin-dependent diabetes mellitus.

Lynch M, Hoffmann NV, Aroney CN: Thrombolytic treatment and proteinuria. Br Heart J 74:354, 1995.
This finding is consistent with the formation of circulating IgG-containing immune complexes that develop immediately after treatment with streptokinase, with their deposition in the renal glomeruli resulting in glomerular proteinuria.

McKenna MJ, Arias C, Feldkamp CS, et al: Microalbuminuria in clinical practice. Arch Intern Med 151:1745, 1991.
Concludes that testing for microalbuminuria is useful for early detection of diabetic nephropathy.

Meyer NL, Mercer BM, Friedman SA, et al: Urinary dipstick protein: A poor predictor of absent or severe proteinuria. Am J Obstet Gynecol 170:137, 1994.
The degree of protein excretion should be confirmed with a 24-hour quantitative study in any classification of pre-eclampsia or other hypertensive disease of pregnancy.

Mitchell SCM, Sheldon TA, Shaw AB: Quantification of proteinuria: A re-evaluation of the protein/creatinine ratio for elderly subjects. Age Ageing 22:443, 1993.
The protein:creatinine ratio is useful as a semiquantitative method for assessing protein excretion in elderly patients.

Roe TF, Costin G, Kaufman FR, et al: Blood glucose control and albuminuria in type 1 diabetes mellitus. J Pediatr 119:178, 1991.
Maintenance of hemoglobin A_{1C} values at 9% or less significantly decreases the risk of diabetic nephropathy.

Schwab SJ, Christensen RL, Dougherty K, et al: Quantitation of proteinuria by the use of protein-to-creatinine ratios in single urine samples. Arch Intern Med 147:943, 1987.
Suggests the use of single urine samples as a reliable way to quantitate proteinuria.

Waller KV, Ward KM, Mahan JD, et al: Current concepts in proteinuria. Clin Chem 35:755, 1989.
Good review of glomerular, tubular, and mixed proteinuria.

Young RA, Buchanan RJ, Kinch RAH: Use of the protein/creatinine ratio of a single voided urine specimen in the evaluation of suspected pregnancy-induced hypertension. J Fam Pract 42:385, 1996.
A ratio less than 0.15 effectively ruled out significant pregnancy-induced hypertension (only two women with proteinuria were missed using this cut-off).

HEMATURIA AND COLORED URINE

Recommendations for hematuria and colored urine are from the medical literature.

1. In patients with hematuria, myoglobinuria, or colored urine, assess the clinical findings, request a complete urinalysis, and measure serum creatinine, urea nitrogen, creatine kinase, and haptoglobin. Obtain a carefully drawn serum specimen for visual inspection.

Hematuria may be either gross (red, red-brown, or brown-black urine) or microscopic (more than one red blood cell [RBC] per high-power field in men and more than three RBCs per high-power field in women). It takes only 1 mL of blood per liter of urine to cause a visible color. It may be caused by a disorder of hemostasis or therapeutic anticoagulation, or it may originate in a lesion located anywhere in the urinary tract. When the urine is red, it is important to determine that the color is caused by blood and not another colored substance such as myoglobin, porphyrins, or the ingestion of beets. Identification of the cause of hematuria depends on clinical findings, radiographs, urologic procedures, and laboratory tests. It helps to know whether the hematuria is painful or painless and whether it is accompanied by other urinary abnormalities such as protein and formed elements in the urine.

In patients with hemoglobinuria, RBCs may be present or absent in the urinary sediment. If RBCs are absent and the urinary reagent test for blood is positive, hemoglobinuria must be distinguished from myoglobinuria. If a carefully drawn serum specimen can be examined (avoiding hemolysis), it often is pink with hemoglobinemia but a normal color with myoglobinemia. Serum myoglobin is rapidly cleared by the kidneys, but serum hemoglobin is not. Additional useful tests are determinations of serum creatine kinase, which often is markedly increased in patients with myoglobinuria secondary to muscle damage, and serum haptoglobin, which is low in patients with hemoglobinuria and normal in those with myoglobinuria.

Hematuria may be present as an isolated finding on urinalysis or may appear together with other abnormal findings. A complete urinalysis can provide clues to a variety of disorders such as urinary tract infection and urinary calculi. Serum creatinine and urea nitrogen measurements are useful to assess renal function.

2. Evaluate the tests.

The usual urine dipstick test relies on the peroxidase-like activity of RBCs and hemoglobin. Both hemoglobin and myoglobin give a positive test result. False-positive results can occur when urine from menstruating women is tested or when the urine is contaminated with residues of strongly oxidizing cleaning agents or with povidone-iodine. False-negative readings can occur when the urine contains large quantities of ascorbic acid (vitamin C) or is preserved with formalin.

Currently available urine dipsticks are capable of detecting two or three RBCs per high-power field with a sensitivity of 97%. Intact RBCs hemolyze on the reagent strip, and the liberated hemoglobin produces a colored dot. Scattered or compacted dots indicate intact RBCs, whereas a uniform green color indicates free hemoglobin, hemolyzed RBCs, or myoglobin.

3. In patients with documented gross or microscopic hematuria, determine the source of the hemoglobin or bleeding.

Hemoglobinuria can be caused by hemolytic disorders, which may be either inherited or acquired. After a race, marathon runners may have hematuria. Myoglobinuria can be caused by rhabdomyolysis, which may occur with the following conditions: primary muscle injury, increased muscle energy consumption (strenuous exercise, status epilepticus), decreased muscle energy consumption (diabetic ketoacidosis), decreased muscle oxygenation, infections, and toxins. Approximately 10% of patients with gross hematuria and 35% with microscopic hematuria have so-called hematuria of unknown cause.

A standard urologic evaluation for asymptomatic hematuria includes urine culture and cytology, a renal ultrasound study or an intravenous urogram, and cystoscopy. Refined urine diagnostic assays, including cytology, may be a less invasive and less costly way to work up patients with asymptomatic hematuria. In patients with idiopathic hematuria, renal biopsy makes no difference therapeutically or prognostically and is therefore unnecessary for routine management of asymptomatic hematuria.

If no pathologic cause of hematuria is present, consider an entity known as *familial hematuria*, in which hematuria is present in other family members and good renal function is maintained during long-term follow-up.

4. In patients with red or brown urine, if the reagent strip (dipstick) test for blood is negative, conclude that a substance other than hemoglobin or myoglobin is responsible for the colored urine.

Red, red-brown, or brown-black urine can result from either ingested substances or substances that originate in the body. Ingested substances include azodyes (phenazopyridine [pyridium]), phenosulfonphthalein, para-aminosalicylic acid, anthraquinones, nitrofurantoin, metronidazole, sulfa compounds, chloroquine, methyldopa, levodopa, phenacetin, salicylates, methocarbamol, cresol, iron sorbitol citrate, and beets (individuals who can absorb betanin). Phenytoin is not a cause of red urine. Substances originating in the body include bilirubin, porphyrin, melanin (in melanoma), homogentisic acid (in alkaptonuria), and the red pigment produced by *Serratia marcescens* (in infection by that organism).

5. In patients with myoglobinuria (acute rhabdomyolysis), the following blood test results may be increased:

- **Uric acid** caused by conversion of muscle purines to uric acid. Renal failure may further increase uric acid.
- **Calcium** from muscle
- **Phosphorus**, probably from muscle. Renal failure may further increase phosphate.

6. In patients with myoglobinuria (acute rhabdomyolysis), the following blood test results may be decreased:

- **Serum urea nitrogen:creatinine ratio** (<10:1) because creatine from injured muscles is rapidly converted into creatinine
- **Calcium** (early) followed by increased calcium (later). Possible deposition of calcium in damaged muscle tissue.

BIBLIOGRAPHY

Britton JP, Dowell AC, Whelan P: Dipstick hematuria and bladder cancer in men over 60: Results of a community study. BMJ 299:1010, 1989.

Discusses hematuria in men with bladder cancer.

Connelly JE: Microscopic hematuria. *In* Panzer RJ, Black ER, Griner PF (eds): Diagnostic Strategies for Common Medical Problems. Philadelphia, American College of Physicians, 1991, p 412.
Recommends strategies for diagnosing the cause of microscopic hematuria.

Culclasure TF, Bray VJ, Hasbargen JA: The significance of hematuria in the anticoagulated patient. Arch Intern Med 154:649, 1994.
Hematuria should not be attributed solely to anticoagulation. Regardless of the prothrombin time, it may indicate significant disease.

Fracchia JA, Motta J, Miller LS, et al: Evaluation of asymptomatic microhematuria. Urology 46:484, 1995.
Refined urine diagnostic assays may be less invasive and less expensive than a standard urologic evaluation.

Gambrell RC, Blount BW: Exercise-induced hematuria. Am Fam Physician 53:905, 1996.
Exercise-induced hematuria is a common, benign condition that should not restrict activity.

Gleeson MJ, Connolly J, Grainger R, et al: Comparison of reagent strip (dipstick) and microscopic hematuria in urological outpatients. Br J Urol 72:594, 1993.
A positive urine dipstick test, despite negative microscopy, may be a clue to an unsuspected urinary tract neoplasm.

Kasinath BS, Stein JH: Sifting the causes of microscopic hematuria. Hosp Pract 31:99, 1996.
Diagnosis is facilitated when hematuria is accompanied by other findings; isolated hematuria presents a more complex challenge.

Laios ID, Caruk R, Wu AHB: Myoglobin clearance as an early indicator for rhabdomyolysis-induced acute renal failure. Ann Clin Lab Sci 25:179, 1995.
The myoglobin clearance ratio may be useful in evaluating patients with rhabdomyolysis for the risk of development of acute renal failure.

Lam MH: False "hematuria" due to bacteriuria. Arch Pathol Lab Med 119:717, 1995.
Bacteriuria can cause a false-positive urine dipstick test due to the presence of microbial peroxidase.

McCarthy JJ: Outpatient evaluation of hematuria: Locating the source of bleeding. Postgrad Med 101:125, 1997.
Discusses the evaluation of patients with red or brown discolorations of the urine.

Paola AS: Hematuria: Essentials of diagnosis. Hosp Pract 25:144, 1990.
Describes differential diagnosis of hematuria.

Sutton JM: Evaluation of hematuria in adults. JAMA 263:2475, 1990.
Gives an approach to adults with hematuria.

Thompson WG: Things that go red in the urine; and others that don't. Lancet 347:5, 1996.
Fourteen percent of people have red urine and feces after consuming beets.

Topham PS, Harper SJ, Furness PN, et al: Glomerular disease as a cause of isolated microscopic hematuria. Q J Med 87:329, 1994.
Gives recommendations for the work-up of patients with microscopic hematuria.

What urine color tells you. Emerg Med 20:155, 1988.
Describes a way to determine the cause of different colored urines: brown or black, yellow or orange, colorless or milky, and blue or green.

• •

URINARY TRACT INFECTION IN WOMEN

Recommendations for urinary tract infection (UTI) in women are from the medical literature.

1. For women with clinical findings of a lower UTI, request a urinalysis. If the clinical findings suggest pyelonephritis (fever, rigors, nausea, vomiting, flank pain, costovertebral angle tenderness), obtain a urinalysis and a urine Gram stain and culture.

   **Patients with findings of lower UTI and possible subclinical pyelo-
nephritis (pregnancy, underlying urinary tract disease, diabetes mellitus, immunosuppression, symptoms for more than 7 days, three or
more UTIs in the past year, history of pyelonephritis, recent use of
antibiotics, poor city neighborhood) should have a urine Gram stain
and culture and a urinalysis.**
   **For sexually active patients with possible chlamydial or gonococ-
cal urethritis, request a urinalysis and obtain a Gram stain and
culture of urethral (or cervical os) discharge. Urethritis in the sexual
partner, a new sexual partner, or mucopurulent endocervical secretions are suggestive findings.**
   **For women with findings of vaginitis (dysuria, itching, discharge,
"fishy" odor), obtain a sample of the vaginal discharge for microscopic examination and possible culture.**

   Because the decision to treat a lower UTI is based on the presence
of pyuria rather than bacteriuria, only a urinalysis is required when
the clinical findings (e.g., dysuria, urgency, and frequency) are limited
to the lower urinary tract.
   Because false-negative results with the urine dipstick nitrite test
can occur when the urine has not been retained in the bladder long
enough for gram-negative bacteria to reduce nitrates in the urine to
nitrites, a first-morning urine specimen is best. Other causes of a false-
negative nitrite test result are deficient dietary nitrate and a urinary
ascorbic acid concentration greater than 75 mg/dL (>4.28 mmol/L).
Factors that can influence test results include hydration (is patient
forcing fluids?), urinary pH, antibiotics, and other drugs.
   Specimens for gonococcal culture should include cervical and
urethral swabs, and the rectum may also be sampled. Maximal recovery of *Chlamydia* is achieved by culture of both cervix and urethra.
These specimens should be collected with synthetic fiber swabs because wooden shafts and calcium alginate swabs are toxic to *Chlamydia* and to a lesser extent to gonococci. Chlamydial cultures require
immediate inoculation of the specimen into a suitable transport medium such as 2SP. Specimens for gonococci taken in a physician's
office should be cultured immediately and placed in an incubator at
95°F (35°C) in 5 to 10% carbon dioxide, and these cultures should be
incubated overnight before being sent to a laboratory for analysis.
Newer tests for *Chlamydia* and *Neisseria* are available, such as the
nucleic acid probe and ligase chain reaction.
   Microscopic examination using a drop of 10% potassium hydroxide to dissolve cellular material is useful to identify the pseudohyphae
and budding forms of *Candida*; a Gram stain is also helpful. A wet
mount of fresh discharge with a drop of warm normal saline solution
can be prepared to identify the motile flagellated *Trichomonas* and
"clue" cells, which are bacilli within epithelial cells often present in
patients with *Gardnerella vaginalis* (formerly *Haemophilus vaginalis*).
Cultures are necessary to diagnose the rare cases of purulent vaginitis
from gonorrhea.

After collection, the urine specimen should be promptly (within 20 minutes) cultured or refrigerated if culture is delayed. The presence of one or more Gram-stained bacterial cells per oil immersion field in at least five fields correlates with more than 100,000 colony forming units/mL—a very useful test in the office or clinic setting.

2. Evaluate the test results.

The most common pathogens in lower urinary tract bacterial infection or subclinical pyelonephritis in women are *Escherichia coli*, other gram-negative enteric bacteria, *Staphylococcus saprophyticus*, and enterococci.

Whenever mixed bacterial species are grown on culture, the likelihood of contamination is high. Moreover, *Staphylococcus epidermidis*, diphtheroids, and lactobacilli are commonly found in the distal urethra and rarely cause infection. If contamination is suspected and culture results are still important, the culture should be repeated.

3. Interpret pyuria, Gram stains, and urine cultures in the context of the clinical findings.

Until recently, the colony count was regarded as the "gold standard" for determining the presence of a real and treatable UTI. Now it appears that there is no single "gold standard" and that the urine bacterial colony count cannot stand alone for diagnosing UTI. It must be evaluated together with other clinical and laboratory data.

Lower Urinary Tract Infection

In patients with findings of lower UTI, the presence of pyuria justifies giving immediate therapy, whereas the absence of pyuria justifies withholding therapy or suspecting vaginitis as a cause. Pyuria is present in 90 to 95% of patients with lower UTI and colony counts greater than 100,000 bacteria/mL of urine, in 70% of patients with lower UTI and colony counts of 100 to 100,000 bacteria/mL, and in only 1% of asymptomatic nonbacteriuric patients. If the patient has pyuria without bacteriuria (by examination of unstained sediment), consider the possibility of chlamydial urethritis, gonococcal urethritis, or urinary infection with gram-positive cocci. Lower UTI caused by yeasts *(Candida* species, *Torulopsis)* may also exhibit pyuria. Urinary tract yeast infections occur more commonly in diabetics.

Pyelonephritis

In patients with findings of acute pyelonephritis or subclinical pyelonephritis, urinalysis typically shows pyuria with possible proteinuria, hematuria, and casts. A urine Gram stain and culture are necessary to isolate the responsible organism and identify the pattern of antibacterial sensitivities. Usually, but not always, the colony count is greater than 100,000 bacteria/mL of urine.

Chlamydial Urethritis

Urethral infection with *Chlamydia trachomatis* accounts for 2 to 20% of cases of acute dysuria in women. The urinalysis shows pyuria without bacteriuria. Hematuria is very unusual, as is proteinuria. Routine urine culture does not isolate *C. trachomatis* and often is negative for other organisms. A variety of methods are available for the laboratory diagnosis of *C. trachomatis*. Of these, culture and nucleic acid probe (sensitivity 60 to 90%) are commonly used. Recently, a urine test, the ligase chain reaction was introduced which, compared with culture, has a sensitivity of 93%.

Gonococcal Urethritis

Neisseria gonorrhoeae typically produces pyuria. Gram stain shows gram-negative intracellular diplococci, and culture on Thayer-Martin or New York City medium isolates the organism. Positive Gram stains of cervical discharge are suggestive but not diagnostic of gonococci. These Gram stains should be interpreted with caution if vaginal epithelial cells are present because anaerobic gram-negative bacteria and coccobacillary bacteria can resemble gonococci. *N. gonorrhoeae* can also be detected with a nucleic acid probe (sensitivity 97%). Recently, a urine test, the ligase chain reaction was introduced which, compared with culture, has a sensitivity of 97 to 100%.

Other Urethral Infections

Urethritis may also be caused by herpes simplex virus, *Trichomonas vaginalis*, and *Candida albicans*. Herpes simplex and *T. vaginalis* produce pyuria, but candidal infection may not.

Vaginitis

Patients with vaginitis may have dysuria (plus frequency and urgency) as their chief complaint. Typically, pyuria is absent except when trichomonal infection involves both the urethra and the vagina. Microscopic examination of the abnormal discharge may reveal budding yeast and pseudohyphae, trichomonads, and clue cells.

Asymptomatic Women with Bacteriuria

The value of identifying asymptomatic bacteriuria (>100,000 bacteria/mL) in asymptomatic, nonpregnant women is controversial. Asymptomatic bacteriuria has been correlated with an increased mortality rate in the elderly, but no evidence indicates that treatment alters the rate. Asymptomatic bacteriuria in pregnant women must be treated because therapy reduces the occurrence of acute pyelonephritis and possibly low-birth-weight babies. Therefore, pregnant women should have regular urinalyses in the prenatal period, with urine cultures if pyuria is noted.

Symptomatic Women without Pyuria

Many women with dysuria have no pyuria, have no recognized pathogen, and do not respond to antimicrobial treatment. These women should have a urinalysis and urine culture. In these women, consider the possibility of urethral inflammation from physical or chemical agents or from trauma.

BIBLIOGRAPHY

Arav-Boger R, Leibovici L, Danon YL: Urinary tract infections with low and high colony counts in young women. Arch Intern Med 154:300, 1994.
  Urinary tract infections with low colony counts frequently progress over several days. Decisions about the duration of therapy should not be guided by the colony count.
Bickley LS: Acute vaginitis. *In* Panzer RJ, Black ER, Griner PF (eds): Diagnostic Strategies for Common Medical Problems. Philadelphia, American College of Physicians, 1991, p 249.
  Recommends diagnostic strategies for acute vaginitis.
Cook RL, Reid G, Pond DG, et al: Clue cells in bacterial vaginosis: Immunofluorescent identification of the adherent Gram-negative bacteria as *Gardnerella vaginalis*. J Infect Dis 160:490, 1989.
  Recent study of clue cells in bacterial vaginosis.
Johnson JR, Stamm WE: Urinary tract infections in women: Diagnosis and treatment. Ann Intern Med 111:906, 1989.
  Reviews recent developments in the diagnosis and management of these infections.
Komaroff AL: Acute dysuria in adult women. *In* Panzer RJ, Black ER, Griner PF (eds): Diagnostic Strategies for Common Medical Problems. Philadelphia, American College of Physicians, 1991, p 239.
  Recommends diagnostic strategies for acute dysuria in women.
Komaroff AL: Urinalysis and urine culture in women with dysuria. *In* Sox HC Jr (ed): Common Diagnostic Tests: Use and Interpretation, 2nd ed. Philadelphia, American College of Physicians, 1990, p 286.
  Good review of the use of urinalysis and urine culture for diagnosing dysuria in women.
Kunin CM: Urinary Tract Infections: Detection, Prevention, and Management, 5th ed. Baltimore, Williams & Wilkins, 1997.
  Good reference text for UTIs.
Kunin CM, White LV, Hua TH: A reassessment of the importance of "low-count" bacteriuria in young women with acute urinary symptoms. Ann Intern Med 119:454, 1993.
  Low-count bacteriuria appears to be common and clinically significant in symptomatic

young women. It may reflect an early phase of infection, possibly localized to the urethra.

Pappas PG: Laboratory in the diagnosis and management of urinary tract infections. Med Clin North Am 75:313, 1991.
Discusses the use of laboratory tests to diagnose UTIs.

Sobel JD: Vaginitis. N Engl J Med 337:1896, 1997.
Neither self-diagnosis nor diagnosis by a physician is reliable without laboratory confirmation.

Wright RA, Blum R: Infectious disease update: Diagnostic imperatives for urinary tract infection. Mod Med 58:46, 1990.
Describes the use of the urine dipstick, examination of the urinary sediment, and in-office culture kits.

ACUTE RENAL FAILURE

Recommendations for acute renal failure are from the medical literature.

1. In patients with clinical findings of acute renal failure, document azotemia by measuring serum urea nitrogen and creatinine.

Clinical findings are nonspecific, such as weight gain and edema. Azotemia is characterized by high serum urea nitrogen and creatinine concentrations. If the renal failure occurs suddenly, over a period of days to weeks, it is acute. If it occurs slowly, over a period of months to years, it is chronic. Division of renal failure into acute and chronic varieties is helpful in arriving at the cause because acute and chronic renal failure have distinct differential diagnoses.

Acute azotemia may be caused by prerenal, renal, or postrenal conditions. Prerenal failure is characterized by azotemia secondary to inadequate perfusion of the kidneys and is reversible within 24 hours if the systemic cause of the renal hypoperfusion is corrected. Postrenal failure is characterized by azotemia resulting from mechanical obstruction distal to the kidneys; in this case renal function may be restored or improved if the obstruction is removed. Renal azotemia is a diagnosis of exclusion. First, prerenal and postrenal causes of azotemia must be excluded; then the exact cause of the renal disease must be determined. Causes of acute renal azotemia include ischemic disorders, nephrotoxicities, diseases of glomeruli and small blood vessels, and diseases of major renal blood vessels.

2. If azotemia is present, request the following studies to help determine its cause: complete blood count; serum sodium, potassium, chloride, bicarbonate, calcium, magnesium, phosphorus, and uric acid; and urinary volume, sediment, osmolality, sodium, urea nitrogen, and creatinine.

Prerenal and postrenal causes of acute renal failure must be vigorously excluded before the diagnosis can be assumed to be intrinsic renal disease, for which immediate specific treatment is only rarely available.

3. Use clinical findings plus serum and urinary test results to diag-

nose postrenal and prerenal causes of acute renal failure. Intrinsic renal disease is a diagnosis of exclusion.

If the laboratory tests establish the presence of acute azotemia (a sudden increase of serum creatinine greater than 2 mg/dL [>177 μmol/L] and urea nitrogen greater than 25 mg/dL [>8.9 mmol/L]), the next step is to exclude a postrenal cause and prerenal cause. A postrenal cause can be excluded by ruling out obstructive uropathy; a prerenal cause can be excluded by clinical information, radiographic studies, and the use of urinary indices as shown below:

Index	Prerenal	Acute Tubular Injury
Urinary osmolality, mOsm/kg water	>500	<350
Urinary sodium (Na), mEq/L	<20	>40
Urinary/plasma creatinine ratio	>40	<20
Fractional sodium excretion*	<1	>1

$$* \frac{\text{Urine/serum (Na)}}{\text{Urine/serum (creatinine)}} \times 100$$

Source: Mitch WE: Acute renal failure. *In* Bennett JC, Plum F (eds): Cecil Textbook of Medicine, 20th ed. Philadelphia, WB Saunders, 1996, p 553.

A postrenal cause for acute azotemia may be excluded by working up the patient for an enlarged prostate, palpable bladder, large residual urinary volume, hydronephrotic kidneys, ureteral obstruction, and a history of renal calculi. Usually no urinary sediment abnormalities are found with postrenal azotemia; however, the sediment may contain white blood cells and RBCs in infected patients. Patients with urinary tract obstruction have urinary indices that are indistinguishable from those of patients with prerenal failure (in patients with obstructions lasting more than 2 days in duration, the indices are similar to those seen with intrarenal tubular injury). If an obstruction is found and if it is relieved, a brisk diuresis ensues, which can be as high as 6 to 8 L/hr. Salt and water losses can be significant and, if not replaced, can result in shock. Hypokalemia can occur.

A prerenal cause for acute azotemia (i.e., volume depletion, congestive heart failure, or severe liver disease) can be excluded by the clinical context and by measuring serum and urine analytes and computing indices.

A rising serum creatinine level greater than 2.5 mg/dL (>221 μmol/L) strongly suggests established renal failure as opposed to prerenal azotemia. The urea nitrogen:creatinine ratio is usually about 10:1 in patients with renal parenchymal disease but is greater than 15:1 in patients with prerenal azotemia and urinary tract obstruction. Urinary sediment abnormalities, except for hyaline casts, are usually not found with prerenal azotemia. In acute azotemia due to renal failure, urinary sediment findings may be helpful; for example, hematuria, proteinuria, red cell casts, and granular casts suggest acute glomerulonephritis.

BIBLIOGRAPHY

Frazee LA, Rutecki GW, Whittier FC: Drug-induced acute renal failure: Recognizing and treating prerenal, postrenal, and pseudorenal injury. Consultant 37:1265, 1997.
Angiotensin-converting enzyme inhibitors and nonsteroidal anti-inflammatory drugs are among the drugs most commonly associated with acute renal failure.

Levin ML: Acute renal failure. *In* Conn RB, Borer WZ, Snyder JW (eds): Current Diagnosis, 9th ed. Philadelphia, WB Saunders, 1997, p 1074.
Describes a diagnostic approach to acute renal failure.

Levy EM, Viscoli CM, Horwitz RI: The effect of acute renal failure on mortality. JAMA 275:1489, 1996.
Renal failure appears to increase the risk of developing severe non-renal complications that lead to death.

Martinez-Maldonado M, Kumjian DA: Acute renal failure due to urinary tract obstruction. Med Clin North Am 74:919, 1990.
Reviews the causes of acute renal failure due to obstruction.

Thadhani R, Pascual M, Bonventre JV: Acute renal failure. N Engl J Med 334:1448, 1996. Simonds RJ, Rogers M: Acute renal failure: A dangerous condition. JAMA 275:1516, 1996.
Reviews the diagnosis and management of acute renal failure.

8

Endocrine and Metabolic Diseases

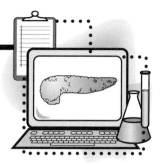

- Hyperthyroidism and Hypothyroidism
- Diabetes Mellitus
- Gestational Diabetes Mellitus
- True Hypoglycemia and the Idiopathic Postprandial Syndrome
- Cushing's Syndrome
- Adrenal Insufficiency

HYPERTHYROIDISM AND HYPOTHYROIDISM

Recommendations for hyperthyroidism and hypothyroidism are from the medical literature. The College of American Pathologists and others have identified groups at risk for thyroid dysfunction.

1. For patients with clinical findings of hyperthyroidism or hypothyroidism or if you wish to screen for these diseases, request a sensitive thyrotropin (S-TSH) test. This strategy is effective for ambulatory patients without pituitary or neuropsychiatric disease. Hospitalized patients may have changes in S-TSH due to stress, nonthyroidal illness, or drug therapy, and increases are more common than decreases. Decreased S-TSH levels may occur secondary to dopamine and glucocorticoid therapy and in terminally ill patients. Individuals at risk for thyroid dysfunction include the following:

- Patients with autoimmune disease
- Persons with a first-degree relative with thyroid disease
- Patients with a history of neck surgery or radiation
- Women over 50 years of age seeking medical care
- All patients entering a geriatric unit at admission and every 5 years thereafter
- Any adult aged 50 years or older who visits a medical facility complaining of anything other than minor transitory ailments
- All adults with newly discovered dyslipidemia

Clinical findings of hyperthyroidism include hyperactivity, sweating, fatigue, heat intolerance, nervousness, palpitations, tremor, frequent stools, weight loss despite a good appetite, tachycardia, proptosis, lid lag, and hyperreflexia. Findings of hypothyroidism include cold intolerance, lethargy, constipation, weight gain, hair loss, dry skin, bradycardia, and hyporeflexia.

2. Evaluate the tests.

First-generation S-TSH assays can measure to 1.0 μU/mL (1.0 mU/L); second-generation (sensitive) assays to 0.1 μU/mL (0.1 mU/L); and third-generation (ultrasensitive) assays to 0.01 μU/mL (0.01 mU/L).

PATIENTS WITHOUT PITUITARY OR NEUROPSYCHIATRIC DISEASE SENSITIVE (SECOND-GENERATION) TSH (μU/mL [mU/L])*

<0.10	0.10–0.29	0.30–5.00	5.10–7.00	>7.00
Hyperthyroid suspect	Borderline hyperthyroid	No metabolic thyroid disease	Borderline hypothyroid	Hypothyroid suspect

*One may wish to start with an ultrasensitive third-generation assay.
Source: Adapted from: Klee GG, Hay ID: Role of thyrotropin measurements in the diagnosis and management of thyroid disease. Clin Lab Med 13:673, 1993.

3. Interpret test results in the context of clinical findings as follows:

This S-TSH testing strategy has some limitations, especially for patients with pituitary disease. Fortunately, such patients are rare. Patients with pituitary tumors that produce TSH generally have multiple endocrine abnormalities and have increased S-TSH levels with hyperthyroidism. Patients with pituitary resection or ablation have decreased S-TSH levels with hypothyroidism.

a. Normal S-TSH
If the S-TSH level is within the reference range, the patient is euthyroid and no further testing is indicated.
b. Borderline hyperthyroidism: S-TSH 0.10 to 0.29 μU/mL (0.10–0.29 mU/L)
Measure free T_4. If free T_4 is not elevated, consider ordering free T_3. Perform a thyrotropin-releasing hormone (TRH) test or follow the patient.
c. Suspect hyperthyroidism: S-TSH less than 0.10 μU/mL (<0.10 mU/L)
Measure free T_4 and a third-generation (ultrasensitive) S-TSH. If free T_4 is not elevated, consider measuring free T_3. If hyperthyroidism is probable, consider ^{131}I uptake.
d. Borderline hypothyroidism: S-TSH 5.10 to 7.00 μU/mL (5.10–7.00 mU/L)
Measure free T_4 and thyroid antibodies. If the patient has hypothyroid symptoms, evaluate hypothyroidism and consider T_4 replacement. If the patient has no hypothyroid symptoms, repeat the S-TSH in 1 year.

e. Suspect hypothyroidism: S-TSH greater than 7.00 μU/ml (>7.00 mU/L)
Measure free T_4 and thyroid antibodies. If the clinical and laboratory findings are consistent, evaluate for hypothyroidism and consider T_4 replacement therapy.

4. In the hyperthyroid patient, the following additional blood test results may be increased:

- **Erythrocyte sedimentation rate**
- **Glucose** from accelerated glycogenolysis secondary to increased catecholamines
- **Urea nitrogen and creatinine** associated with excessive protein catabolism
- **Sodium** caused by hypercalcemic diabetes insipidus
- **Calcium** due to bone dissolution by osteoclasts
- **Phosphorus** with increased bone dissolution and increased renal reabsorption
- **Alkaline phosphatase** from stimulation of osteoclasts by thyroid hormones
- **Bilirubin** caused by hemolysis

5. In the hyperthyroid patient, the following additional blood test results may be decreased:

- **Partial pressure of oxygen (Po_2)**
- **Partial pressure of carbon dioxide (Pco_2)** with respiratory alkalosis
- **Mild anemia**, typically normocytic
- **Moderate neutropenia**
- **Idiopathic thrombocytopenic purpura** in Graves' disease and Hashimoto's thyroiditis
- **Potassium**, possible periodic paralysis
- **Magnesium**
- **Amylase** in thyrotoxicosis
- **Albumin**, possibly related to rapid turnover
- **Bilirubin** related to decreased red blood cell mass and low albumin
- **Cholesterol and triglycerides**

6. In the hypothyroid patient, the following additional blood test results may be increased:

- **Erythrocyte sedimentation rate**
- **Glucose**
- **Slightly high creatinine, urea nitrogen, and uric acid**, which are related to lower glomerular filtration and which return to normal with replacement therapy; uric acid is frequently high and may lead to attacks of gout.
- **Bicarbonate** related to increased CO_2
- **Calcium**

- **Magnesium**
- **Creatine kinase, aspartate aminotransferase, and lactate dehydrogenase** caused by skeletal muscle myopathy
- **Albumin**
- **Cholesterol**
- **Triglyceride**

7. In the hypothyroid patient, the following additional blood test results may be decreased:

- **Anemia, mild and typically normocytic, but may be macrocytic;** sometimes pernicious anemia with Hashimoto's thyroiditis
- **Po$_2$** with dyspnea secondary to pleural effusion
- **Sodium**, with or without the inappropriate antidiuretic hormone syndrome; may also be caused by psuedohyponatremia associated with hyperlipidemia
- **Alkaline phosphatase** caused by low osteoblastic activity
- **Ferritin**, presumably because of low protein turnover

8. If you diagnose hypothyroidism and decide to treat the patient with thyroid replacement hormone, measure S-TSH to monitor therapy 2 to 6 months after the full replacement dose is achieved.

In one study, more than one half of the elevated S-TSH values were attributed to non-compliance, and the S-TSH values normalized on subsequent visits without a change of T_4 dosage. So, be sure to consider the issue of noncompliance before changing T_4 dosages.

BIBLIOGRAPHY

Bauer DC, Brown AN: Sensitive thyrotropin and free thyroxine testing in outpatients. Arch Intern Med 156:2333, 1996.
> *Use the S-TSH test for outpatients and save 20% of costs by eliminating free T_4 tests when S-TSH results are normal.*
Behnia M, Gharib H: Primary care diagnosis of thyroid disease. Hosp Pract 31:121, 1996.
> *Recommends guidelines for thyroid tests, beginning with an S-TSH assay.*
Braverman LE, Dworkin HJ, MacIndoe JH II: Thyroid disease: When to screen, when to treat. Patient Care 31:18, 1997.
> *Discusses diagnosis and management.*
Brody MB, Reichard RA: Thyroid screening: How to interpret and apply the results. Postgrad Med 98:54, 1995.
> *The ultrasensitive third-generation assay for thyrotropin is now the gold standard for measuring thyroid activity.*
Burnett JR, Crooke MJ, Delahunt JW, et al: Serum enzymes in hypothyroidism. N Z Med J 107:355, 1994.
> *Three patients without clinically apparent hypothyroidism had elevations in the serum enzymes creatine kinase, aspartate aminotransferase, and lactate dehydrogenase at 10 to 15, 2 to 6, and 2 to 3 times the upper reference limits, respectively.*
Check W: Polishing thyroid testing practices. CAP Today 11:1, 1997.
> *A sensitive TSH assay, also called a second-generation TSH assay, is typically defined as one that measures TSH to a lower limit of 0.1 μU/mL (mU/L) with a coefficient of variation of 20% or less.*
Costa AJ: Interpreting thyroid tests. Am Fam Physician 52:2325, 1995.

Provides an update on laboratory tests used to diagnose common thyroid disorders and also provides a practical framework for interpreting test results.

Danese MD, Powe NR, Sawin CT, et al: Screening for mild thyroid failure at the periodic health examination: A decision and cost-effectiveness analysis. JAMA 276:285, 1996.
A reasonable case for using a low threshold for serum TSH screening, or perhaps even adopting treatment of mild thyroid failure as routine therapy for patients aged 35 and older.

Dayan CM, Daniels GH: Chronic autoimmune thyroiditis. N Engl J Med 335:99, 1996.
Reviews the diagnosis and management of chronic autoimmune thyroiditis.

Felicetta JV: The aging thyroid: Its effects—and how it affects diagnosis and therapy. Consultant 36:837, 1996.
Hypothyroidism, common in older persons, raises cholesterol and triglyceride levels; hyperthyroidism may be masked by the severity of the cardiac problems it causes.

Hayward RSA, Steinberg EP, Ford DE, et al: Preventive care guidelines: 1991. Ann Intern Med 114:758, 1991.
Recommendations about wellness screening using thyroid function testing.

Helfand M, Crapo LM: Testing for suspected thyroid disease. *In* Sox HC Jr (ed): Common Diagnostic Tests: Use and Interpretation, 2nd ed. Philadelphia, American College of Physicians, 1990, p 148.
Reviews the use of thyroid function tests to diagnose thyroid dysfunction.

Kassirer JP, Kopelman RI: Case 5—A hit after a miss. *In* Learning Clinical Reasoning. Baltimore, Williams & Wilkins, 1991, p 63.
Discusses clinical reasoning in the diagnosis and management of a patient with hypothyroidism in whom hypercholesterolemia is the initial clue.

Keffer JH: Thyroid function testing: Toward efficiency and effectiveness. Arch Pathol Lab Med 120:913, 1996.
  Valenstein P, Shifman RB: Duplicate laboratory orders: A College of American Pathologists Q-Probes study of thyrotropin requests in 502 institutions. Arch Pathol Lab Med 120:917, 1996.
Reviews the S-TSH testing strategy and the issue of duplicate S-TSH tests.

Klee GC, Hay ID: Role of thyrotropin measurements in the diagnosis and management of thyroid disease. Clin Lab Med 13:673, 1993.
Recommends a strategy based on S-TSH testing.

Lazarus JH: Hyperthyroidism. Lancet 349:339, 1997.
Reviews the diagnosis and management of hyperthyroidism.

LeMar HJ Jr, West SG, Garrett CR, et al: Covert hypothyroidism presenting as a cardiovascular event. Am J Med 91:549, 1991.
Increased creatine kinase concentration may be a clue to hypothyroidism in patients with cardiovascular findings.

Lindsay RS, Toft AD: Hypothyroidism. Lancet 349:413, 1997.
Reviews the diagnosis and management of hypothyroidism.

Masters PA, Simons RJ: Clinical use of sensitive assays for thyroid-stimulating hormone. J Gen Intern Med 11:115, 1996.
Reviews the optimal use of S-TSH assays by clinicians.

Pittman JG: Evaluation of patients with mildly abnormal thyroid function tests. Am Fam Physician 54:961, 1996.
Subclinical hypothyroidism, subclinical hyperthyroidism, and the sick euthyroid syndrome are three conditions that can be effectively assessed using newer tests.

Sawin CT: Thyroid dysfunction in older persons. Adv Intern Med 37:223, 1991.
Discusses the problem of undiagnosed or misdiagnosed thyroid disease in the elderly.

Sundbeck G, Jagenburg R, Johansson P-M, et al: Clinical significance of low serum thyrotropin concentration by chemiluminometric assay in 85-year-old women and men. Arch Intern Med 151:549, 1991.
Approximately 2% of elderly asymptomatic persons have low TSH levels with new sensitive assays, but the majority of these patients are not hyperthyroid.

Suzuki S, Ichikawa K, Nagai M, et al: Elevation of serum creatine kinase during treatment with antithyroid drugs in patients with hyperthyroidism due to Graves' disease. Arch Intern Med 157:693, 1997.
Describes four patients with Graves' disease who had abnormal increases of serum creatine kinase concentrations during treatment with antithyroid medications.

Symposium on sensitive TSH assays: Introduction, Parts I, II, and III. Mayo Clin Proc
   63:1026, 1988.
   Reviews the role of S-TSH assays in patient care.
Woeber KA: Subclinical thyroid dysfunction. Arch Intern Med 157:1065, 1997.
   *Subclinical thyroid dysfunction may be defined as an abnormal serum thyrotropin
   concentration in an asymptomatic patient with a normal serum free thyroxine concen-
   tration.*
Wynne AG, Gharib H, Scheithauer BW, et al: Hyperthyroidism due to inappropriate
   secretion of the thyrotropin in 10 patients. Am J Med 92:15, 1992.
   Reports 10 cases of secondary hyperthyroidism from the Mayo Clinic.

DIABETES MELLITUS

Recommendations for diabetes mellitus are from the American Diabetes Association and are agreed to by other groups.

**1. Screen all asymptomatic adults aged 45 and older and all younger
individuals with risk factors by measuring the fasting serum glucose
concentration after a fast (at least 8 hr). A value greater than 126
mg/dL (>6.99 mmol/L) is diagnostic and must be confirmed by repeating the test on another day. Values between 110 and 125 mg/dL
(6.11 to 6.94 mmol/L) indicate impairment, and values less than
110 mg/dL (<6.11 mmol/L) are considered normal. Hemoglobin A_{1c}
(HbA_{1c}) measurement is not currently recommended for the diagnosis of diabetes. Follow-up individuals with impaired glucose levels
and encourage them to lose weight, exercise, stop smoking, and treat
hypertension, if present. Individuals at risk for diabetes mellitus
include the following:**

- Those who are obese (more than 20% over desirable body weight)
- Those who have a close relative with diabetes
- Members of high-risk groups like African Americans, Hispanics,
  and Native Americans
- Women who have delivered a baby weighing more than 9 pounds
  or who have been given a diagnosis of gestational diabetes
- Those who have high blood pressure, 140/90 mm Hg or higher
- Those with low levels of high-density lipoprotein cholesterol (35
  mg/dL [0.91 mmol/L] or lower) or high triglyceride levels (250 mg/
  dL [2.83 mmol/L] or higher)
- Those who on previous testing had impaired glucose tolerance or
  impaired fasting glucose

**2. In patients with obvious features of diabetes mellitus such as
rapid weight loss, polyuria, polydypsia, and ketonuria, immediately
measure serum glucose—fasting or nonfasting. A value of equal to
or greater than 200 mg/dL (≥11.0 mmol/L) is diagnostic of diabetes.**

  A 2-hour postprandial glucose level equal to or greater than 200
mg/dL (≥11.0 mmol/L) during an oral glucose tolerance test using
the equivalent of 75 g of glucose dissolved in water is also diagnostic
of diabetes, but this test is not recommended for routine use. A
diagnostic test result should be confirmed by repeat testing on another day. The tolerance test is more sensitive for diagnosis than the
fasting test.

The oral glucose tolerance test may be compromised if the protocol is not closely followed and the results correctly interpreted. It may be more convenient to perform the oral glucose tolerance test in the morning after the person has fasted at least 8 hours. The individual should not be ill or taking a medication known to affect the blood sugar and should have had normal physical activity and carbohydrate intake greater than 150 grams/day for at least 3 days before the test. The individual should remain seated and should not eat, smoke, or drink coffee, tea, or alcohol during the test. First, draw a fasting blood glucose sample, and afterward give 75 grams of glucose orally. A 2-hour value less than 140 mg/dL (<7.8 mmol/L) is normal, and a value greater than 140 mg/dL (>7.8 mmol/L) and less than 200 mg/dL (<11.0 mmol/L indicates impaired glucose tolerance.

The following drugs and chemical agents are known to affect glucose tolerance:

- **Diuretics and antihypertensive agents:** chlorthalidone, clonidine, diazoxide, flurosemide, thiazides
- **Hormonally active agents:** corticotropin, glucagon, glucocorticoids, oral contraceptives, somatotropin, thyroid hormones
- **Psychoactive agents:** Chlorprothixene, haloperidol, lithium carbonate, phenothiazines, tricyclic antidepressants
- **Catecholamines and other neurologically active agents:** epinephrine, isoproterenol, levodopa, norepinephrine, phenytoin
- **Analgesic, antipyretic, and anti-inflammatory agents**
- **Antineoplastic agents:** alloxan, L-asparaginase, streptozocin
- **Miscellaneous agents:** encainide, isoniazid, nicotinic acid

3. Evaluate the tests.

Use a laboratory with an accurately standardized glucose method. Enzymatic methods for measuring serum glucose such as hexokinase and glucose oxidase are best because they give the most accurate results. Reduction methods using substances such as ferricyanide and neocuproine are obsolete and tend to overestimate the serum glucose concentration because of non–glucose-reducing substances in the blood. In patients with uremia, serious errors can occur using reduction methods because of overestimation of serum glucose up to 40 mg/dL (2.22 mmol/L) as a result of increased uric acid and creatinine levels. Patients taking vitamin C have erroneously low glucose values when measured with the glucose oxidase method.

4. If the diagnosis of diabetes is confirmed, begin therapy and monitor the patient to include the detection of the six most common complications: uncontrolled diabetes, retinopathy, nephropathy, cardiovascular disease, peripheral vascular disease and neuropathy leading to amputations, and adverse outcomes of pregnancy. Treatment goals are fasting glucose less than 120 mg/dL (<6.66 mmol/L) and HbA$_{1c}$ less than 7%. For an example of guidelines for following these patients, see the schedules developed for the Ohio State University Health Plan.

As indicated in the schedules, regular monitoring of serum glucose and glycated hemoglobin (HbA_{1c}) provides far better identification of patients with poor glycemic control, leading to appropriate changes in therapy. Patients taking insulin should monitor their glucose at home at regular intervals. Patients should be monitored for microalbuminuria and frank proteinuria (see the discussion of proteinuria in Chapter 7).

5. In diabetic patients, the following test results may be increased:

- **Platelets**
- **Urea nitrogen, creatinine, and uric acid** with renal failure
- **Creatinine** due to high glucose and acetone interference with the test
- **Potassium** related to metabolic acidosis
- **Calcium** from hyperalbuminemia with dehydration
- **Phosphorus** caused by glucose intolerance with hyperglycemia
- **Creatine kinase, lactate dehydrogenase, and transaminase levels** caused by effects on skeletal muscle and fatty liver
- **Alkaline phosphatase**
- **Protein and high albumin** caused by dehydration
- **Cholesterol and triglyceride** caused by disturbed carbohydrate metabolism
- **Ferritin**

6. In diabetic patients, the following test results may be decreased:

- **Uric acid** caused by hyperuricosuria
- **Sodium** caused by hyperglycemia
- **Total carbon dioxide** from ketoacidosis
- **Calcium, potassium, sodium, and chloride** from osmotic diuresis caused by hyperglycemia
- **Albumin**

DIABETES MELLITUS TYPE 1 (INSULIN-DEPENDENT) AND TYPE 2 (NON–INSULIN-DEPENDENT) INITIAL AND ONGOING EVALUATION AND CARE: ANNUAL FLOW SHEET AND CARE GUIDELINES

Elements of Care	Initial	Months 3	6	9	12	As Needed
Comprehensive evaluation* (may require frequent contact until stable)	X				X	X
Routine examination; stable patients may require examination only every 6 months		X	X	X		X
Nutrition evaluation and teaching	X				X	X

DIABETES MELLITUS TYPE 1 (INSULIN-DEPENDENT) AND TYPE 2 (NON–INSULIN-DEPENDENT) INITIAL AND ONGOING EVALUATION AND CARE: ANNUAL FLOW SHEET AND CARE GUIDELINES *Continued*

| Elements of Care | Initial | Months | | | | As Needed |
		3	6	9	12	
Eye examination (visual acuity, intraocular pressure, ophthalmic examination through dilated pupil in darkened room)	X				X	X
Foot examination	X	X	X	X	X	X
Dental examination	X		X		X	
Gynecologic examination					X	
Preconception counseling and obstetric care						X
Home glucose monitoring: Continuously 2–8 times per day; record mean glucose at each visit	X	X	X	X	X	
Fasting plasma glucose	X					X
Hemoglobin A$_{1c}$	X	X	X	X	X	
Fasting lipid profile (total cholesterol, high-density lipoproteins, triglycerides)	X				X	X
Electrolytes, hemoglobin and hematocrit, white blood cells, blood urea nitrogen, creatinine	X				X	
Urinalysis per dipstick; protein, ketones, leukocytes, etc.	X	X	X	X	X	
Electrocardiogram	X				X	
24-hr urine albumin and creatinine clearance (5 yrs after diagnosis, then annually)	X				X	X

*According to American Diabetes Association guidelines, annual visit to diabetes specialist is encouraged.

Source: OSU Health Plan Clinical Notes, vol 1, no 3, Spring 1991.

DIABETES MELLITUS TYPE 2 (NON–INSULIN-DEPENDENT) INITIAL AND ONGOING EVALUATION AND CARE: ANNUAL FLOW SHEET AND CARE GUIDELINES

| Elements of Care | Initial | Months | | | | As Needed |
		3	6	9	12	
Comprehensive evaluation* (may require frequent contact until stable)	X				X	X

Table continued on following page

DIABETES MELLITUS TYPE 2 (NON–INSULIN-DEPENDENT) INITIAL AND ONGOING EVALUATION AND CARE: ANNUAL FLOW SHEET AND CARE GUIDELINES *Continued*

Elements of Care	Initial	Months 3	6	9	12	As Needed
Routine examination			X			X
Nutrition evaluation and teaching	X				X	X
Eye examination (visual acuity, intraocular pressure, ophthalmic examination through dilated pupil in darkened room)	X				X	
Foot examination	X		X		X	X
Dental examination	X		X		X	
Gynecologic examination					X	X
Preconception counseling and obstetric care						X
Fasting plasma glucose	X					X
Hemoglobin A$_{1c}$	X		X		X	X
Fasting lipid profile (total cholesterol, high-density lipoproteins, triglycerides)	X				X	X
Electrolytes, hemoglobin and hematocrit, white blood cells, blood urea nitrogen, creatinine	X				X	
Urinalysis per dipstick	X		X		X	
Electrocardiogram (in adults)	X				X	
24-hr urine albumin and creatinine clearance	X				X	

*According to American Diabetes Association guidelines, annual visit to diabetes specialist is encouraged.

Source: OSU Health Plan Clinical Notes, vol 1, no 3, Spring 1991.

BIBLIOGRAPHY

Borch-Johnsen K, Wenzel H, Viberti GC, et al: Is screening and intervention for microalbuminuria worthwhile in patients with insulin-dependent diabetes? BMJ 306:1722, 1993.
   Screening diabetics for albuminuria is cost-effective.
Burge MR, Schade DS: Diabetes mellitus: Managing type II disease. Hosp Pract 31:51, 1996.
   Discusses recommendations for the diagnosis and management of type II disease.
Cohen K: Diabetes mellitus: Practical ways to achieve tight control. Consultant 36:1179, 1996.
   Optimal control of diabetes involves home blood glucose monitoring and—most important—self-adjustment of insulin doses.
Expert Committee on the Diagnosis and Classification of Diabetes Mellitus: Report of the Expert Committee on the diagnosis and classification of diabetes mellitus. Diabetes Care 20:1183, 1997.

Grady D: Newer guidelines redefine diabetes in broader terms. New York Times, June 24, 1997, p A1.
Discusses the new recommendations about the diagnosis and classification of diabetes.

Hayward RSA, Steinberg EP, Ford DE, et al: Preventive care guidelines: 1991. Ann Intern Med 114:758, 1991.
Authoritative recommendations about wellness screening for diabetes mellitus using fasting serum glucose.

Hirsch IB: Glycemic control and complications of diabetes mellitus. West J Med 162:430, 1995.

Grady D: Newer guidelines redefine diabetes in broader terms. New York Times, June 24, 1997, p A1.
Normal or nearly normal serum glucose levels are desirable.

Israngkun PP, Speicher CE: Glucose: Review of methods. Chicago, American Society of Clinical Pathologists, Core chemistry no. PTS 91-3 (PTS-53), 1991.
Extensively reviews methodology for measuring glucose.

Jaspan JB: Taking control of diabetes. Hosp Pract 30:55, 1995.
Strict glycemic control can protect against the complications of diabetes.

Kaye TB, Guay AT, Simonson DC: Non–insulin-dependent diabetes mellitus and elevated serum ferritin level. J Diabetes Complications 7:246, 1993.
Serum ferritin was increased in about one third of patients.

Klein CE, Oboler SK, Prochazka A, et al: Home blood glucose monitoring: Effectiveness in a general population of patients who have non–insulin-dependent diabetes mellitus. J Gen Intern Med 8:597, 1993.
Home blood glucose monitoring has limited value in treating non–insulin-dependent diabetes mellitus in the primary care setting.

Krolewski AJS, Laffel LMB, Krolewski M, et al: Glycosylated hemoglobin and the risk of microalbuminuria in patients with insulin-dependent diabetes mellitus. N Engl J Med 332:1251, 1995.
Maintaining glycated hemoglobin levels below 10.1%—equivalent to HbA_{1c} levels below 8.1%—can reduce the occurrence of microalbuminuria and diabetic nephropathy.

McCance DR, Hanson RL, Charles M-A, et al: Comparison of tests for glycated haemoglobin and fasting and two hour plasma glucose concentrations as diagnostic methods for diabetes. BMJ 21:308, 1994.
Fasting plasma glucose, glycated hemoglobin, and 2-hour postprandial glucose tests perform similarly in detecting diabetes that is destined to produce end-organ complications within 5 years.

Nathan DM: Long-term complications of diabetes mellitus. N Engl J Med 328:1676, 1993.
Reviews the relationship between glycemic control and the long-term complications of diabetes mellitus.

Ohio State Faculty: Diabetes mellitus. Columbus, Ohio State University Health Plan Clinical Notes, vol 1, no 3, Spring 1991.
Medical practice guidelines for diabetes mellitus.

Peters AL, Davidson MB, Schriger DL, et al: A clinical approach for the diagnosis of diabetes mellitus. JAMA 276:1246, 1996.

Stewart M: Will glycosylated haemoglobin replace the oral glucose-tolerance test? Lancet 349:223, 1997.
Measurement of glycated hemoglobin levels may represent a reasonable approach to identifying treatment-requiring diabetes.

Reichard P, Nilsson B-Y, Rosenqvist U: The effect of long-term intensified insulin treatment on the development of microvascular complications of diabetes mellitus. N Engl J Med 329:304, 1993.
The value of tight control in type I diabetes is worthwhile.

Sazama K, Robertson EA, Chesler RA: Is antiglycolysis required for routine glucose analysis? Clin Chem 25:2038, 1979.
Use tubes with fluoride for patients with leukocytosis or when delays longer than 90 minutes are anticipated.

Singer DE, Coley CM, Samet JH, et al: Tests of glycemia in diabetes mellitus: Their use in establishing a diagnosis and in treatment. *In* Sox HC Jr (ed): Common Diagnostic Tests: Use and Interpretation, 2nd ed. Philadelphia, American College of Physicians, 1990, p 121.

Recommendations by the American College of Physicians for using tests to diagnose and manage diabetes mellitus.

Speicher CE: The bottom line: Can portable blood glucose monitoring improve the outcomes of diabetic patients? Am J Clin Pathol 95:112, 1991.
Discussion of the role of portable blood glucose monitoring in the management of diabetes.

Susman JL, Helseth LD: Reducing the complications of type II diabetes: A patient-centered approach. Am Fam Physician 55:471, 1997.
Evidence strongly suggests that improved glycemic control may reduce the morbidity, mortality, and treatment costs of type II diabetes.

Westphal SA, Palumbo PJ: The trouble with glycosylated hemoglobin. Patient Care 29:95, 1995.
Describes situations in which glycated hemoglobin results are falsely elevated.

GESTATIONAL DIABETES MELLITUS

Recommendations for gestational diabetes mellitus are from the American Diabetes Association and the American College of Obstetricians and Gynecologists.

1. Screen all pregnant women for gestational diabetes mellitus between the 24th and 28th weeks of pregnancy with a 50-gram oral glucose load without regard to the time of the last meal or the time of day, and obtain a serum glucose level and a glucose concentration at 1 hour. If a pregnant woman has clinical findings suggestive of diabetes, screen her in the same manner at the time of the initial visit. Gestational diabetes mellitus is defined as glucose intolerance or diabetes mellitus diagnosed for the first time during pregnancy. It occurs in approximately 4% of all pregnancies. However, in certain minority populations, such as Hispanics, African-Americans, and Native Americans, the incidence can run as high as 10 to 12%.

Twenty-four to 28 weeks of pregnancy is the optimal time for screening for gestational diabetes mellitus because at this time its frequency peaks and there is still sufficient time for appropriate therapy. Clinical findings include polyuria, nocturia, polydipsia, recurrent vaginal infections, and failure to gain expected weight. The specimen collection and handling and methodologic considerations are the same as for diagnosing diabetes in nonpregnant individuals.

Other findings that should trigger testing at the first visit include women who (1) are obese or overweight, (2) have diabetes in the family, (3) have had miscarriages or stillbirths without a specific reason, (4) have had a baby that weighed 9 pounds or more (about 4000 grams or more), (5) have had gestational diabetes in a previous pregnancy, (6) have hypertension and/or hyperlipidemia, (7) have had a baby with anomalies, or (8) are 30 years old or more.

Recognition and treatment of gestational diabetes prevent both maternal mortality and morbidity (hypertension, hydramnios, cesarean section) and perinatal mortality and morbidity (intrauterine death, macrosomia, birth trauma, neonatal hypoglycemia, hyperbilirubinemia, hypocalcemia, polycythemia).

2. If the 1-hour serum glucose level is more than 140 mg/dL (7.77 mmol/L), perform the 100-gram pregnancy oral glucose tolerance test.

Perform the oral glucose tolerance test the same way as in screening for diabetes in the nonpregnant individual with these exceptions: give 100 grams of glucose orally instead of 75 grams, and draw blood samples every hour for 3 hours instead of once at 2 hours. The specimen collection concerns are the same as for diabetes mellitus, as discussed in the preceding section.

3. Evaluate the tests and the results.

DIAGNOSTIC ORAL GLUCOSE TOLERANCE TEST IN PREGNANCY

Time	Findings*
Fasting	>105 mg/dL (>5.83 mmol/L)
1 hr	>190 mg/dL (>10.55 mmol/L)
2 hr	>165 mg/dL (>9.16 mmol/L)
3 hr	>145 mg/dL (>8.05 mmol/L)

*Any two or more values exceeding these concentrations are diagnostic.

The methodologic considerations are the same as for diabetes mellitus. Because glucose methodology has changed from reduction methods to more specific enzymatic methods, some authorities advocate revising these criteria levels to fasting, greater than 95 mg/dL (>5.27 mmol/L); 1 hour, greater than 180 mg/dL (>9.99 mmol/L); 2 hours, greater than 155 mg/dL (>8.60 mmol/L); and 3 hours, greater than 140 mg/dL (>7.77 mmol/L).

4. If the oral glucose tolerance test is diagnostic, the patient has gestational diabetes mellitus. Re-examine the patient after the pregnancy, using the strategy for the non-pregnant adult.

After pregnancy terminates, the woman must be re-examined to determine whether she has normal, diabetic, or impaired glucose tolerance. In the majority of patients with gestational diabetes mellitus, glucose tolerance returns to normal after delivery, and the individual can be classified as having a previous abnormality of glucose tolerance. Approximately 40% of women with gestational diabetes mellitus become diabetic within 15 years after delivery, and the risk increases with obesity. Once a woman has had the condition, a 90% probability exists for recurrence with future pregnancies.

5. If the oral glucose tolerance test is not diagnostic of gestational diabetes mellitus but one value is increased, some authorities recommend repeating the test in 3 to 4 weeks.

Up to one third of women having one increased value on the oral glucose tolerance test have a diabetic glucose tolerance test on repeat testing. These women are at increased risk for fetal macrosomia and pre-eclampsia or eclampsia.

BIBLIOGRAPHY

Corcoy R, Cabero L, de Leiva A: Gestational diabetes: What are the implications? Postgrad Med 91:393, 1992.
Discusses gestational diabetes and the merits of screening tests for all pregnant women.
Cousins L, Baxi L, Chez R, et al: Screening recommendations for gestational diabetes mellitus. Am J Obstet Gyecol 165:493, 1991.
Ninety-six percent of maternal-fetal medicine subspecialists and 84% of fellows of the American College of Obstetricians and Gynecologists use these guidelines in their practice.
Davidson JA, Roberts VL: Gestational diabctes: Ensuring a successful outcome. Postgrad Med 99:165, 1996.
Discusses incidence of gestational diabetes and outlines guidelines for testing.
De Veciana M, Major CA, Morgan MA, et al: Postprandial versus preprandial blood glucose monitoring in women with gestational diabetes mellitus requiring insulin therapy. N Engl J Med 333:1237, 1995.
Dornhorst A, Girling JC: Management of gestational diabetes mellitus. N Engl J Med 333:1281, 1995.
Better glycemic control achieved with postprandial monitoring improves short-term outcomes for mothers and infants.
Do gestational diabetes criteria need revision? Emerg Med 24:266, 1992.
Because glucose measurements have changed from reduction methods to enzymatic methods, the criteria need downward revision.
Expert Committee on the Diagnosis and Classification of Diabetes Mellitus: Report of the Expert Committee on the diagnosis and classification of diabetes mellitus. Diabetes Care 20:1183, 1997.
Reviews the diagnosis of gestational diabetes mellitus.
Garner P: Type I diabetes mellitus and pregnancy. Lancet 346:157, 1995.
Patients with insulin-dependent diabetes mellitus are one of the greatest challenges of obstetric medicine.
Gribble RK, Meier PR, Berg RL: The value of urine screening for glucose at each prenatal visit. Obstet Gynecol 86:405, 1995.
Routine urine glucose screening in the third trimester of pregnancy is of questionable value.
Kurishita M, Nakashima K, Kozu H: A retrospective study of glucose metabolism in mothers of large babies. Diabetes Care 17:649, 1994.
Based on high levels of HbA$_{1c}$ reflecting maternal hyperglycemia, a group of women were found who exhibit mild hyperglycemia in late pregnancy with resulting heavy-for-dates infants who are undetected by current antenatal screening tests for gestational diabetes mellitus.
Lewis GF, McNally C, Blackman JD, et al: Prior feeding alters the response to the 50-g glucose challenge test in pregnancy. Diabetes Care 16:1551, 1993.
Prior feeding reduces plasma glucose responses to oral glucose loading for at least 2 hours after a meal and may affect the sensitivity and specificity of the 1 hour 50-gram screening test.
Lindsay MK, Graves W, Klein L: The relationship of one abnormal glucose tolerance test value and pregnancy complications. Obstet Gynecol 73:103, 1989.
Pregnant women with one abnormal value in the oral glucose tolerance test are at increased risk for fetal macrosomia and pre-eclampsia/eclampsia.
McElduff A, Goldring J, Gordon P, et al: A direct comparison of the measurement of a random plasma glucose and a post–50-g glucose load in the detection of gestational diabetes. Aust NZ Obstet Gynecol 34:28, 1994.

Although it is only 85.7% sensitive, data support using the 50-gram glucose load to screen for gestational diabetes.

Naylor CD, Sermer M, Chen E, et al: Selective screening for gestational diabetes mellitus. N Engl J Med 337:1591, 1997.
Consideration of women's clinical characteristics allows efficient selective screening for gestational diabetes.

Naylor CD, Sermer M, Chen E, et al: Cesarean delivery in relation to birth weight and gestational glucose tolerance: Pathophysiology or practice style? JAMA 275:1165, 1996.
Recognition of gestational diabetes mellitus may lead to a lower threshold for surgical delivery that mitigates the potential benefits of treatment.

Neiger R, Coustan DR: The role of repeat glucose tolerance tests in the diagnosis of gestational diabetes. Am J Obstet Gynecol 165:787, 1991.
Suggest repeating the oral glucose tolerance test if one value is abnormal.

Position Statement: Gestational diabetes mellitus. Diabetes Care 14(Suppl 2):5, 1991.
Recommendations of the American Diabetes Association for the screening, diagnosis, and management of gestational diabetes mellitus.

van Turnhout HEW, Lotgering FK, Wallenburg HCS: Poor sensitivity of the 50-g 1 hour glucose screening test for hyperglycemia. Eur J Obstet Gynecol Reprod Biol 53:7, 1994.
The 1-hour glucose screen after a 50-gram oral glucose challenge that is recommended for detecting gestational diabetes at a threshold of 140 mg/dL (7.8 mM/L) is not a reliable indicator of hyperglycemia in a normal group of women at increased risk for gestational diabetes because it offers many false negatives and false positives.

TRUE HYPOGLYCEMIA AND THE IDIOPATHIC POSTPRANDIAL SYNDROME

Recommendations for hypoglycemia and the idiopathic postprandial syndrome are from the medical literature.

1. In patients with clinical findings of hypoglycemia, measure serum glucose. Draw an additional 10 to 20 mL of blood for studies determined by clues from the clinical findings.

In healthy persons, postabsorptive levels of serum glucose concentration are maintained between 60 mg/dL (3.33 mmol/L) and 100 mg/dL (5.6 mmol/L) despite the intermittent ingestion of food. The only unequivocal diagnostic test for true hypoglycemia is documentation of a low serum glucose concentration **during the time the patient experiences spontaneously developed symptoms.**

True Hypoglycemia Syndrome

The *true hypoglycemia syndrome* refers to the presence of adrenergic or neuroglycopenic signs and symptoms in the presence of a low serum glucose concentration—generally less than 40 mg/dL (<2.22 mmol/L)—in which the signs and symptoms can be relieved by the administration of glucose (Whipple's triad). Patients with type 1 diabetes mellitus who have had repeated episodes of hypoglycemia may develop an unawareness of subsequent hypoglycemic episodes. In these patients, careful avoidance of hypoglycemia may restore hypoglycemia awareness. Caffeine appears to increase awareness of hypoglycemia.

Adrenergic symptoms of hypoglycemia are induced by epinephrine secretion and consist of sweating, tremor, tachycardia, anxiety, weakness, and hunger. Neuroglycopenic findings are caused by low central nervous system glucose and consist of dizziness, headache, clouded vision, blunted mental acuity, confusion, abnormal behavior, convulsions, and coma. Persistent, very low central nervous system glucose values can cause features of decortication or decerebration and focal abnormalities, particularly hemiplegia. Without glucose administration, these defects may become permanent. Interestingly, the peripheral nervous system is seldom affected by hypoglycemia.

Idiopathic Postprandial Syndrome

Idiopathic postprandial syndrome is a term applied to the adrenergic signs and symptoms (often reduced by glucose administration), for which the cause frequently is unclear, that occur in many individuals 2 to 5 hours after a meal. The serum glucose, if measured, is normal.

In the work-up of a patient with hypoglycemia, a detailed history is essential and should include information about every medication (prescription and nonprescription) and alcohol ingestion. For patients who have underlying disease, the results of the history and the physical examination should determine the direction of the investigation.

Be alert for artifactual hypoglycemia, which can occur in patients with leukemia, polycythemia, and hemolytic anemia with excessive nucleated red blood cells. Serum should be separated promptly from blood cells, or blood should be preserved with fluoride because blood cells metabolize glucose and decrease the serum glucose concentration.

2. Evaluate the serum glucose result.

A low serum glucose concentration is generally one that is less than 40 mg/dL (<2.22 mmol/L). Normally, at glucose concentrations of 40 mg/dL (2.22 mmol/L) or less, little or no insulin is released. Vitamin C ingestion can depress values measured with the glucose oxidase method. The methodologic considerations are the same as for diagnosing diabetes, which were discussed in the previous problem.

Serum glucose concentrations do not always correlate with an individual's signs and symptoms. Symptoms of hypoglycemia usually occur at serum glucose values less than 40 mg/dL (<2.22 mmol/L), but some persons show no findings with values as low as 30 mg/dL (1.67 mmol/L). Other persons may show findings at values up to 100 mg/dL (5.55 mmol/L) when the serum glucose rapidly falls from a previously high concentration. Adrenergic signs and symptoms apparently are related to a rapidly falling glucose concentration. If glucose falls rapidly but central nervous system levels remain adequate, adrenergic findings can occur in the absence of neuroglycopenic findings. If the glucose concentration falls slowly to very low levels, neuroglycopenic findings can occur in the absence of adrenergic findings.

3. If a patient has adrenergic signs and symptoms and a normal serum glucose concentration in the postprandial state, consider the idiopathic postprandial syndrome. Never use the 5-hour oral glucose tolerance test to diagnose the idiopathic postprandial syndrome.

In healthy individuals, ingestion of a meal provokes a rise in serum glucose and a brisk insulin release, followed by a falling serum glucose concentration and a decrease in insulin. Frequently the falling glucose value drops below baseline, even below 40 mg/dL (2.22 mmol/L), but these persons usually have no symptoms. Insulin is the primary hypoglycemic hormone. Other hormones that affect serum glucose (i.e., cortisol, growth hormone, glucagon, epinephrine) tend to increase the serum concentration.

Patients in the postprandial state with clinical findings suggestive of hypoglycemia usually do not have a low serum glucose concentration. The 5-hour oral glucose tolerance test produces so many false-positive results that it has become completely discredited. If the patient has adrenergic signs and symptoms and the serum glucose concentration is normal, the diagnosis is the idiopathic postprandial syndrome. Treatment is controversial; however, a high-protein, low-carbohydrate diet frequently is prescribed for patients with the idiopathic postprandial syndrome and may relieve symptoms.

4. If a patient has a low serum glucose concentration in the postprandial state, consider the following.

Alimentary Hypoglycemia

Alimentary hypoglycemia is the most common cause of postprandial hypoglycemia. After certain procedures such as gastrectomy, gastrojejunostomy, pyloroplasty, or vagotomy, patients may have rapid postprandial gastric emptying with rapid absorption of glucose and excessive release of insulin. Because blood glucose values tend to fall faster than insulin values, hypoglycemia may ensue.

Other Causes of Postprandial Hypoglycemia

In certain children with fructose intolerance or galactosemia, ingestion of fructose or galactose causes hypoglycemia. Rarely leucine causes hypoglycemia in susceptible infants. In Jamaica, extreme hypoglycemia after ingestion of unripe ackee fruit is called the *toxic hypoglycemic syndrome.* True postprandial hypoglycemia of unknown cause or idiopathic hypoglycemia in which the patient has adrenergic signs and symptoms relieved by glucose administration is rare.

5. If a patient has a low serum glucose concentration in the fasting state, consider the following causes:

- **Hyperinsulinism:** too much insulin in a diabetic patient; islet cell hyperplasia or tumor; factitious administration of insulin or sulfonylureas
- **Drugs:** alcohol; salicylates in children; propranolol; disopyramide; sulfamethoxazole-trimethoprim in a patient with renal failure; pentamidine and quinine when used to treat cerebral malaria; chlorpropamide (may stimulate beta cells, producing hyperinsulinemia); fluoxetine; angiotensin-converting enzyme inhibitors; and miscellaneous drugs (see the references for a review article on this subject)
- **Acquired liver disease:** hepatic congestion; severe hepatitis; cirrhosis; Reye's syndrome; secondary to uremia or sepsis
- **Renal failure:** low gluconeogenic substrate and/or glucagon deficiency
- **Hormone deficiencies:** hypopituitarism; adrenal insufficiency
- **Extrapancreatic tumors:** large mesenchymal tumors; carcinomas of liver, gastrointestinal tract, and adrenal gland
- **Substrate deficiency:** severe malnutrition; late pregnancy
- **Enzyme defects:** glucose-6-phosphatase; pyruvate carboxylase
- **Insulin antibodies**
- **Miscellaneous disorders:** diffuse carcinomatosis; rampant leukemia

6. To diagnose hyperinsulinism secondary to an insulinoma or insulin administration, proceed as follows.

Hypoglycemia in a diabetic who is taking insulin or a sulfonylurea is perhaps the most common cause of fasting hypoglycemia. The diagnosis is obvious.

Hypoglycemia secondary to islet cell hyperplasia or tumor can be provoked by fasting. Start with a 12-hour overnight fast, but remember that a longer fast may be required (exercise such as walking up and down stairs for an hour can help provoke hypoglycemia). Twenty-nine percent become hypoglycemic in 12 hours, 71% in 24 hours, 92% in 48 hours, and 98% in 72 hours. When hypoglycemia occurs (glucose level <45 mg/dL [<2.50 mmol/L]), measurement of serum insulin, C peptide, and proinsulin in simultaneous samples shows inappropriately increased values in most patients with an insulinoma.

Factitious hypoglycemia caused by insulin administration may be diagnosed by measuring serum insulin and C peptide. In patients with factitious hypoglycemia, the serum insulin level is increased and the C peptide level is decreased because insulin is administered directly instead of being produced in the islet beta cells where proinsulin normally gives rise to increased serum levels of both insulin and C peptide. Insulin antibodies may also be present. Patients with factitious hypoglycemia are often suicidal; consider consulting a psychiatrist before confronting these patients with the evidence.

Diagnosis of insulinoma is supported by a plasma C peptide of at least 0.6 ng/mL (0.2 nmol/L) and insulin of at least 6.1 μU/mL (42 pmol/L) at the time Whipple's triad develops during a prolonged fast. The concentrations of insulin and C peptide are reported in conventional units of microunits per milliliter for insulin and nanograms per milliliter for C peptide, an insulin:C peptide ratio greater than 47.17 μU/ng implies that exogenous insulin has been administered.

7. In patients with hypoglycemia, the following blood test results may be decreased:

- **Potassium and phosphorus** caused by intracellular shifts after administration of glucose and insulin

BIBLIOGRAPHY

Axelrod L: Insulinoma: Cost-effective care in patients with a rare disease. Ann Intern Med 123:311, 1995.
  Assays for serum insulin, C peptide, and proinsulin have dramatically improved our ability to diagnose an insulinoma.
Boyle PJ, Kempers SF, O'Connor AM, et al: Brain glucose uptake and unawareness of hypoglycemia in patients with insulin-dependent diabetes mellitus. N Engl J Med 333:1726, 1995.
  Cranston I, Lomas J, Maran A, et al: Restoration of hypoglycaemia awareness in patients with long-duration insulin-dependent diabetes. Lancet 344:283, 1994.
  Discusses unawareness of hypoglycemia in patients with type 1 diabetes mellitus.
Boyle PJ, Schwartz NS, Shah SD, et al: Plasma glucose concentrations at the onset of hypoglycemic symptoms in patients with poorly controlled diabetes and in nondiabetics. N Engl J Med 318:1487, 1988.
  Poorly controlled diabetics may have symptoms of hypoglycemia at plasma levels that are normal or even above normal.
Deeg MA, Lipkin EW: Hypoglycemia associated with the use of fluoxetine. West J Med 164:262, 1996.
  Describes another drug associated with hypoglycemia.
Herings RMC, de Boer A, Stricker BH, et al: Hypoglycaemia associated with use of inhibitors of angiotensin converting enzyme. Lancet 345:1195, 1995.
  Angiotensin-converting enzyme inhibitors may account for almost 14% of hospital admissions for hypoglycemia in diabetic patients.
Kerr D, Sherwin RS, Pavalkis F, et al: Effect of caffeine on the recognition of and responses to hypoglycemia in humans. Ann Intern Med 119:799, 1993.
  Caffeine seems to heighten awareness of hypoglycemia.
Lebowitz MR, Blumenthal SA: The molar ratio of insulin to C-peptide. Arch Intern Med 153:650, 1993.
  When the concentrations of insulin and C peptide are reported in conventional units of microunits per milliliter for insulin and nanograms per milliliter for C peptide, an insulin:C peptide ratio greater than 47.17 μU/ng implies that exogenous insulin has been administered.
Nelson RL: Drug-induced hypoglycemias. In Service FJ (ed): Hypoglycemic Disorders: Pathogenesis, Diagnosis, and Treatment. Boston, GK Hall, 1983, p 97.
  Many drugs have been implicated as a cause of hypoglycemia.
Service FJ: Hypoglycemic disorders. N Engl J Med 332:1144, 1995.

Authoritative and comprehensive review of the diagnosis and management of hypogly-cemia.

Service FJ, O'Brien PC, McMahon MM, et al: C-peptide during the prolonged fast in insulinoma. J Clin Endocrinol Metab 76:655, 1993.
Discusses serum insulin and C peptide levels in diagnosis of insulinoma.

Snorgaard O, Binder C: Monitoring of blood glucose concentration in subjects with hypoglycemia symptoms during everyday life. BMJ 300:16, 1990.
Functional hypoglycemia more likely is due to something other than low blood sugar.

Toxic hypoglycemic syndrome: Jamaica, 1989–1991. MMWR 41:53, 1992.
In Jamaica, extreme hypoglycemia can follow ingestion of unripe ackee fruit.

• •

CUSHING'S SYNDROME

Recommendations for Cushing's syndrome are from the medical literature.

1. In patients with clinical findings suggesting Cushing's syndrome, measure 24-hour urinary free cortisol excretion. If the results are equivocal, perform an overnight dexamethasone suppression test.

Clinical findings of Cushing's syndrome include weakness/fatigue, weight gain, dermatologic changes, depression, gonadal dysfunction, central obesity with supraclavicular fullness (buffalo hump), facial rounding with plethora (moonface), hypertension, proximal muscular weakness, hirsutism and acne, and glucose intolerance.

Measure 24-hour urinary free cortisol by collecting a 24-hour urine sample in a clear container into which 25 mL of 50% acetic acid as preservative is added at the start of the collection.

Perform an overnight dexamethasone test by giving the patient 1.0 mg of dexamethasone orally at 10:00 PM (2200 h), and measure serum cortisol at 8:00 AM (0800 h) the next day.

2. Evaluate the test results.

Reference ranges vary among different laboratories.

REFERENCE RANGES FOR CORTISOL

Test	Specimen	Conventional Units	International Units
Free cortisol	Urine	20–90 μg/d	55–248 nmol/d
Dexamethasone suppression test	Serum	<5 μg/dL (typically <1–2 μg/dL) >10 μg/dL in patients with Cushing's syndrome	<138 nmol/L (typically <28–53 nmol/L) >275 nmol/L

3. Interpret test results in the context of clinical findings.

A 24-hour urine free cortisol level less than 100 μg/24 h (<276 nmol/24 h) excludes the diagnosis of Cushing's syndrome, and a level greater than 150 μg/24 h (>414 nmol/24 h) strongly suggests the diagnosis. False-negative results are rare, and false-positive results are seldom seen except in stress and chronic alcoholism. False-positive results (e.g., stress, obesity, estrogen therapy) occur more with the overnight dexamethasone suppression test. Therefore, if a single test is to be done to "rule out" Cushing's syndrome, the 24-hour urinary free cortisol is preferred.

In a recent study, a single midnight serum cortisol level drawn within 2 minutes of waking the patients—without previously informing the patients that this would be done—had 100% sensitivity for the diagnosis of Cushing's syndrome. Every patient with Cushing's syndrome had a detectable midnight serum level between 0.9 and 26.2 μg/dL (70 to 2000 nmol/L). In control subjects the level was less than 1.8 μg/dL (<50 nmol/L).

4. In patients with Cushing's syndrome, the following test results may be increased:

- **Hemoglobin and hematocrit**
- **Leukocytes**
- **Glucose**

5. In patients with Cushing's syndrome, the following test results may be decreased:

- **Lymphocytes**
- **Potassium**

BIBLIOGRAPHY

Faulkner WR: Laboratory diagnosis of Cushing's syndrome. Lab Report Physicians 18:9, 1996.
  Reviews the laboratory diagnosis of Cushing's syndrome.
Newell-Price J, Trainer P, Perry L, et al: A single sleeping midnight cortisol has 100% sensitivity for the diagnosis of Cushing's syndrome. Clin Endocrinol 43:545, 1995.
  Single inpatient midnight cortisol level detects all cases of Cushing's syndrome.
Watts NB, Keffer JH (eds): Practical Endocrinology, 4th ed. Philadelphia, Lea & Febiger, 1989, p 99.
  Recommends test strategies for the initial evaluation of Cushing's syndrome.
Yanovski JA, Cutler GB Jr, Chrousos GP, et al: Corticotropin-releasing hormone stimulation following low-dose dexamethasone administration. JAMA 269:2232, 1993.
  Suggests corticotropin-releasing hormone stimulation following low-dose dexamethasone administration as the most sensitive and specific strategy for diagnosing Cushing's syndrome.

ADRENAL INSUFFICIENCY

Recommendations for adrenal insufficiency are from the medical literature.

1. In patients with clinical findings of adrenal insufficiency, if the

findings are severe, draw a blood sample for serum cortisol and adrenocorticotropic hormone (ACTH) levels before treating with glucocorticoids. If the findings are early or mild, perform a rapid ACTH test.

Clinical findings include weakness and fatigue, anorexia, nausea and vomiting, abdominal pain, salt craving, postural dizziness, weight loss, hypotension, and hyperpigmentation, especially of scars and nipples.

To perform the rapid ACTH test, draw a baseline blood sample for a serum cortisol determination and give ACTH, 250 µg, intramuscularly or intravenously. Then draw additional blood samples for serum cortisol measurements at 30 minutes and 60 minutes.

2. Evaluate the test results.

Reference ranges may vary among different laboratories.

REFERENCE RANGES FOR SERUM CORTISOL

Test	Specimen	Conventional Units	International Units
Cortisol	Serum	0800 hr: 5–23 µg/dL	138–635 nmol/L
		1600 hr: 3–16 µg/dL	83–441 nmol/L
		2000 hr: ≤50% of concentration at 0800 hr	≤50% of concentration at 0800 hr
Adrenocorticotropic hormone (ACTH)	Plasma (with heparin)	0800 hr: <120 pg/mL 1600–2000 hr: <85 pg/mL	<26 pmol/L <19 pmol/L
Rapid ACTH test	See below		

3. Interpret test results in the context of clinical findings.

In severe cases, a low serum cortisol level in the presence of an increased ACTH level indicates primary adrenal insufficiency, whereas a low cortisol level with a low or inappropriately "normal" level of ACTH indicates secondary adrenal insufficiency.

In early or mild cases, using the rapid ACTH test, a peak serum cortisol level equal to or greater than 20 µg/dL (≥552 nmol/L) is a good indicator of normal adrenal function. It is reassuring also to see a rise in the serum cortisol level of equal to or greater than 7 µg/dL (≥193 nmol/L) above the baseline level.

If the cortisol response to ACTH stimulation is low or subnormal, additional testing is necessary to diagnose primary versus secondary adrenal insufficiency, and an endocrinologist should be consulted.

4. In patients with adrenal insufficiency, the following test results may be increased:

- **Eosinophils**, in 10 to 20% of patients
- **Lymphocytes**
- **Urea nitrogen and creatinine** related to dehydration and hypotension with prerenal impairment of renal function
- **Potassium**
- **Calcium**
- **Magnesium**
- **Protein** due to dehydration and hemoconcentration

5. In patients with adrenal insufficiency, the following test results may be decreased:

- **Hemoglobin and hematocrit** with low reticulocytes
- **Leukocytes**
- **Neutrophils**
- **Blood pH** with high potassium level and metabolic acidosis
- **Glucose** and increased glucose tolerance with a flat curve
- **Sodium**
- **Chloride**
- **Carbon dioxide**
- **Phosphorus**

BIBLIOGRAPHY

Grinspoon SK, Bilezikian JP: HIV disease and the endocrine system. N Eng J Med 327:1360, 1992.
  The most important endocrine abnormality in human immunodeficiency virus infection is adrenal insufficiency.
Hsu Werbel SS, Chin R Jr: Acute adrenal insufficiency. *In* Conn RB, Borer WZ, Snyder JW (eds): Current Diagnosis, 9th ed. Philadelphia, WB Saunders, 1997, p 771.
  Discusses the diagnosis of acute adrenal insufficiency.
Oelkers W: Adrenal insufficiency. N Engl J Med 335:1206, 1996.
  Reviews the diagnosis and management of adrenal insufficiency.

9

Hematologic Diseases

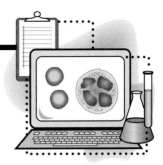

- Classifying Blood Cell Disorders by a Complete Blood Count With Differential
- Microcytic Anemia Without Reticulocytosis
- Macrocytic Anemia Without Reticulocytosis
- Normocytic Anemia Without Reticulocytosis
- Anemia With Reticulocytosis
- Classifying Bleeding Disorders by Laboratory Tests

CLASSIFYING BLOOD CELL DISORDERS BY A COMPLETE BLOOD COUNT WITH DIFFERENTIAL

Recommendations for wellness screening for anemia are from the medical literature.

1. For patients with clinical findings of a blood disorder or to screen for a blood disorder, request a complete blood count (CBC) with differential. For patients with clinical findings or an abnormal CBC, carefully review the peripheral blood smear.

Even though anemia is common in a typical US community, several groups do not recommend wellness screening for anemia, but some endorse selective screening for individuals at increased risk—such as infants—especially cow's milk–fed infants; persons of low socioeconomic status; institutionalized elderly persons; pregnant women; and recent immigrants from Third World countries. A recent study concluded that iron deficiency and iron deficiency anemia are still relatively common in toddlers, adolescent girls, and women of childbearing age.

A Wright-stained peripheral blood smear can show helpful red blood cell (RBC), white blood cell (WBC), and platelet changes: sickling and targeting suggest Hb SS (sickle cell anemia) or Hb S plus thalassemia minor; targeting and stippling suggest complications of thalassemia minor; marked targeting suggests Hb E, Hb C, or obstructive liver disease; RBC fragments and polychromatophilia suggest hemolysis; rouleaux suggest increased globulins and/or decreased albumin; and hypersegmented neutrophils with or without macrocytes suggest megaloblastic anemia. WBCs can be differentiated and the changes of the reactive disorders and leukemias noted. Any "left shift" (increased bands) can be noted. Unusual forms such as the bilobed neutrophils and eosinophils of the Pelger-Hüet anomaly or the large purple cytoplasmic granules of the Alder-Reilly anomaly may be present. The platelet count can be estimated, and abnormal forms such as small platelets, large platelets, or platelets with bizarre shapes and forms can be noted.

2. Evaluate the tests.

A CBC performed on an automated hematology analyzer is widely available and provides hemoglobin (Hb) and hematocrit (Hct) values, RBC count, RBC indices, WBC values—and often the platelet count and an electronic WBC differential as well. The report from automated hematology analyzers such as the Coulter STKR (Coulter Electronics, Inc) is expressed in a blood cell hemogram (modified for reproduction) as follows:

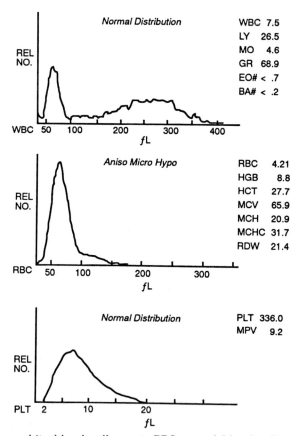

Key: WBC = white blood cell count; RBC = red blood cell count; PLT = platelets; Aniso = anisocytosis; Micro = microcytosis; Hypo = hypochromia; LY = % lymphocytes; MO = % monocytes; GR = % granulocytes; EO# = absolute number of eosinophils (× 10⁹/L); BA# = absolute number of basophils (× 10⁹/L); HBG = hemoglobin; HCT = hematocrit; MCV = mean corpuscular volume; MCH = mean corpuscular hemoglobin; MCHC = mean corpuscular hemoglobin concentration; RDW = red cell distribution width; MPV = mean platelet volume; REL NO = relative number; fL = femtoliters.

In this hemogram the microcytic, hypochromic RBCs with anisocytosis (high RBC distribution width [RDW]) are consistent with iron deficiency anemia. Not only are the numerical results seen for the CBC, including WBC differential and RBC indices, but so are graphic displays of WBCs, RBCs, and platelets. The RBC indices are calculated as follows:

Mean corpuscular volume (MCV) (fL) =
$$\frac{\text{Hct (\%)} \times 10}{\text{RBC (in millions/}\mu\text{L)}} \text{ or } \frac{\text{Hct (vol. fr.)} \times 1000}{\text{RBC (in millions/}\mu\text{L)}}$$

Mean corpuscular hemoglobin (MCH) (pg) =
$$\frac{\text{Hb (g/dL)} \times 10}{\text{RBC (in millions/}\mu\text{L)}} \text{ or } \frac{\text{Hb (g/L)}}{\text{RBC (in millions/}\mu\text{L)}}$$

Mean corpuscular hemoglobin concentration (MCHC) (g/dL) =
$$\frac{\text{Hb (g/dL)} \times 100}{\text{Hct (\%)}} \text{ or } \frac{\text{Hb (g/dL)}}{\text{Hct (vol. fr.)}}$$

The RDW is an estimate of RBC size variability (anisocytosis) and is calculated as follows:

$$\text{RDW} = \frac{\text{SD}}{\text{Mean}} \times 100 \ (13 \pm 1.5\%)$$

The deficiency anemias (iron, vitamin B_{12}, folic acid) tend to have higher RDWs (greater anisocytosis) than anemias caused by genetic defects (e.g., thalassemia) or primary bone marrow disorders.

3. Interpret test results in the context of clinical findings.

Classifying Red Blood Cell Disorders

Anemia. In patients with anemia, review the CBC with differential, determine the reticulocyte count, and examine the peripheral blood smear.

Pay attention to abnormal RBC indices, even when no anemia is present. A high MCV without anemia may be a clue to chronic alcoholism or an early vitamin B_{12} deficiency. Similarly, a low MCV without anemia may be a clue to heterozygous α- or β-thalassemia.

CRITERIA FOR ANEMIA IN MEN AND WOMEN

	Women	Men
Red blood cells	<4 × 10^6 cells/μL (<4 × 10^{12} cells/L)	<4.5 × 10^6 cells/μL (<4.5 × 10^{12} cells/L)

Table continued on following page

CRITERIA FOR ANEMIA IN MEN AND WOMEN *Continued*

	Women	Men
Hemoglobin	<12 g/dL (<120 g/L)	<13.5 g/dL (<135 g/L)
Hematocrit	<35% (<0.36 volume fraction)	<40% (<0.40 volume fraction)

Reticulocyte Count. The reticulocyte count is a key value that should be determined as part of the initial work-up of every anemic patient. Reticulocytes are 1- to 2-day-old young RBCs in the peripheral blood. They are macrocytic (MCV >100 fL) and contain aggregates of ribosomes that take up supravital stain (methylene blue). The reticulocyte count is expressed as the percentage of reticulocytes per 500 or 1000 RBCs counted. The reference ranges for the reticulocyte count follow:

Test	Specimen	Conventional Units	International Units
Percent reticulocytes	Peripheral blood smear	0.5–1.5% of RBCs	0.005–0.015 (number fraction)
Absolute reticulocyte count	Peripheral blood smear	<100 × 10³/ μL	<100 × 10⁹/L

Use the reticulocyte production index (RPI [normal = 1]) to correct for anemia for the longer presence of reticulocytes in the peripheral blood.

$$RPI = \% \text{ Reticulocytes} \times \frac{\text{Patient Hct}}{\text{Normal Hct}} \times \frac{1}{\text{Maturation time (days)}}$$

Maturation times (days) for Hct of 45%, 35%, 25%, and 15% are 1.0, 1.5, 2.0, and 2.5, respectively.

Characterize the anemia as having either a normal to low reticulocyte count or a high reticulocyte count. Classify anemia with a normal to low reticulocyte count according to whether the RBCs are microcytic, macrocytic, or normocytic. Examination of a peripheral blood smear may be helpful. Many patients with anemia do not require examination of the bone marrow. Classification of anemia according to RBC size and reticulocyte count has exceptions; nevertheless, it provides a useful overall format for the differential diagnosis of anemia.

Anemia occurs secondary to decreased production of RBCs, increased loss, or a combination of the two. Classification of anemia according to RBC size and reticulocyte count is a useful first step toward finding a cause. For example, iron deficiency anemia, thalassemia minor, and anemia of chronic disease typically are seen as microcytic anemia with a normal or low reticulocyte count, whereas anemia caused by vitamin B_{12} or folate deficiency typically is seen as macrocytic anemia with a normal to low reticulocyte count. In contrast, anemia due to blood loss or hemolysis usually exhibits normocytic RBCs with a high reticulocyte count.

A bone marrow examination is not required in all patients with anemia. For example, a 65-year-old woman with microcytic anemia, a high RDW, and a low serum ferritin concentration has obvious iron deficiency anemia and does not require bone marrow aspiration to evaluate iron stores. Similarly, patients with obvious hemolytic anemias should be examined by other means and do not require bone marrow aspiration.

Polycythemia. Polycythemia is a condition in which the patient has an increased RBC volume, Hb concentration, Hct value, and RBC count. It may be primary (polycythemia vera) or secondary to another disorder such as chronic cardiac or pulmonary disease. See the references at the end of this section for a discussion of strategies for diagnosis.

Classifying White Blood Cell Disorders

In patients with an abnormal WBC count, review the CBC with differential and examine the peripheral blood smear. Characterize the WBC count as normal, low, or high according to leukocyte differentials expressed in absolute numbers. You may wish to ask your laboratory to express leukocyte differentials in percentages as well as absolute counts.

Leukopenia. When the WBC count is low, neutropenia (absolute neutrophilic granulocyte count [ANC] $<1.5 \times 10^3$ cells/μL ($<1.5 \times 10^9$ cells/L) is a major concern. The ANC is calculated by multiplying the total WBC count by the percentage of bands and mature neutrophils (ANC = WBC × [% bands + % mature neutrophils] × 0.01). Susceptibility to infections in neutropenic patients is particularly related to the ANC. Once the ANC is documented as low, the cause should be determined. Drugs are an important common cause that should be ruled out by stopping medications and obtaining weekly WBC counts for 8 weeks. Patients with significant infections and those who are still neutropenic after 8 weeks should be thoroughly examined.

Leukocytosis. When the WBC count is high, a major concern is whether the high count is due to a reactive process or to a leukemia. A reactive process with a WBC count exceeding 50×10^3 cellsμL (50×10^9 cells/L) is referred to as a *leukemoid reaction.*

A high WBC count may be due to neutrophilia, eosinophilia, basophilia, monocytosis, or lymphocytosis. Some causes follow:

- **Neutrophilia:** infections, leukemia, rheumatic and autoimmune disorders, neoplastic disorders, chemicals, trauma, endocrine and metabolic disorders, hematologic disorders, miscellaneous (e.g., drugs)
- **Eosinophilia:** infectious diseases, parasitic infections, allergic diseases, myeloproliferative and neoplastic diseases, cutaneous diseases, gastrointestinal diseases, miscellaneous (e.g., long-term peritoneal dialysis)
- **Basophilia:** allergic reactions, chronic myeloid leukemia, myeloid metaplasia, polycythemia vera, ionizing radiation, hypothyroidism, chronic hemolytic anemia, splenectomy
- **Monocytosis:** infections, neoplastic disorders, gastrointestinal disorders, sarcoidosis, drug reactions, recovering from marrow suppression
- **Lymphocytosis:** viral infections, lymphocytic leukemia, other infectious diseases, neoplastic disorders, other disorders (e.g., Graves' disease)

Useful tests for differentiating a leukemoid reaction from chronic granulocytic leukemia follow:

Test	Leukemoid Reaction	Chronic Granulocytic Leukemia
WBC $\times$ 10^3/μL (WBC $\times$ 10^9/L)	<100	May be 30–500
Percent PMNs	Up to 95%	May be normal (60–70%)
Immature granulocytes	To myelocyte	Usually includes occasional progranulocytes or blasts
Eosinophils, basophils	Normal or decreased	Slightly increased
Nucleated red blood cells	Occasional	Late; may be common
Bone marrow M:E ratio	6–8:1	$\geq$15:1
LAP	>100	<10

PMN, polymorphonuclear leukocytes; M:E, myeloid:erythroid ratio; LAP, leukocyte alkaline phosphatase.

Source: Kjeldsberg C, Beutler E, Bell C, et al (eds): Practical Diagnosis of Hematologic Disorders. Chicago, American Society of Clinical Pathologists, 1989, p 235.

Infectious mononucleosis is a lymphocytic leukocytosis that may be confused with leukemia and other disorders. The presence of heterophil antibodies (Monospot test) in the context of the appropriate clinical and hematologic findings is diagnostic for infectious mononucleosis. False-positive reactions are rare. Atypical lymphocytes usually account for more than 10% of the leukocytes in the peripheral blood smear. Detection of viral capsid antigen antibody IgM (VCA-IgM) is the most accurate test for confirming acute infection.

Infectious conditions that may cause an infectious mononucleosis–like syndrome include streptococcal or gonococcal pharyngeal infection, cytomegalovirus infection, viral hepatitis, toxoplasmosis, human immunodeficiency virus infection, and adenovirus infection.

4. In patients with infectious mononucleosis, the following test results may be increased:

- **Autoimmune hemolytic anemia** caused by cold agglutinins against i antigens
- **White blood cell count** may be high, normal, or low; a relative and absolute neutropenia is present in many patients
- **Thrombocytopenia** is common
- **Uric acid** caused by accelerated lymphocyte nucleic acid turnover
- **Transaminase levels** in most patients, related to hepatic involvement
- **Lactate dehydrogenase** in most patients
- **Alkaline phosphatase** in some patients, related to hepatic involvement
- **Serum globulins** caused by antibodies to Epstein-Barr virus; first IgM, then IgG
- **Bilirubin,** usually mild and only occasionally 6 mg/dL (103 µmol/L) or greater; rarely bilirubin levels of 10.2 to 23 mg/dL (174 to 393 µmol/L) are encountered

5. In patients with infectious mononucleosis, the following test results may be decreased:

- **Serum albumin** related to decreased synthesis

BIBLIOGRAPHY

Anía BJ, Suman VJ, Fairbanks VF, et al: Prevalence of anemia in medical practice: Community versus referral patients. Mayo Clin Proc 69:730, 1994.
  This study confirms that anemia is common in a typical US community and often may go undiagnosed in the general population.
Ardron MJ, Westengard JC, Dutcher TF: Band neutrophil counts are unnecessary for the diagnosis of infection in patients with normal total leukocyte counts. Am J Clin Pathol 102:646, 1994.
  The band count adds no information to the leukocyte differential for diagnosing infection.
Brigden ML, Horak MG: Incidence and clinical significance of unsuspected eosinophilia discovered by automated WBC differential counting. Lab Med 24:173, 1993.
  The cause of unsuspected eosinophilia includes allergic processes, asthma, eczema/dermatitis, parasitic disease, drug allergy, cancer, and collagen disease.
Buss DH, Cashell AW, O'Connor ML, et al: Occurrence, etiology, and clinical significance of extreme thrombocytosis: A study of 280 cases. Am J Med 96:247, 1994.
  The most common causes of reactive thrombocytosis were infection, post-splenectomy

hyposplenism, malignancy, and trauma; the most common myeloproliferative disorders were chronic granulocytic leukemia and primary thrombocythemia.

Conley CL: Polycythemia vera. JAMA 263:2481, 1990.

Djulbegovic B, Hadley T, Joseph G: A new algorithm for the diagnosis of polycythemia. Am Fam Physician 44:113, 1991.

Two articles that discuss polycythemia vera, including strategies for diagnosis.

Dalal BI, Nyokong AM: Hyperthrombocytosis: A clinicohematological study. Lab Med 23:811, 1992.

The causes were acute and chronic infections, malignant neoplasms, severe trauma, immediate postoperative status, massive acute hemorrhage or thrombotic episodes, and neonatal respiratory distress syndrome.

Dale DC: A new look at an old laboratory test: The WBC count. J Gen Intern Med 6:264, 1991.

Chang R, Wong GY: Prognostic significance of marked leukocytosis in hospitalized patients. J Gen Intern Med 6:199, 1991.

Discusses the WBC count and the prognostic significance of a neutrophilic leukocytosis greater than 20×10^3 cells/μL ($>20 \times 10^9$ cells/L).

Goldstein KH, Abramson N: Efficient diagnosis of thrombocytopenia. Am Fam Physician 53:915, 1996.

Discusses the clinical findings and differential diagnosis of thrombocytopenia.

Griner PF: Infectious mononucleosis. *In* Panzer RJ, Black ER, Griner PF (eds): Diagnostic Strategies for Common Medical Problems. Philadelphia, American College of Physicians, 1991, p 196.

Recommends strategies for the diagnosis of infectious mononucleosis.

Hayward RSA, Steinberg EP, Ford DE: Preventive care guidelines: 1991. Ann Intern Med 114:758, 1991.

Authoritative recommendations for wellness screening for iron deficiency anemia.

Jones AR, Twedt D, Hellman R: Absolute versus proportional differential leukocyte counts. Clin Lab Haematol 17:115, 1995.

The absolute cell count is more likely to provide diagnostic support than the proportional cell count.

Lambore S, McSherry J, Kraus AS: Acute and chronic symptoms of mononucleosis. J Fam Pract 33:33, 1991.

Discusses the clinical findings of infectious mononucleosis.

Looker AC, Dallman PR, Carroll MD, et al: Prevalance of iron deficiency in the United States. JAMA 277:973, 1997.

Iron deficiency and iron deficiency anemia are still relatively common in toddlers, adolescent girls, and women of childbearing age.

Mates M, Heyd J, Souroujon M, et al: The hematologist as watchdog of community health by full blood count. Q J Med 88:333, 1995.

Routine CBC for a high-risk ambulatory population may be an effective screen for serious clinical problems.

Messinezy M, Westwood NB, Woodcock SP, et al: Low serum erythropoietin: A strong diagnostic criterion of primary polycythemia even at normal hemoglobin levels. Clin Lab Haematol 17:217, 1995.

Suggests that low serum erythropoietin in one or both of two samples taken on different occasions be considered a diagnostic criterion for primary polycythemia.

Payne SK, Wheby MS: Anemia: How to streamline the diagnosis, identify reversible causes. Consultant 36:1685, 1995.

Use the RBC size to guide the work-up. The absolute reticulocyte count is also useful.

Rice L: Anemia: Using a rational approach to diagnosis. Consultant 30:39, 1990.

Believes that therapeutic trials are inappropriate.

Rockey DC, Cello JP: Evaluation of the gastrointestinal tract in patients with iron-deficiency anemia. N Engl J Med 329:1691, 1993.

Sixty-two percent of patients had a gastrointestinal source; peptic ulcer and colorectal cancer were the most common lesions.

Rotenberg Z, Harell D, Weinberger I, et al: Total lactate dehydrogenase and its isoenzymes in serum of patients with infectious mononucleosis. Clin Chem 37:116, 1991.

Recommends lactate dehydrogenase studies for every patient with clinical suspicion of infectious mononucleosis.

Shapiro MF, Greenfield S: The complete blood count and leukocyte differential count. *In* Sox HC Jr (ed): Common Diagnostic Tests: Use and Interpretation, 2nd ed. Philadelphia, American College of Physicians, 1990, p 183.
   Discusses the American College of Physicians guidelines for the complete blood count.
Simel DL: Is the RDW-MCV classification of anemia useful? Clin Lab Haematol 9:349, 1987.
   Discusses the use of RDW and MCV for diagnosing microcytic anemia.
Welborn JL, Meyers FJ: A three-point approach to anemia. Postgrad Med 89:179, 1991.
   Gives a three-step approach to evaluate patients with anemia.
Wheby MS: A rational approach to the anemia workup. Patient Care 30:158, 1996.
   Recommends a step-by-step approach. An extensive work-up often is not necessary.
Young NS: Agranulocytosis. JAMA 271:935, 1994.
   Discusses the clinical presentation and differential diagnosis of agranulocytosis.

• •

MICROCYTIC ANEMIA WITHOUT RETICULOCYTOSIS

Recommendations for microcytic anemia without reticulocytosis are from the medical literature.

1. In patients with microcytic anemia (mean cell volume [MCV] <80 fL) and a normal to low reticulocyte count, causes include iron deficiency anemia, thalassemia minor, anemia of chronic disease, and sideroblastic anemia. Consider the following studies: examination of a peripheral blood smear, serum iron, total iron-binding capacity, percent saturation, ferritin, free erythrocyte protoporphyrin, and hemoglobin electrophoresis. A bone marrow examination occasionally is necessary.

Useful findings include the following: (1) in an otherwise healthy woman, anemia is usually caused by iron deficiency (probability, 80 to 90%); (2) microcytic red blood cells (RBCs) with little or no anemia are usually caused by thalassemia minor (probability >90%); and (3) in individuals with early or mild iron deficiency, anemia of chronic disease, and sideroblastic anemia, the RBCs may be normocytic instead of microcytic. Iron loss may be physiologic (e.g., menstruation, pregnancy) or pathologic (e.g., colon cancer). A complete gastrointestinal work-up is necessary in men and postmenopausal women in whom iron deficiency has been discovered. A recent study suggests that iron supplementation may improve cognition in nonanemic, iron-deficient girls.

A practical approach in the absence of an obvious chronic disease is to determine initially whether the anemia is caused by iron deficiency. Determinations of the serum iron, total iron-binding capacity, and iron saturation are generally more easily available than that for serum ferritin, and if they are diagnostic, there is no need to measure serum ferritin. When the probability of uncomplicated anemia caused by iron deficiency is high on clinical grounds alone, the values for serum iron, total iron-binding capcity, and percent saturation are approximately equal to that for ferritin in confirming the diagnosis of iron deficiency anemia, but when the clinical probability is low, determining the ferritin value is the better test. Another approach to the diagnosis of iron deficiency anemia is a therapeutic trial: determine whether iron therapy produces reticulocytosis. Clues to the diagnosis of thalassemia minor are a normal RDW and an MCV less than 80 fL in patients with normal or borderline iron studies and no evidence of other causes of microcytosis. An MCV less than 70 fL is almost always due to iron deficiency or thalassemia.

Serum for iron studies should be drawn in the morning because of the diurnal variation (peak value, 7 to 10 AM) in iron values and the fact that reference ranges are for morning samples.

2. Evaluate the tests.

Reference ranges may vary among different laboratories.

REFERENCE RANGES

Test	Specimen	Conventional Units	International Units
Iron	Serum	M: 65–175 µg/dL F: 50–170 µg/dL	11.6–31.3 µmol/L 9.0–30.4 µmol/L
Total iron-binding capacity	Serum	250–450 µg/dL	44.8–80.6 µmol/L
Iron saturation	Serum	M: 20–50% F: 15–50%	0.20–0.50 saturation 0.15–0.50 saturation
Ferritin	Serum	M: 20–250 ng/mL F: 10–120 ng/mL	20–250 µg/L 10–120 µg/L
Free erythrocyte protoporphyrin	Whole blood (EDTA or heparin)	30–80 µg/dL	0.534–1.424 µmol/ dL packed cells
Hemoglobin electrophoresis	Whole blood (EDTA, citrate, or heparin)	Hb A >95% Hb A₂ 1.5–3.5%	Hb A >0.95 (mass fraction) Hb A₂ 0.015–0.035 (mass fraction)

3. Interpret test results in the context of clinical findings.

The common anemias show characteristic patterns of test results.

COMMON ANEMIAS

Test	Iron Deficiency Anemia	Anemia of Chronic Disease	Thalassemia Minor	Sideroblastic Anemia
Peripheral blood smear	Normocytic to microcytic, hypochromic RBCs	Normocytic to microcytic, hypochromic RBCs	Normocytic to micro- cytic RBCs, target cells, basophilic stippling	Dimorphic; hypochromic, microcytic, and macrocytic RBCs with Pappenheimer bodies

COMMON ANEMIAS *Continued*

Test	Iron Deficiency Anemia	Anemia of Chronic Disease	Thalassemia Minor	Sideroblastic Anemia
RBC distribution width (RDW)	High (>16)	Usually normal	Normal	High
Iron	Low	Low	Normal to high	Normal to high
Total iron-binding capacity	High	Normal to low	Normal	Normal to low
Iron saturation	Low	Normal to low	Normal to high	High
Ferritin	Low	Normal to high	Normal to high	Normal to high
Free erythrocyte protoporphyrin	High	High	Normal	Normal to high
Hemoglobin electrophoresis	Normal	Normal	High Hb A_2 in β-thalassemia but normal in α-thalassemia	Normal
Bone marrow	Iron absent	Normal to high iron Low number of sideroblasts	Normal to high iron	High iron Ringed sideroblasts

Iron Deficiency Anemia

Although iron deficiency anemia is typically a microcytic anemia, in mild cases of iron deficiency the RBCs may be normocytic. Initially there is a loss of stainable bone marrow iron and a decrease in the serum ferritin level, which is followed by a decrease in the serum iron level and an increase in the total iron-binding capacity. Then anemia occurs, with a decreasing MCV, increasing anisocytosis, poikilocytosis, and hypochromia, but no basophilic stippling. Indices are often normal until the hemoglobin (Hb) concentration falls below 10 g/dL (100 g/L). A decreasing RBC count and increasing RDW are early changes. The fall in the erythrocyte count usually is less than the fall in Hb. Generally, examination of the bone marrow is not required to establish a diagnosis of iron deficiency anemia. An exception is the clinical situation in which iron deficiency co-exists with a chronic disease. A normal serum iron and iron-binding capacity do not exclude iron deficiency when the Hb concentration is greater than 9 g/dL (90 g/L) in women and 11 g/dL (110 g/L) in men.

Anemia of Thalassemia Minor

The anemia of thalassemia minor (α- or β-thalassemia minor) and Hb E is typically microcytic and, in contrast to iron deficiency anemia, is characterized by a normal or increased RBC count. For example, at a hemoglobin level of 9 g/dL (90 g/L), an iron-deficient patient typically has an RBC count of approximately 3×10^6 cells/μL (3×10^{12} cells/μL), whereas a patient with thalassemia minor has a count of approximately 5×10^6 cells/L (5×10^{12} cells/L). The variation in size is no more than normal, and the RDW is usually normal. There may be basophilic stippling. If the Hb value is greater than 10 g/dL (100 g/L) but the MCV is decreased, thalassemia is more likely than iron deficiency anemia. In the case of β-thalassemia minor, the diagnosis is established by demonstrating an increased concentration of Hb A_2 using Hb A_2 quantitation and Hb electrophoresis. Sometimes the diagnosis is difficult; with α-thalassemia minor, Hb A_2 is not increased. With Hb E disease, however, the abnormal Hb is identified by Hb electrophoresis.

Anemia of Chronic Disease

The anemia of chronic disease is typically normocytic. In approximately 25% of cases the anemia is microcytic, but the MCV rarely falls below 78 fL. Because this form of anemia is specifically related to acute or chronic inflammation rather than chronic disease, the term *anemia of inflammation* has been suggested for this disorder. In contrast to iron deficiency anemia, the serum iron level is low, total iron-binding capacity is normal or low, and the serum ferritin value is usually greater than 100 ng/mL (>100 μg/L). Iron deficiency and anemia of chronic disease may occur together, such as in patients with inflammatory bowel disease or rheumatic diseases treated with aspirin or other nonsteroidal anti-inflammatory drugs. With these conditions, the iron saturation (iron and total iron-binding capacity) may be quite low, even without iron deficiency. If the saturation is greater than 30%, iron deficiency is excluded. A serum ferritin level less than 50 ng/mL (<50 μg/L) in patients with these inflammatory conditions suggests iron deficiency because serum ferritin is an acute-phase reactant and usually is increased in these inflammatory states. In patients with rheumatoid arthritis, a red cell MCV less than 80 fL and a serum ferritin concentration less than 50 ng/mL (<50 μg/L) are 79% sensitive but 100% specific for iron deficiency. A serum ferritin concentration less than 50 ng/mL (<50 μg/L) is a good indicator of iron deficiency anemia in hospitalized geriatric patients. When serum ferritin values are borderline (i.e., 50 ng/mL [50 μg/L]), a bone marrow aspirate for iron stain can settle the question.

Sideroblastic Anemia

Sideroblastic anemia constitutes a group of refractory anemias with erythroid hyperplasia of the marrow. The cause may be either hereditary (sex-linked or autosomal recessive) or acquired. If acquired, it may be drug induced (e.g., lead, alcohol, isoniazid) or idiopathic (myelodysplastic syndromes). The peripheral blood smear exhibits hypochromic microcytic RBCs; but the picture is dimorphic, and macrocytes may prevail, making the MCV normal or high. There may be coarse basophilic stippling. Typically the serum iron and ferritin levels are normal to high, and the serum total iron-binding capacity is normal to low with a high saturation. Free erythrocyte porphyrin levels may be normal or high. The bone marrow contains increased iron stores and ringed sideroblasts. The Hb A_2 level is normal.

BIBLIOGRAPHY

Beutler E: The common anemias. JAMA 259:2433, 1988.
Excellent discussion of thalassemia, iron deficiency anemia, and anemia of chronic disease.
Bick RL, Baker WF: Iron deficiency anemia. Lab Med 21:641, 1990.
Good discussion of iron deficiency anemia and its differentiation from other microcytic anemias.
Brown RG: Determining the cause of anemia: General approach, with emphasis on microcytic hypochromic anemias. Postgrad Med 89:161, 1991.
Recommends strategies for diagnosis.
Bruner AB, Duggan AK, Casella JF, et al: Randomised study of cognitive effects of iron supplementation in non-anemic iron-deficient girls. Lancet 348:992, 1996.
Iron may improve cognition in nonanemic adolescent girls.
Finch CA, Bellotti V, Stray S, et al: Plasma ferritin determination as a diagnostic tool. West J Med 145:657, 1986.
Review of the use of plasma ferritin to diagnose iron deficiency and iron overload.
Griner P: Microcytic anemia. *In* Panzer RJ, Black ER, Griner PF (eds): Diagnostic Strategies for Common Medical Problems. Philadelphia, American College of Physicians, 1991, p 448.
Suggests strategies for the differential diagnosis of microcytic anemia.
Guyatt GH, Oxman AD, Ali M, et al: Laboratory diagnosis of iron-deficiency anemia: An overview. J Gen Intern Med 7:145, 1992.
Suggests serum ferritin radioimmunoassay as the most powerful test for iron deficiency anemia.
Hallberg L, Bengtsson C, Lapidus L, et al: Screening for iron deficiency: An analysis based on bone marrow examinations and serum ferritin determinations in a population sample of women. Br J Haematol 85:787, 1993.
The best discriminator of iron deficiency in women was ferritin levels below 16 ng/mL (16 µg/L), but iron-deficient erythropoiesis starts at ferritin levels of 25 to 40 ng/mL (25 to 40 µg/L).
Holyoake TL, Stott DJ, McKay PJ, et al: Use of plasma ferritin concentration to diagnose iron deficiency in elderly patients. J Clin Pathol 46:857, 1993.
The results show that the clinical use of plasma ferritin of 45 ng/mL (45 µg/L) or lower indicates likely iron deficiency.
Joosten E, Hiele M, Ghoos Y, et al: Diagnosis of iron-deficiency anemia in a hospitalized geriatric population. Am J Med 90:653, 1991.
Ferritin is best to diagnose iron deficiency anemia in hospitalized geriatric patients.
Kalantar-Zadeh K, Höffken B, Wünsch H, et al: Diagnosis of iron deficiency in renal failure patients during the post-erythropoietin era. Am J Kidney Dis 26:292, 1995.
Using both the serum ferritin and the transferrin saturation provides for excellent specificity and acceptable sensitivity for diagnosing iron deficiency anemia in patients with renal failure, excluding those patients with transferrin of less than 150 mg/dL (<1.50 g/L).
Kario K, Matsuo T, Kodama K, et al: Clinical significance of red blood cell distribution

width in the elderly: A potential indicator of bone marrow stimulation by erythropoi-etin. Clin Lab Haematol 15:185, 1993.
The results suggest that the RDW is useful in distinguishing iron deficiency anemia from senile anemia and may reflect erythropoietin stimulation of bone marrow.
Saxena S, Shulman IA, Johnson C: Effect of blood transfusion on serum iron and trans-ferrin saturation. Arch Pathol Lab Med 117:622, 1993.
Blood transfusion can affect diagnostic serum iron studies for 24 to 36 hours.
Schilling RF: Anemia of chronic disease: A misnomer. Ann Intern Med 115:572, 1991.
Suggests the term anemia of inflammation *instead of* anemia of chronic disease.
Wallerstein RO Jr: Laboratory evaluation of anemia. West J Med 146:443, 1987.
Good strategy for the laboratory evaluation of anemia using RBC size, reticulocyte count, and other selected studies.

MACROCYTIC ANEMIA WITHOUT RETICULOCYTOSIS

Recommendations for macrocytic anemia without reticulocytosis are from the medical literature.

1. In patients with macrocytic anemia (mean cell volume [MCV] >100 fL) and a normal to low reticulocyte count, causes include macrocytic megaloblastic anemia and macrocytic nonmegaloblastic anemia. Consider performing the following studies: examination of a peripheral blood smear and bone marrow aspirate; serum vitamin B$_{12}$ and folate determinations; thyroid function tests; and liver func-tion tests.

2. Evaluate the tests.

Reference ranges may vary among different laboratories.

REFERENCE RANGES

Test	Specimen	Conventional Units	International Units
Peripheral blood smear	Presence of oval macrocytes, hypersegmented neutrophils (>5% neutrophils with five lobes or any neutrophil with six lobes), and giant platelets is consistent with megaloblastic anemia. Round macrocytes are consistent with other causes. Target cells occur with liver disease.		
Bone marrow	Presence of megaloblasts separates megaloblastic causes from nonmegaloblastic causes.		
Vitamin B$_{12}$	Serum	100–700 pg/mL	74–516 pmol/L
Folate	Serum	3–16 ng/mL	7–36 nmol/L
	erythrocytes	130–628 ng/mL packed cells	294–1422 nmol/L packed cells
Thyroid function		See Chapter 8	
Liver function		See Chapter 6	

3. Interpret test results in the context of clinical findings.

Macrocytic Megaloblastic Anemia

In patients with macrocytic megaloblastic anemia, macrocytic red blood cells (RBCs) are found in the peripheral blood and megaloblasts in the marrow. Causes include vitamin B_{12} deficiency, folate deficiency, antimetabolite drugs, and antifolate drugs. If drugs are excluded as a cause, the most likely diagnosis is either vitamin B_{12} deficiency or folate deficiency. The distinction between these two causes is very important for two reasons: (1) folate does not correct the neuropsychiatric abnormalities caused by vitamin B_{12} deficiency; and (2) a diagnosis of vitamin B_{12} deficiency commits the patient to parenteral therapy for life.

Vitamin B_{12} Deficiency. In addition to serum vitamin B_{12} and folate levels, serum methylmalonic acid and homocysteine levels are useful in distinguishing between vitamin B_{12} and folate deficiency. The serum methylmalonic acid concentration is high in patients with vitamin B_{12} deficiency (>95% sensitive) and normal in those with folate deficiency. In contrast, serum homocysteine concentrations are high with both vitamin B_{12} and folate deficiency. A therapeutic trial of intramuscular vitamin B_{12}, 1 μg per day for 10 days, may be useful. This dose produces reticulocytosis in patients with vitamin B_{12} deficiency but not in patients with folate deficiency. Once vitamin B_{12} deficiency is diagnosed, the cause must be determined. Useful ancillary tests include examination of parietal cell and intrinsic factor antibodies, a gastrin test, and a Schilling test.

Folate Deficiency. Serum folate is low in patients with megaloblastic anemia due to folate deficiency but is usually normal in patients with vitamin B_{12} deficiency. A low serum folate concentration precedes low RBC or tissue folate values. RBC folate is a better test of tissue stores than serum folate; however, the RBC folate concentration is also low in the majority of cases of vitamin B_{12} deficiency, so vitamin B_{12} deficiency must be excluded. A therapeutic trial of oral folate, 100 μg per day for 10 days, is useful. This dose produces reticulocytosis in patients with folate deficiency but not in patients with vitamin B_{12} deficiency. Once folate deficiency is diagnosed, the cause must be determined.

Macrocytic Nonmegaloblastic Anemia

In patients with macrocytic nonmegaloblastic anemia, macrocytic RBCs are present in the peripheral blood, but no megaloblasts are in the marrow (i.e., the marrow shows normoblasts). Causes include reticulocytosis, alcoholism, liver disease, hypothyroidism, aplastic anemia, and sideroblastic anemia. Because a normal to low reticulocyte count excludes reticulocytosis as a cause, only the other causes are considered here.

Alcoholism and Liver Disease. In alcoholic individuals, macrocytic RBCs (MCV usually 100 to 110 fL) that are not due to reticulocytosis or a vitamin deficiency are seen in the peripheral blood smear. It is unclear whether this represents a nonspecific effect of marrow damage or a direct effect of alcohol on RBCs or RBC precursors. Macrocytic RBCs may also occur in patients with liver disease.

Patients with alcoholism may have a variety of causes for anemia: toxic suppression of the marrow, folate deficiency, iron deficiency, decreased RBC survival, abnormal iron metabolism, and hemodilution.

Hypothyroidism. There is a tendency to develop macrocytic RBCs with hypothyroidism and microcytic RBCs with hyperthyroidism. Typically, however, the anemia of hypothyroidism or hyperthyroidism is normocytic. These changes can occur even in the presence of adequate amounts of vitamins and iron.

Aplastic Anemia. In patients with aplastic and hypoplastic anemia, the peripheral blood count may show pancytopenia. Macrocytic RBCs may be seen.

Sideroblastic Anemia. In patients with sideroblastic anemia, the peripheral blood shows a dimorphic picture: hypochromic microcytes and macrocytes. If macrocytes prevail, the MCV may be high. See additional information about sideroblastic anemia in the discussion of microcytic anemia without reticulocytosis.

4. In patients with macrocytic anemia, the following test results may be increased:

- **Indirect bilirubin** in megaloblastic anemia due to hemolysis of some abnormal RBCs
- **Lactate dehydrogenase** in megaloblastic anemia due to intramedullary destruction of red cells
- **Gastrin** in pernicious anemia

BIBLIOGRAPHY

Brown RG: Normocytic and macrocytic anemias. Postgrad Med 89:125, 1991.
    Good discussion of the differential diagnosis of normocytic and macrocytic anemias.
Carmel R: Prevalence of undiagnosed pernicious anemia in the elderly. Arch Intern Med 156:1097, 1996.
    Undiagnosed pernicious anemia is a common finding in the elderly, especially among black and white women.
Carmel R, Green R, Jacobsen DW, et al: Neutrophil nuclear segmentation in mild cobalamin deficiency. Am J Clin Pathol 106:57, 1996.

Neutrophil hypersegmentation is not a sensitive test for mild cobalamin deficiency.

Kassirer JP, Kopelman RI: Case 19—Searching for a pony. *In* Learning Clinical Reasoning. Baltimore, Williams & Wilkins, 1991, p 124.
Discusses clinical reasoning in a patient with vitamin B$_{12}$ deficiency.

Mahmoud MY, Lugon M, Anderson CC: Unexplained macrocytosis in elderly patients. Age Ageing 25:310, 1996.
The causes for the macrocytosis in the patients for whom noninvasive studies were sufficient included hypothyroidism, ethanol intake, folic acid deficiency, vitamin B$_{12}$ deficiency, combined vitamin B$_{12}$ and folate deficiency, chronic liver disease, antiepileptic drugs, and malignant disease.

Rapoport AP, Rowe JM: Macrocytosis. *In* Panzer RJ, Black ER, Griner PF (eds): Diagnostic Strategies for Common Medical Problems. Philadelphia, American College of Physicians, 1991, p 458.
Suggests strategies for the differential diagnosis of macrocytic anemias.

Scates S, Glaspy J: The macrocytic anemias. Lab Med 21:736, 1990.
Good discussion of the differential diagnosis of the macrocytic anemias.

Sumner AE, Chin MM, Abrahm JL, et al: Elevated methylmalonic acid and total homocysteine levels show high prevalance of vitamin B$_{12}$ deficiency after gastric surgery. Ann Intern Med 469:124, 1996.
The data support both frequent screening and vitamin B$_{12}$ replacement therapy in patients who have had gastric surgery and have serum vitamin B$_{12}$ levels less than 299 pg/mL (<221 pmol/L).

Wymer A, Becker DM: Recognition and evaluation of red blood cell macrocytosis in the primary care setting. J Gen Intern Med 5:192, 1990.
Macrocytosis is common in outpatients. Treatable causes include alcohol abuse, vitamin B$_{12}$ deficiency, folate deficiency, and hypothyroidism.

NORMOCYTIC ANEMIA WITHOUT RETICULOCYTOSIS

Recommendations for normocytic anemia without reticulocytosis are from the medical literature.

1. In patients with normocytic anemia and a normal to low reticulocyte count, causes include primary and secondary bone marrow failure and other miscellaneous disorders. Consider the following studies: examination of a peripheral blood smear and bone marrow aspirate; determinations of serum iron, total iron-binding capacity, percent saturation, and ferritin; creatinine determination; liver function tests; and tests of endocrine function—especially thyroid function tests.

Before considering bone marrow failure as a cause, remember that normocytic anemia with a normal or low reticulocyte count may have other miscellaneous causes: early stages of iron deficiency anemia, anemia of chronic disease, acquired sideroblastic anemia, and dilutional anemia due to hypervolemia. Moreover, mixed anemias (e.g., from folate and iron deficiency) may be normocytic.

The anemias of primary bone marrow failure include the aplastic and hypoplastic anemias and the bone marrow replacement disorders.

The anemias of secondary bone marrow failure include uremia, endocrinologic causes, and human immunodeficiency virus (HIV) infection.

2. Interpret test results in the context of clinical findings.

Miscellaneous Causes

Early Stages of Microcytic Anemia. Mild cases of iron deficiency anemia, anemia of chronic disease, and sideroblastic anemia may be seen as normocytic anemia without reticulocytosis.

Dilutional Anemia. Normocytic anemia can occur with an increased plasma volume. This happens in alcoholic patients who have splenomegaly and with the use of drugs such as alpha-adrenergic blockers.

Primary Bone Marrow Failure

Aplastic and Hypoplastic Anemia. Aplastic and hypoplastic anemias are typically normocytic but may be macrocytic. Hereditary forms of these anemias can occur in children, and acquired forms can occur at any age. Acquired anemias include acquired aplastic anemia (from drugs, toxins, infections, miscellaneous conditions) and acquired pure red blood cell aplasia (from thymoma, drugs, toxins, neoplasms, autoimmune disorders, viral infections).

Bone Marrow Replacement Disorders. Bone marrow replacement patients have normocytic anemia because of failure of hematopoiesis secondary to replacement of the bone marrow by fibrosis, neoplastic cells, or nonneoplastic cells (e.g., Gaucher's cells). Pancytopenia may be present.

Secondary Bone Marrow Failure

Normocytic anemia can occur in patients with uremia, liver disease, endocrinologic disease, and HIV infection. Normocytic anemia occurs with chronic renal insufficiency, and its severity is roughly proportional to the degree of renal failure. It is caused by erythropoietin deficiency and other metabolic abnormalities that accompany uremia. It does not depend on the presence of inflammation. Normocytic anemia frequently occurs with diseases of the thyroid, adrenal glands, and gonads. With endocrinologic disease, especially hypothyroidism, a decreased hemoglobin concentration is related to reduced oxygen consumption. Decreased erythropoietin production may also be a factor in endocrinologic disorders. The prevalence of anemia in HIV-infected persons increases as the disease worsens. The anemia is typically normocytic.

BIBLIOGRAPHY

Björkholm M: Aplastic anemia: Pathogenetic mechanisms and treatment with special reference to immunomodulation. J Intern Med 231:575, 1992.
  Reviews the disease and emphasizes immune mechanisms.
Brown RB: Normocytic and macrocytic anemias. Postgrad Med 89:125, 1991.
  Good discussion of the differential diagnosis of normocytic and macrocytic anemia.
Schilling RF: Anemia of chronic disease: A misnomer. Ann Intern Med 115:572, 1991.
  Scholarly discussion of anemia due to inflammation, iron deficiency anemia, hypothyroidism, and malignancy.

ANEMIA WITH RETICULOCYTOSIS

Recommendations for anemia with reticulocytosis are from the medical literature.

1. In patients with anemia and a high reticulocyte count, causes include acute blood loss and hemolytic anemia. First consider acute blood loss.

A high reticulocyte count may cause some of these patients to have a high mean cell volume (MCV). Others have a normal MCV.

Acute Blood Loss

After acute blood loss, it may take a few days for the onset of reticulocytosis. In the bleeding patient, reticulocytosis continues until iron stores are depleted. Usually the source of bleeding is obvious (gastrointestinal or genitourinary), but it may be occult (into a fractured hip or into the retroperitoneum). Even though a bleeding source is obvious, it is still advisable to do an adequate work-up (i.e., there may be other co-existing causes for anemia).

2. If acute blood loss is not the cause, consider hemolytic anemia. Consider obtaining the following studies: examination of a peripheral blood smear, and determinations of plasma haptoglobin, serum unconjugated bilirubin and lactate dehydrogenase, and urinary hemoglobin and hemosiderin.

A Wright-stained peripheral blood smear may show helpful red blood cell (RBC) changes: spherocytes suggest hereditary spherocytosis; elliptocytes suggest hereditary elliptocytosis; abnormal RBC shapes and increased target cells suggest hemoglobinopathies; and fragmented cells suggest intravascular coagulation and a variety of other disorders that may cause mechanical fragmentation of RBCs.

Hemolytic anemias are less common than those caused by marrow failure or blood loss. Two questions should be addressed in the diagnosis:

1. Is hemolysis present?

2. What is its cause?

COMMONLY USED TESTS INDICATING PRESENCE OF HEMOLYSIS

Test	Result
Plasma haptoglobin	Decreased
Urine hemosiderin	Present
Urine hemoglobin	Present
Serum unconjugated bilirubin	Increased
Serum lactate dehydrogenase	Increased

Source: Lindenbaum J: An approach to the anemias. *In* Bennett JC, Plum F (eds): Cecil Textbook of Medicine, 20th ed. Philadelphia, WB Saunders, 1996, p 829.

The above tests detect hemolysis in an indirect manner. Although rarely needed, a direct estimate of RBC survival is available using radioactive chromium (^{51}Cr). Reference range for the normal RBC half-life is 25 to 32 days (elution of ^{51}Cr from RBCs at 1% per day produces this reference range instead of 60 days).

The following table lists some causes of congenital and acquired hemolytic anemia.

Mechanism	Examples
Congenital	
• Enzyme deficiency	Glucose-6-phosphate dehydrogenase, pyruvate kinase
• Membrane skeletal protein abnormalities (e.g., spectrin)	Hereditary spherocytosis, hereditary elliptocytosis
• Hemoglobinopathies	Hemoglobin SS, SC, CC, S-thalassemia
Acquired	
• Antibody induced	Autoimmune hemolysis (warm antibodies), cold agglutinin disease, hemolytic transfusion reaction
• Mechanical fragmentation	Intravascular coagulation, malignant hypertension, cancer chemotherapy, malfunctioning valve prosthesis, thrombotic thrombocytopenic purpura
• Membrane protein anchoring abnormality	Paroxysmal nocturnal hemoglobinuria

Source: Lindenbaum J: An approach to the anemias. *In* Bennett JC, Plum F (eds): Cecil Textbook of Medicine, 20th ed. Philadephia, WB Saunders Company, 1996, p 830.

3. If there is evidence of hemolysis, perform appropriate studies as indicated by the clinical findings and peripheral blood smear.

The causes of hemolysis are many, and the list of available tests is long. Therefore, testing should be based on clues discovered in the clinical findings and peripheral blood smear. Testing strategies for some causes of hemolytic anemia follow.

Congenital Causes

Enzyme Deficiency. Glucose-6-phosphate dehydrogenase (G6PD) deficiency is a prevalent X-linked genetic abnormality that can cause hemolytic anemia. The anemia can be induced by drugs, chemicals, infections, and fava beans. The fluorescent screening test for G6PD deficiency is reliable for detecting the disease. A quantitative G6PD assay is also available.

Pyruvate kinase deficiency is a less prevalent autosomal recessive abnormality that can cause hemolytic anemia. A fluorescent screening test for pyruvate kinase deficiency is available, and RBC enzyme levels can also be measured.

Membrane Skeletal Protein Abnormalities. Hereditary spherocytosis is the most prevalent hemolytic anemia among individuals of Northern European origin. It has an autosomal dominant inheritance, although some recessive forms may exist. The peripheral blood smear shows spherocytes. Laboratory tests include the osmotic fragility test and the autohemolysis test.

Hereditary elliptocytosis is another hemolytic anemia with an autosomal dominant inheritance. The peripheral blood smear shows at least 25% elliptocytes.

Hemoglobinopathies. Hemolytic anemias can occur with RBC hemoglobin defects such as Hb SS, SC, CC, and S-thalassemia. These defects can be diagnosed using Hb electrophoresis and other tests: sickle cell test, solubility test for Hb S, alkali denaturation test for Hb F, quantitation of Hb A_2 by chromatography, acid elution test for hemoglobin in RBCs, test for Hb H inclusion bodies, and other ancillary tests (Heinz bodies, crystal cells of Hb C disease, and RBC inclusions in Hb H disease).

Acquired Causes

Antibody-Induced Anemia. Antibody-induced anemia can be caused by autoimmune hemolysis (warm antibodies), cold agglutinin disease, or a hemolytic transfusion reaction. The direct antiglobulin test (Coombs' test) is useful for detecting antibodies attached to RBCs.

In patients with warm antibody–induced hemolysis, the antibodies are usually IgG, react best at body temperature, usually do not activate complement, and never cause agglutination. The antibodies are usually nonspecific, panspecific for Rh antigens, or drug induced. Women are affected more than men; 55% of cases are idiopathic, 20 to 25% drug induced, 15 to 20% associated with lymphoproliferative disorders, and 5 to 10% other.

In patients with cold agglutinin–induced hemolysis, the antibodies are usually IgM, are highly reactive at 0°C (32°F), activate complement, and cause agglutination. Specificity against I antigen is 95% and against i, 5%. Anti-I is associated with *Mycoplasma pneumoniae* and anti-i with infectious mononucleosis. These antibodies can occur with lymphoproliferative disorders or may be idiopathic. Another rare hemolytic disorder is paroxysmal cold hemoglobinuria.

Membrane Protein Anchoring Abnormality. Paroxysmal nocturnal hemoglobinuria is a rare cause of chronic hemolytic anemia due to an abnormality of the RBC membrane. The sucrose hemolysis test and the test for urinary hemosiderin are useful for screening, and the acid hemolysis test is the definitive diagnostic test.

Mechanical Fragmentation. In mechanical fragmentation traumatic hemolysis occurs because of shear forces on RBCs in turbulent flow, producing schistocytes, triangular cells, and helmet cells. In addition to occurring with intravascular coagulation, malignant hypertension, cancer, cardiac valve prosthesis, and thrombotic thrombocytopenic purpura, traumatic hemolysis can occur in patients with the hemolytic-uremic syndrome, vasculitis, and giant hemangioma.

Infections. Various infections can cause hemolysis, and different tests are necessary for diagnosis: blood cultures for *Clostridium perfringens*, wound cultures for *Escherichia coli* sepsis, stool cultures for cholera, and examination of RBCs in a peripheral blood smear for malaria.

Physiochemical Injuries. Burns, chemical toxins, and drugs can cause hemolytic anemia.

BIBLIOGRAPHY

Hoffman GC: The sickling disorders. Lab Med 21:797, 1990.
> *Good discussion not only of sickle cell trait and sickle cell anemia but also of the combinations of sickle hemoglobin with thalassemia and other structurally abnormal hemoglobins.*

Spivak JL: Hemolytic anemia; Paroxysmal nocturnal hemoglobinuria; Sickle cell anemia. *In* Spivak JL, Barnes HV (eds): Manual of Clinical Problems in Internal Medicine, 4th ed. Boston, Little, Brown & Co, 1990, pp 321, 345, 367.
> *Good discussion of diagnosis and management, with annotated key references.*

CLASSIFYING BLEEDING DISORDERS BY LABORATORY TESTS

Recommendations for screening patients for bleeding disorders by laboratory tests are from the American College of Physicians, the University Hospital Consortium, and the medical literature.

1. For patients with clinical findings of a bleeding disorder or to screen for such a disorder, request appropriate tests: complete blood count (CBC), examination of a peripheral blood smear, and determinations of bleeding time, prothrombin time (PT), and activated partial thromboplastin time (APTT). Routine screening of medical or surgical patients who have no clinical findings of a bleeding disorder is inappropriate.

In patients with clinical findings of a bleeding disorder, these tests provide a useful initial work-up. Most experts believe that routine screening tests for a bleeding disorder in asymptomatic medical patients or healthy patients about to undergo surgery are unnecessary. Occasionally a patient with a history of bleeding has normal screening test results (e.g., mild von Willebrand's disease, Factor XIII deficiency). In this situation, additional special tests can demonstrate the abnormality.

Clinical findings, if present, should be scrutinized to determine any family history of bleeding, the age and circumstances of onset, and the presence or absence of any underlying disorder. Bleeding due to thrombocytopenia (petechiae and purpura) should be distinguished from bleeding due to defective fibrin clot formation. Platelet disorders are caused by either decreased platelets or functional platelet disorders, which may be acquired or hereditary. Defective fibrin clot disorders can also be hereditary or acquired.

Platelet-type bleeding is characterized by mucocutaneous and post-traumatic bleeding. Patients with petechiae and purpura usually lack a sex-linked hereditary history, and affected individuals may be males or females. Bleeding episodes may follow dental procedures and operations, but the bleeding starts immediately at the time of the operation and often can be controlled by pressure. Epistaxis and gastrointestinal bleeding are often major problems.

Defective fibrin clot bleeding is commonly associated with hemarthrosis and intramuscular hematoma formation. Defective fibrin clot disorders are often sex-linked recessive diseases of males (hemophilia A and B), and almost 50% of patients have a sex-linked history of the disorder. The milder forms of hemophilia A and B resemble von Willebrand's disease. Bleeding frequently follows surgery or trauma such as venipuncture, dental procedures, surgical wounds, and bruises. Hematuria and hemarthroses may occur.

2. Evaluate the tests.

The CBC is useful to determine any quantitative blood cell abnormalities such as anemia and thrombocytopenia, and the peripheral blood smear is valuable for detecting morphologic changes such as RBC fragments, which may be a clue to disseminated intravascular coagulation, and large platelets, which may be a clue to immune thrombocytopenia. Any WBC abnormalities can be evaluated.

The bleeding time is useful to evaluate platelet function. A prolonged bleeding time may be due to either thrombocytopenia, a functional platelet disorder (e.g., aspirin ingestion), or a poorly done test. The combination of a long bleeding time and a platelet count greater than $100 \times 10^3/\mu L$ ($>100 \times 10^9/L$) is indicative of abnormal platelet function. The combination of a long bleeding time and APTT with a normal PT and platelet count suggests von Willebrand's disease. The response of platelets to a variety of aggregating agents (adenosine diphosphate [ADP], collagen, epinephrine) is useful to diagnose functional platelet disorders.

The PT and APTT are useful to detect abnormalities of the extrinsic and intrinsic pathways, respectively. Both tests are sensitive to defects in the common pathway. When the PT and/or APTT is prolonged, mixing experiments of normal plasma and the abnormal plasma determine whether the problem is a simple deficiency of a coagulation factor(s) (in which case the abnormal test result is corrected) or an inhibitor of coagulation (in which case the abnormal test result is not corrected). In a patient with a factor deficiency, the diagnosis can be established by mixing studies, using a series of plasmas with specific factor deficiencies.

3. In patients with clinical findings of platelet-type bleeding (i.e., mucocutaneous and post-traumatic bleeding), consider a platelet disorder. When the platelet count is less than $50 \times 10^3/\mu L$ ($50 \times 10^9/L$), determining a bleeding time is unnecessary because it is greatly prolonged. In a patient with thrombocytopenia, decreased platelet production can be distinguished from increased platelet destruction by a bone marrow aspirate, which also provides information about primary bone marrow disease such as leukemia. A normal PT and a normal APTT exclude an associated coagulation abnormality such as a lupus anticoagulant. Occasionally purpura is caused by a vascular or connective tissue abnormality.

Clinical bleeding and purpura do not occur unless the platelet count is less than 50 to $70 \times 10^3/\mu L$ (50 to $70 \times 10^9/L$) or an associated qualitative platelet defect is present. When the count decreases to less than 10 to $20 \times 10^3/\mu L$ (10 to $20 \times 10^9/L$), major spontaneous bleeding may occur.

Causes of nonthrombocytopenic purpura include connective tissue disorders (Marfan's syndrome, Ehlers-Danlos syndrome, osteogenesis imperfecta); vasculitis (drug hypersensitivity, Henoch-Schönlein syndrome); infections (bacterial, viral, rickettsial); and miscellaneous diseases (Cushing's syndrome, systemic lupus erythematosus).

Quantitative Platelet Disorders

Quantitative platelet disorders may be due to either too few platelets (thrombocytopenia) or too many platelets (thrombocytosis). Thrombocytosis may be reactive (secondary) or primary. Interestingly, bleeding or thrombosis is usually seen only in patients with primary thrombocytosis (e.g., essential thrombocythemia, chronic myelocytic leukemia, polycythemia vera).

Qualitative Platelet Disorders

Qualitative platelet disorders may be either hereditary or acquired.

Hereditary Disorders. Hereditary disorders are due to problems with platelet adhesion, secretion or release, or aggregation. Von Willebrand's disease, the most common hereditary bleeding disorder, is due to abnormal platelet adhesion caused by a quantitative or qualitative abnormality of von Willebrand's factor. Because this factor also acts as a carrier for factor VIII, the APTT and the bleeding time are also prolonged. Other functional platelet disorders are rare and can be differentiated with special platelet aggregation studies.

Acquired Disorders. Acquired platelet disorders commonly cause abnormal platelet function. The most prevalent of them is drug therapy, but there are additional causes (e.g., platelet antibodies, renal disease, myeloproliferative disorders). A variety of different drugs can interfere with platelet function (e.g., anti-inflammatory agents [commonly aspirin], antibiotics, tricylic antidepressants, beta-blockers, calcium channel blockers, lipid-lowering drugs, antihistamines, and miscellaneous agents [ethanol, hydrocortisone]). Diagnosis can be made using the clinical history and the demonstration of a prolonged bleeding time. Platelet aggregation studies are not usually necessary.

4. In patients with clinical findings of defective fibrin clot bleeding (i.e., hemarthrosis, intramuscular bleeding), consider a disorder of fibrin clot formation. Any or all of the initial bleeding disorder tests may be abnormal: the CBC, the peripheral blood smear, the bleeding time, the PT, and the APTT.

The differential for abnormal screening tests of fibrin clot formation follows:

Prolonged APTT	Prolonged PT	Prolonged PT and APTT
Common		
Heparin	Vitamin K	Vitamin K deficiency
Lupus anticoagulants	deficiency	Oral anticoagulants
Hemophilia A	Oral	Liver disease
Hemophilia B	anticoagulants	Consumptive
VWD (plus long BT)	Liver disease	coagulopathies

Table continued on following page

Prolonged APTT	Prolonged PT	Prolonged PT and APTT
Uncommon		
Specific factor inhibitors	Factor VII deficiency	Factor II, V, or X deficiency
Factor XI or XII deficiency		Hereditary dysfibrinogenemia
Prekallikrein deficiency		Afibrinogenemia
High-molecular-weight kininogen deficiency		Specific factor inhibitors
		Amyloidosis

APTT, activated partial thromboplastin time; PT, prothrombin time; VWD, von Willebrand's disease; BT, bleeding time.

Source: Brandt JT; Hemostasis. *In* Howanitz JH, Howanitz PJ (eds): Laboratory Medicine: Test Selection and Interpretation. New York, Churchill Livingstone, 1991, p 518.

Disorders of fibrin clot formation may be hereditary or acquired.

Hereditary Disorders. Hereditary disorders usually are seen initially as soft tissue bleeding in childhood. Hemophilia A (factor VIII deficiency) and hemophilia B (factor IX deficiency), together with von Willebrand's disease, constitute the vast majority of these conditions. The diagnosis is established by demonstrating the specific defect by factor assays.

Acquired Disorders. A number of acquired disorders can affect fibrin clot formation. There are two kinds of disorders that can be differentiated with special studies.

Acquired Deficiency States	Inhibition of Clot Formation
Liver disease	Heparin
Vitamin K deficiency	Lupus anticoagulants*
Oral anticoagulants	Neutralizing factor inhibitors
Amyloidosis	Non-neutralizing factor inhibitors
Consumptive coagulopathies	Macromolecules (e.g., dextran)
Hematin	Dysfibrinogenemia
Snake venoms	

*Generally not associated with bleeding.

Source: Brandt JT: Hemostasis. *In* Howanitz JH, Howanitz PJ (eds): Laboratory Medicine: Test Selection and Interpretation. New York, Churchill Livingstone, 1991, p 517.

Some acquired disorders are complex and may be seen initially with simultaneous bleeding and microvascular thrombosis.

Disorder	Laboratory Manifestations
Disseminated intravascular coagulation	Thrombocytopenia, low fibrinogen, long PT, long APTT, increased FDPs, low AT III
Thrombotic thrombocytopenic purpura; hemolytic-uremic syndrome	Thrombocytopenia, microangiopathic peripheral blood film, normal fibrinogen, normal AT III
Liver disease	Long PT, normal to low fibrinogen, low AT III

PT, prothrombin time; APTT, activated partial thromboplastin time; FDPs, fibrin degradation products; AT III, antithrombin III.

Source: Brandt JT: Hemostasis. *In* Howanitz JH, Howanitz PJ (eds): Laboratory Medicine: Test Selection and Interpretation. New York, Churchill Livingstone, 1991, p 522.

BIBLIOGRAPHY

AbuRahma AF, Boland JP, Witsberger T: Diagnostic and therapeutic strategies of white clot syndrome. Am J Surg 162:175, 1991.
Describes two kinds of heparin-induced thrombocytopenia and makes management recommendations.

Brody JE: von Willebrand's disease, a clotting disorder, afflicts millions, but few know they have it. The New York Times, August 23, 1995, p B6.
Von Willebrand's disease may affect as many as 1 in 100 persons, often causing frequent nosebleeds, bleeding gums, easy bruising, and excessive menstrual flow.

Burns ER, Lawrence C: Bleeding time: A guide to its diagnostic and clinical utility. Arch Pathol Lab Med 113:1219, 1989.
Concludes that determining a preoperative bleeding time is necessary only in the presence of a positive history of bleeding.

Colon-Otero G, Cockerill KJ, Bowie EJ: How to diagnose bleeding disorders. Postgrad Med 90:145, 1991.
Recommends practical strategies.

Erban SB, Kinman JL, Schwartz JS: Routine use of the prothrombin and partial thromboplastin times. JAMA 262:2428, 1989.
Believe that routine screening using the PT and APTT is inappropriate.

Konkle BA: Laboratory evaluation of von Willebrand disease. Clin Chem 41:489, 1995.
Ermens AAM, de Wild PJ, Vader HL, et al: Four agglutination assays evaluated for measurement of von Willebrand factor (ristocetin cofactor activity). Clin Chem 41:510, 1995.
Discusses testing strategies for von Willebrand disease.

Kugelmass AD, Oia A, Monahan K, et al: Activation of human platelets by cocaine. Circulation 88:876, 1993.
Suggests that cocaine causes myocardial infarction and other cardiovascular syndromes by activating platelets. Aspirin is unlikely to provide protection.

Remaley AT, Kennedy JM, Laposata M: Evaluation of the clinical utility of platelet aggregation studies. Am J Hematol 31:188, 1989.
Concludes that platelet aggregation studies are rarely useful in the diagnosis of specific bleeding disorders.

Santhosh-Kumar CR, Yohannan MD, Higgy KE, et al: Thrombocytosis in adults: Analysis of 777 patients. J Intern Med 229:493, 1991.
Studied the causes of thrombocytosis found on routine blood counts.

Spivak JL: Disseminated intravascular coagulation; Nonthrombocytopenic purpura;

Thrombocytopenia; Thrombocytosis; Thrombotic thrombocytopenic purpura. *In* Spivak JL, Barnes HV (eds): Manual of Clinical Problems in Internal Medicine, 4th ed. Boston, Little, Brown & Co, 1990, pp 306, 342, 377, 382, 385.
Good discussion of diagnosis and management, with annotated key references.
Suchman AL, Griner PF: Coagulation disorders. *In* Panzer RJ, Black ER, Griner PF (eds): Diagnostic Strategies for Common Medical Problems. Philadelphia, American College of Physicians, 1991, p 478.
Believe that no coagulation tests are indicated before surgery in asymptomatic individuals without risk factors.
Suchman AL, Griner PF: Common uses of the activated partial thromboplastin time and prothrombin time. *In* Sox HC Jr (ed): Common Diagnostic Tests: Use and Interpretation, 2nd ed. Philadelphia, American College of Physicians, 1990, p 227.
Technology Assessment: Routine Preoperative Diagnostic Evaluations. University Hospital Consortium Technology Advancement Center, Oak Brook, IL, June, 1994.
Recommends against routine screening of medical or surgical patients who have no clinical findings of a bleeding disorder.

10

Acid-Base, Fluid Volume, Osmolality, and Electrolyte Diseases

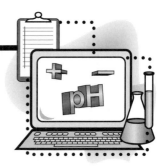

CLASSIFYING ACID-BASE, FLUID VOLUME, OSMOLALITY, AND ELECTROLYTES BY LABORATORY TESTS

Recommendations for diseases of acid-base, fluid volume, osmolality, and electrolytes are from the medical literature.

1. In patients with clinical findings of an acid-base, fluid volume, and/or electrolyte disease, assess the patient's hydration (hypervolemia, normovolemia, hypovolemia) and request appropriate laboratory tests: arterial blood gas analysis and determinations of serum electrolytes and serum osmolality.

The American College of Physicians does not recommend arterial blood gas analysis and determinations of serum electrolytes and serum osmolality for screening but does recommend these tests to diagnose and manage patients with a serious illness in which these analytes may be affected. Canadian researchers developed guidelines for cost-efficient use of blood gas analyses in the intensive-care unit with no adverse effects or outcomes. The guidelines stipulated 12-hour monitoring with special triggers for more frequent determinations, such as arterial oxygenation by oximetry less than 85%, dyspnea, respiratory rate greater than 30/min, mean blood pressure equal to or less than 70 mm Hg, and hourly urine output equal to or less than 0.5 mL/kg. In the emergency department, 10 clinical criteria are helpful in deciding which patients need serum electrolyte determinations: poor oral intake, vomiting, chronic hypertension, taking a diuretic, recent seizure, muscle weakness, age 65 years or older, alcoholism, abnormal mental status, and recent history of an electrolyte abnormality. Inability to communicate has been suggested as an additional criterion. Unfortunately, these criteria do not work very well for elderly patients.

Acid-base and electrolyte diseases occur in the context of fluid volumes that are increased (hypervolemic diseases), normal (normovolemic diseases), or decreased (hypovolemic diseases). The history and physical examination are the mainstays of evaluating the existence and causes of volume diseases.

Clinical findings of hypervolemia include edema, shortness of breath, paroxysmal nocturnal dyspnea, orthopnea, and hypertension. Clinical findings of normovolemia include well-being and alertness and normal vital signs, skin turgor, thirst, sweating, and urination. Clinical findings of hypovolemia include increased thirst, decreased sweating and skin turgor, decreased mucous membrane secretions, oliguria with increased urine concentration, central nervous system depression, weakness and muscle cramps, decreased blood pressure, increased pulse rate, and decreased central venous pressure.

2. Evaluate the tests.

Arterial blood gas and serum electrolyte and osmolality tests should be evaluated with an understanding of the body fluid compartments. Body water comprises approximately 60% of body weight and is divided into two compartments: the intracellular fluid (ICF) compartment and the extracellular fluid (ECF) compartment. The ICF compartment contains two thirds of the body water and the ECF compartment one third. The ECF, in turn, is divided into two parts: the intravascular part (blood) and the extravascular part. Thus, in a healthy 70-kg man, total body water is approximately 40 L, of which 25 L are intracellular and 15 L extracellular, of which 5 L is blood. Because the normal hematocrit value is 40 to 45%, total plasma (serum) volume is 2.75 to 3 L. Arterial blood gas and serum electrolyte analyses are determined using whole blood and serum, respectively. Assumptions about changes in the ICF are based on blood and serum gas and electrolyte concentrations interpreted in the context of a clinical assessment of body fluid volume. In addition to acid-base and electrolyte balance, serum osmolality must be considered. Besides the maintenance of normal pH and electrolyte concentrations, the serum osmolality is maintained in a narrow range of 275 to 295 mOsmol/kg. Serum osmolality is either measured directly or calculated using the following formula:

Calculated osmolality (mOsm/kg) =

$$2 \times \text{Sodium (mEq/L)} + \frac{\text{Glucose (mg/dL)}}{18} + \frac{\text{Urea nitrogen (mg/dL)}}{2.8}$$

OR

Calculated osmolality (mOsm/kg) = 2 × Sodium (mmol/L) +
Glucose (mmol/L) + Urea nitrogen (mmol/L)

3. Interpret arterial blood gas, serum electrolyte, and serum osmolality test results in the context of fluid volume status.

Arterial blood gas, electrolyte, and serum osmolality test results should be interpreted in the context of a clinical assessment of fluid volume status. This is especially true of serum sodium, which is the principal cation of the ECF, in which 95% of total body sodium is located. For example, hyponatremic diseases can occur with increased extracellular volume (congestive heart failure, cirrhosis, nephrotic syndrome), normal extracellular volume (adrenal or thyroid insufficiency, redistribution of sodium), or decreased extracellular volume. Potassium is the principal cation of the ICF, which contains nearly 90% of total body potassium.

BIBLIOGRAPHY

Bany-Mohammed FM, Macknin ML, van Lente F, et al: The effect of prolonged tourniquet application on serum bicarbonate. Cleve Clin J Med 62:68, 1995.
Applying a tourniquet for up to 5 minutes prior to blood collection does not reduce the serum bicarbonate or significantly change the lactate concentration.

Beck LH, Kassirer JP: Serum electrolytes, serum osmolality, blood urea nitrogen, and serum creatinine; and Raffin TA: Indications for arterial blood gas analysis. *In* Sox HC Jr (ed): Common Diagnostic Tests: Use and Interpretation, 2nd ed. Philadelphia, American College of Physicians, 1990, pp 367, 100.
Reviews of arterial blood gas analysis, serum electrolytes, serum osmolality, blood urea nitrogen, and serum creatinine with American College of Physicians' guidelines for appropriate use.

Kapsner CO, Tzamaloukas AH: Understanding serum electrolytes: How to avoid mistakes. Postgrad Med 90:151, 1991.
Discusses pitfalls in the interpretation of serum electrolytes.

Low LL, Harrington GR, Stoltzfus DP: The effect of arterial lines on blood-drawing practices and costs in intensive care units. Chest 108:216, 1995.
Presence of an arterial line promotes an increase in arterial blood gas and CBC studies and contributes to anemia.

Lowe RA, Arst HF, Ellis BK: Rational ordering of electrolytes in the emergency department. Ann Emerg Med 20:16, 1991.
Summarizes 10 clinical criteria that should trigger a request for serum electrolytes.

Roberts D, Ostryzniuk P, Loewen E, et al: Control of blood gas measurements in intensive-care units. Lancet 337:1580, 1991.
Canadian guidelines for blood gas analysis in intensive care units that produced favorable outcomes and decreased costs.

Singal BM, Hedges JR, Succop PA: Prediction of electrolyte abnormalities in elderly emergency patients. Ann Emerg Med 20:964, 1991.
Points out that criteria for ordering electrolytes in the emergency department do not work very well for elderly patients.

ACID-BASE DISEASES

Recommendations for acid-base diseases are from the medical literature.

1. For patients with clinical findings of an acid-base disease, request arterial blood gas studies and serum electrolyte determinations.

Perform blood gas studies within 30 minutes of drawing the sample. Use glass syringes placed on ice for patients with thrombocytosis, leukocytosis, reticulocytosis, or a high Po_2.

2. Evaluate the test results.

a. Determine pH status: A pH greater than 7.45 indicates alkalosis, and a pH less than 7.35 indicates acidosis.

b. Determine whether the primary process is respiratory or metabolic (or both): Consider whether the pH is above or below 7.4. The process or processes that caused it to shift to that side are the primary abnormalities.

	Primary Uncompensated Alkalosis	**Primary Uncompensated Acidosis**
Respiratory	**Alkalosis:** pH >7.45 and partial pressure of carbon dioxide (Pco_2) <35 mm Hg	**Acidosis:** pH <7.35 and Pco_2 >45 mm Hg
Metabolic	**Alkalosis:** pH >7.45 and bicarbonate >23 mEq/L (>23 mmol/L)	**Acidosis:** pH <7.35 and bicarbonate <18 mEq/L (<18 mmol/L)

c. Calculate the serum anion gap. Use the anion gap reference range established by your laboratory.

Anion gap = Sodium − (Chloride + Bicarbonate)

An anion gap that is increased more than 15 mEq/L (15 mmol/L) may indicate metabolic acidosis. An anion gap that is increased more than 25 mEq/L (25 mmol/L) always indicates metabolic acidosis.

d. Check the degree of compensation: In a patient with metabolic acidosis, compensation is evidenced by a decreasing arterial Pco_2 and an increasing arterial pH, whereas in a patient with metabolic alkalosis compensation is shown by an increasing arterial Pco_2 and a decreasing arterial pH.

e. Determine whether there is a 1:1 relationship between anions in blood.

Pure Metabolic Acidosis

Increased anion gap	Every one-point increase in anion gap should be accompanied by a 1 mEq/L (1 mmol/L) decrease in bicarbonate.
Normal anion gap	Every 1 mEq/L (1 mmol/L) increase in chloride should be accompanied by a 1 mEq/L (1 mmol/L) decrease in bicarbonate.

3. Interpret test results in the context of clinical findings.

Simple Acid-Base Diseases

Respiratory Alkalosis. With respiratory alkalosis, the pH is greater than 7.45 and the Pco_2 is less than 35 mm Hg. A normal bicarbonate concentration means lack of metabolic compensation, which indicates an acute respiratory alkalosis, whereas a low bicarbonate concentration with a normal pH value means metabolic compensation, which indicates chronic respiratory alkalosis.

The causes of acute respiratory alkalosis include anxiety; lung disease, with or without hypoxia; drug use (salicylates, catecholamines, progesterone); mechanical ventilation; central nervous system (CNS) disease; pregnancy; sepsis; and hepatic encephalopathy.

Metabolic Alkalosis. With metabolic alkalosis, the pH is greater than 7.45 and the serum bicarbonate concentration is greater than 23 mEq/L (>23 mmol/L). The Pco_2 can rise modestly in compensation for metabolic alkalosis, with a concomitant decrease in pH, but Pco_2 greater than 55 mm Hg probably is not just compensatory, and an additional primary respiratory abnormality should not be excluded.

The causes of metabolic alkalosis with respiratory compensation include disorders in which the urinary chloride level is low and disorders in which the urinary chloride concentration is normal or high. Conditions in which the urinary chloride concentration is low include vomiting; nasogastric suction; diuretic use in the past; and posthypercapnia. Conditions in which the urinary chloride level is normal or high include excess mineralocorticoid activity (Cushing's syndrome, Conn's syndrome, exogenous steroids, licorice ingestion, increased renin states, Bartter's syndrome); current or recent diuretic use; and excess alkali administration.

Respiratory Acidosis. With respiratory acidosis, the pH is less than 7.35 and the Pco_2 is greater than 45 mm Hg. A normal bicarbonate concentration means lack of metabolic compensation, which indicates acute respiratory acidosis, whereas a high bicarbonate concentration with a normal pH level means metabolic compensation, which indicates chronic respiratory acidosis.

The causes of acute respiratory acidosis include CNS depression (drugs, CNS event); acute airway obstruction (in upper airway, laryngospasm, bronchospasm, severe pneumonia, pulmonary edema); thoracic cage injury (flail chest, ventilator dysfunction); neuromuscular disorders (myopathies, neuropathies); and impaired lung motion (hemothorax, pneumothorax).

The causes of chronic respiratory acidosis with metabolic compensation include chronic lung disease (obstructive or restrictive); chronic respiratory center depression (central hypoventilation); and chronic neuromuscular disorders.

Metabolic Acidosis. With metabolic acidosis, the pH is less than 7.35 and the serum bicarbonate concentration is less than 18 mEq/L (<18 mmol/L). Low P_{CO_2} with a normal pH level indicates respiratory compensation.

The causes of metabolic acidosis are divided into those with an increased anion gap and those without an increased anion gap. Those with an increased anion gap include ketoacidosis (diabetic, alcoholic); renal failure; lactic acidosis (anion gap not always increased); rhabdomyolysis; and toxins (methanol, ethylene glycol, paraldehyde, salicylates). Those without an increased anion gap include gastrointestinal bicarbonate loss (diarrhea, ureteral diversions); renal bicarbonate loss (renal tubular acidosis, early renal failure, carbonic anhydrase inhibitors, aldosterone inhibitors); hydrochloric acid administration; and hypocapnia.

Mixed Acid-Base Diseases

See the article by Haber listed in the references for a discussion of the following mixed acid-base diseases:

- Respiratory alkalosis and metabolic acidosis
- Metabolic acidosis and metabolic alkalosis
- Respiratory alkalosis, metabolic acidosis, and metabolic alkalosis
- Respiratory acidosis, metabolic acidosis, and metabolic alkalosis
- Anion gap and nonanion gap metabolic acidoses

BIBLIOGRAPHY

Badrick T, Hickman PE: The anion gap: A reappraisal. Am J Clin Pathol 98:249, 1992.
    Only extremes of abnormality of the anion gap may be clinically useful. The diagnosis of the underlying abnormalities can be made more reliable by clinical parameters and other laboratory measurements.
Blanke RV: High anion-gap acidosis with high osmolal gap. *In* Tietz NW, Conn RB, Pruden EL (eds): Applied Laboratory Medicine. Philadelphia, WB Saunders, 1992, p 335.

Case discussion of the use of anion and osmolar gaps in a patient with ethylene glycol poisoning.

Delclaux B, Orcel B, Housset B, et al: Arterial blood gases in elderly persons with chronic obstructive pulmonary disease. Eur Respir J 7:856, 1994.
The probable normal PaO₂ for all subjects older than 65 years, regardless of age, is 80 to 85 mm Hg.

Flanagan NG, Ridway JC, Irving AG: The anion gap as a screening procedure for occult myeloma in the elderly. J R Soc Med 81:27, 1988.
A low anion gap can be used to detect myeloma.

Haber RJ: A practical approach to acid-base disorders. West J Med 155:146, 1991.
Excellent discussion of how to diagnose simple and complex acid-base disorders.

Iberti TJ, Leibowitz AB, Papadakos PJ, et al: Low sensitivity of the anion gap as a screen to detect hyperlactatemia in critically ill patients. Crit Care Med 18:275, 1990.
Increased anion gap is not always present in patients with lactic acidosis.

Liss HP, Payne CP Jr: Stability of blood gases in ice and at room temperature. Chest 103:1120, 1993.
It is not necessary to place arterial blood on ice if the blood gas studies can be done within 30 minutes. However, glass syringes should be used and placed on ice for patients with severe thrombocytosis, leukocytosis, reticulocytosis, or a very high PO₂.

Roberts WL, Johnson RD: The serum anion gap: Has the reference interval really fallen? Arch Pathol Lab Med 121:568, 1997.
Results suggest that although it may be appropriate to lower the anion gap reference interval to 5 to 10 mEq/L (5 to 10 mmol/L) for some analyzers, as suggested by earlier reports, 9 to 14 mEq/L (9 to 14 mmol/L) may be a more appropriate reference interval for other analyzers.

Rutecki GW, Whittier FC: Acid-base interpretation: Five rules, and how they help in everyday cases. Consultant 31:44, 1991.

Rutecki GW, Whittier FC: Acid-base interpretation: Five rules, and how they simplify complex cases. Consultant 31:19, 1991.
Two short practical articles on acid-base interpretation.

Sasse SA, Chen PA, Mahutte CK: Variability of arterial blood gas values over time in stable medical ICU patients. Chest 106:187, 1994.
The substantial variation of arterial blood gas values in medically stable ICU patients, with mean coefficients of variation of 6.1% for PO₂ and 4.7% for PCO₂, should be considered when making clinical decisions based on arterial blood gas values.

Williamson JC: Acid-base disorders: Classification and management strategies. Am Fam Physician 52:584, 1995.
Simple acid-base disorders can be diagnosed by clinical findings and determinations of electrolyte levels, anion gap, and pH.

Winter SD, Pearson JR, Gabow PA, et al: The fall of the serum anion gap. Arch Intern Med 150:311, 1990.
Found that modern analyzers often generate anion gaps that are significantly lower than in the past (e.g., 3 to 11 mEq/L [3 to 11 mmol/L], compared with 8 to 16 mEq/L [8 to 16 mmol/L]).

HYPERNATREMIA

Recommendations for hypernatremia are from the medical literature.

1. For patients at risk for hypernatremia or with clinical findings of hypernatremia, request measurements of serum sodium and serum and urinary osmolality.

Hypernatremia is a hypertonic disorder caused by an increased serum sodium concentration above 146 mEq/L (146 mmol/L). The clinical features are produced by brain shrinkage secondary to an increased extracellular fluid (ECF) osmolality. Causes include too little dietary water, too much dietary salt, and excessive water loss from the body. Clinical findings of hypernatremia progress from somnolence, confusion, and coma to respiratory paralysis and death as the hypernatremia worsens.

A serum sodium determination can be used to verify the presence of hypernatremia, and serum and urinary osmolality measurements are helpful to determine the cause of the hypernatremia. Using serum or heparinized plasma for the test is satisfactory, but avoid collection tubes containing sodium, for example, sodium fluoride, sodium citrate, sodium ethylenediaminetetraacetic acid, and sodium heparin. When obtaining the blood specimen, avoid significant hemolysis, which can decrease the serum sodium concentration because of a dilutional effect from the erythrocyte fluid. Lipemia or hyperproteinemia can artifactually decrease the serum sodium concentration, causing a normal serum sodium value to appear decreased.

2. Evaluate the test results.

The severity of the clinical findings correlates with the degree of hypernatremia and the rate at which it develops. In a patient with acute hypernatremia, symptoms may appear when serum osmolality exceeds 320 to 330 mOsm/kg, and respiratory arrest may occur when osmolality exceeds 360 to 380 mOsm/kg.

In diabetics, nonketotic hyperglycemic hyperosmolality can produce clinical findings similar to those of hypernatremia. In patients with this syndrome, the serum sodium concentration is initially low, but as hyperglycemia rapidly depletes extracellular water, the serum sodium concentration becomes normal or increases. Depressed consciousness is uncommon when serum osmolality is less than 350 mOsm/kg, whereas virtually all patients with serum osmolalities exceeding 400 mOsm/kg are comatose.

3. Interpret test results in the context of clinical findings. Antidiuretic hormone (ADH) levels may be normal or low.

Hypernatremic States With Normal ADH Levels

Hypovolemia With Excessive Water Loss

- Impaired water intake: if water intake is impaired and falls behind normal insensitive loss through the skin, lungs, and gastrointestinal tract, the ECF volume contracts, and the serum sodium concentration increases. The individual is appropriately thirsty, and the urine is highly concentrated.
- Excessive water loss: excessive water loss can occur through the skin (excessive sweating, burns), the lungs (hyperventilation), and the gastrointestinal tract (vomiting, diarrhea). The ECF volume

contracts, the serum sodium concentration increases, and the urine is highly concentrated.

- Osmotic diuresis: osmotic diuresis secondary to glucose, urea, mannitol, or radiocontrast dye excretion can result in a contracted ECF volume and a high serum sodium concentration.

Normovolemia With Altered Regulation of Osmolality. Diseases of the hypothalamus and pituitary can alter the regulation of thirst and ADH secretion, causing a high serum sodium concentration. The ECF volume is normal.

Hypervolemia With Excessive Sodium Loads. A high serum sodium concentration and an expanded extracellular volume can occur with excessive salt intake either by ingestion or parenteral administration. Also, in patients with primary hyperaldosteronism and Cushing's syndrome, the serum sodium concentration may be high with an expansion of the ECF volume.

Hypernatremic States With Low ADH Levels

Central Diabetes Insipidus. A variety of diseases (traumatic, neoplastic, infiltrative, infectious, vascular) and drugs (ethanol, opiate antagonists, α-adrenergic agents, phenytoin) can affect the hypothalamus and cause an ADH deficiency, which results in polyuria with dilute urine. If the ADH deficiency is severe enough, the serum sodium concentration can increase.

Nephrogenic Diabetes Insipidus. Unresponsiveness of the kidneys to ADH can be either congenital or acquired. The congenital form is X-linked and rare. The acquired forms (electrolyte disorders, drugs, tubulointerstitial nephropathies) are common.

BIBLIOGRAPHY

Beck LH, Kassirer JP: Serum electrolytes, serum osmolality, blood urea nitrogen, and serum creatinine. *In* Sox HC Jr (ed): Common Diagnostic Tests: Use and Interpretation, 2nd ed. Philadelphia, American College of Physicians, 1990, p 367.
  American College of Physicians guidelines for measuring serum sodium.
Borra SI, Beredo R, Kleinfeld M: Hypernatremia in the aging: Causes, manifestations, and outcomes. J Natl Med Assoc 87:220, 1995.
  Mortality associated with hypernatremia is high, but outcomes are improved when serum sodium is normalized within a 72-hour period.
Felig P, Johnson C, Levitt M, et al: Hypernatremia induced by maximal exercise. JAMA 248:1209, 1982.
  Intense exercise can cause hypernatremia.
Klosinski DD: Troubleshooting elevated sodium levels. Lab Med 28:369, 1997.
  Discusses preanalytic causes of hypernatremia.
Palevsky PM, Bhagrath R, Greenberg A: Hypernatremia in hospitalized patients. Ann Intern Med 124:197, 1996.

Hypernatremia is frequently iatrogenic, caused by inappropriate prescription of fluids and diuretics for patients with increased water loss, impaired thirst, and restricted free-water intake.

Snyder NA, Feigal DW, Arieff AI: Hypernatremia in elderly patients: A heterogeneous, morbid, and iatrogenic entity. Ann Intern Med 107:309, 1987.

Beck LH, Lavizzo-Mourey R: Geriatric hypernatremia. Ann Intern Med 107:768, 1987. *Discusses the increased susceptibility to hypernatremia in the elderly.*

HYPONATREMIA

Recommendations for hyponatremia are from the medical literature.

1. In patients at risk for hyponatremia or with clinical findings of hyponatremia, exclude pseudohyponatremia before proceeding with the work-up. Request measurements of serum sodium and osmolality and urinary sodium.

Hyponatremia is a hypotonic disorder caused by a depressed serum sodium concentration, below 136 mEq/L (136 mmol/L). The clinical features are produced by brain swelling secondary to a decreased extracellular fluid osmolality. Causes include excessive total body water and sodium depletion. When evaluating hyponatremia, it is important to assess whether the patient is hypervolemic, hypovolemic, or euvolemic. Usually, hyponatremia is modest, the patient is asymptomatic, and if the cause is removed (e.g., diuretic therapy), the condition improves. On the other hand, severe symptomatic hyponatremia (serum sodium <120 mEq/L [<120 mmol/L]) is rare and constitutes a medical emergency. The findings progress from lethargy, weakness, and somnolence to seizures, coma, and death as the hyponatremia worsens. Hyponatremic infants may have seizures.

Hyponatremia is the most common serum electrolyte abnormality in hospitalized patients. It often occurs in patients in the intensive care unit. A serum sodium determination can be used to detect or verify hyponatremia, and serum osmolality and urinary sodium measurements are useful to determine the cause of hyponatremia. The specimen collection and handling issues are the same as for hypernatremia. Dietary sodium, excessive water intake, and drugs may be contributing factors.

2. Evaluate the test results.

Exclude pseudohyponatremia (euosmolar hyponatremia) caused by severe hyperlipidemia or hyperproteinemia. If the serum is lipemic or the proteins are high (>10 g/dL [>100 g/L]), determine whether there is a significant osmolar gap, according to the following formula:

Osmolar gap = Measured osmolality − Calculated osmolality*

---

*All units are in milliosmoles per kilogram (mOsm/kg). See the first problem in this chapter for the formula for calculated osmolality.

If the measured osmolality is normal and the osmolar gap is significant, the low serum sodium concentration is probably an artifact caused by lipemia or hyperproteinemia. This is true only if there are no unusual osmotically active substances (ethanol, methanol, mannitol) in the serum because these substances can also cause an increased osmolar gap (see the discussion of alcoholism in Chapter 1).

The occurrence of pseudohyponatremia is method dependent; that is, it is observed when the serum sodium concentration is measured by flame photometry but not when sodium is measured in undiluted serum using an ion-specific electrode. It is important to recognize pseudohyponatremia because it requires no therapy.

A high serum glucose concentration (an osmotically active, low-molecular solute) can also contribute to a low serum sodium value because every 100 mg/dL (5.55 mmol/L) rise in the serum glucose concentration produces a decrease of approximately 1.6 mEq/L (1.6 mmol/L) in the serum sodium value. This phenomenon can also occur with mannitol. Increased serum immunoglobulins, particularly IgG (but also IgA), can behave as cations and cause a decreased serum sodium value and a low anion gap (anion gap = $Na - [Cl + HCO_3]$). Normally the gap is 8 to 16 mEq/L (8 to 16 mmol/L) and is composed of phosphate, sulfate, organic acids, and proteinate. Myeloma patients have a mean anion gap of 6.8, whereas the mean gap of controls is 9.4. Patients with monoclonal gammopathy of undetermined significance have a mean anion gap of 9.1.

In a patient with true hyponatremia, the severity of the clinical findings correlates with the degree of hyponatremia and the rate at which it develops. With acute hyponatremia, the clinical features generally appear when the serum sodium concentration falls to 120 mEq/L (120 mmol/L) or less. With chronic hyponatremia clinical manifestations are far less common, even when the serum sodium concentration is below 120 mEq/L (120 mmol/L).

According to a recent study, neither hyponatremic encephalopathy nor its therapy is commonly associated with central pontine myelinolysis. Another study suggests that myelinolysis, if it occurs, is more commonly associated with the rapid correction of chronic hyponatremia.

3. Interpret test results in the context of clinical findings.

Hypervolemic Hyponatremia

Edematous patients often have hypervolemic hyponatremia (congestive heart failure, cirrhosis, nephrotic syndrome, renal failure). In patients with cardiac failure, cirrhosis, and the nephrotic syndrome, the urinary sodium concentration is less than 10 mEq/L (<10 mmol/L); in patients with acute or chronic renal failure, the urinary sodium concentration is greater than 20 mEq/L (>20 mmol/L).

An additional cause of hypervolemic hyponatremia is transurethral resection of the prostate: 5 to 10% of patients develop hypervolemic hyponatremia because of absorption of the irrigate solution used to clear the operative field.

Normovolemic Hyponatremia

Certain drugs can cause normovolemic hyponatremia and severe emotional stress (acute psychosis), and **physical stresses** (trauma, surgery) are additional causes. Two endocrine disorders, hypothyroidism and hypopituitarism, may be seen initially as normovolemic hyponatremia. The syndrome of inappropriate antidiuretic hormone (SIADH) secretion can also cause normovolemic hyponatremia. This syndrome is characterized by hyponatremia, volume expansion without edema, natriuresis, hypouricemia, normal or reduced creatinine level, and normal thyroid and adrenal function. Causes of SIADH include the following:

Malignant Neoplasia	Central Nervous System Disorders	Pulmonary Disorders
Carcinoma: bronchogenic, pancreatic, ureteral, prostatic, bladder	Trauma Infection Tumors Porphyria	Tuberculosis Pneumonia Ventilators with positive pressure
Lymphoma and leukemia Thymoma and mesothelioma		

Source: Andreoli TE: Disorders of fluid volume, electrolyte, and acid-base balance. *In* Wyngaarden JB, Smith LH Jr, Bennett JC (eds): Cecil Textbook of Medicine, 19th ed. Philadelphia, WB Saunders, 1992, p 509.

Fluoxetine (Prozac) is an additional cause of SIADH.
  In a patient with normovolemic hyponatremia, the urinary sodium concentration is typically greater than 20 mEq/L (>20 mmol/L).

Hypovolemic Hyponatremia

Gastrointestinal and renal loss of fluid and electrolytes can lead to hypovolemic hyponatremia. **Gastrointestinal disorders** include external loss (diarrhea, vomiting, external fistula) or internal loss (pancreatitis, peritonitis, internal fistula). **Renal disorders** include excessive diuretic use, osmotic diuresis, postobstructive diuresis, bicarbonaturia, renal salt wasting, ketonuria, and adrenocortical hormone deficiency.
  The skin can be a site of substantial loss of fluid and electrolytes

in long-distance runners and patients with severe burns or widespread skin diseases.

A urinary sodium concentration greater than 20 mEq/L (>20 mmol/L) is characteristic of renal causes of hypovolemic hyponatremia, and a urinary sodium concentration less than 10 mEq/L (<10 mmol/L) occurs with extrarenal diseases (gastrointestinal or skin diseases).

BIBLIOGRAPHY

Beck LH, Kassirer JP: Serum electrolytes, serum osmolality, blood urea nitrogen, and serum creatinine. *In* Sox HC Jr (ed): Common Diagnostic Tests: Use and Interpretation, 2nd ed. Philadelphia, American College of Physicians, 1990, p 367.
American College of Physicians' guidelines for measuring serum sodium.
DeVita MV, Gardenswartz MH, Konecky A, et al: Incidence and etiology of hyponatremia in an intensive care unit. Clin Nephrol 34:163, 1990.
Patients in the intensive care unit often develop hyponatremia.
Ellis RE, Carmichael JK: Hyponatremia and volume overload as a complication of transurethral resection of the prostate. J Fam Pract 33:89, 1991.
Awareness of this complication of prostate surgery is important.
Epstein M: Renal sodium retention in liver disease. Hosp Pract 30:33, 1995.
Most patients with liver disease and edema are prone to dilutional hyponatremia.
Flanagan NG, Ridway JC, Irving AG: The anion gap as a screening procedure for occult myeloma in the elderly. J R Soc Med 81:27, 1988.
A low anion gap can be used to detect myeloma.
Hyponatremic seizures among infants fed with commercial bottled drinking water—Wisconsin, 1993. MMWR 43:641, 1994.
Infants who drink bottled water risk water intoxication and hyponatremia.
Kassirer JP, Kopelman RI: Case 36—Leaving no stone unturned. *In* Kassirer JP, Kopelman RI: Learning Clinical Reasoning. Baltimore, Williams & Wilkins, 1991, p 192.
Discusses clinical reasoning in a patient with confusion and disorientation secondary to hyponatremia.
Laureno R, Karp BI: Myelinolysis after correction of hyponatremia. Ann Intern Med 126:57, 1997.
Myelinolysis is more likely to occur after the treatment of chronic rather than acute hyponatremia and is more likely to occur with a rapid rate of correction.
Miller M, Hecker MS, Friedlander DA, et al: Apparent idiopathic hyponatremia in an ambulatory geriatric population. J Am Geriatr Soc 44:404, 1996.
In the elderly, hyponatremia due to the syndrome of inappropriate antidiuretic hormone secretion may develop with no apparent underlying cause.
Moran SM, Jamison RL: The variable hyponatremic response to hyperglycemia. West J Med 142:49, 1985.
High serum glucose concentration can cause hyponatremia.
Schrier RW, Briner VA: The differential diagnosis of hyponatremia. Hosp Pract 25:29, 1990.
Review of the differential diagnosis and management of patients with hyponatremia.
Steele A, Gowrishankar M, Abrahamson S, et al: Postoperative hyponatremia despite near-isotonic saline infusion: A phenomenon of desalination. Ann Intern Med 126:20, 1997.
Hyponatremia was generally caused by generation of electrolyte-free water during excretion of hypertonic urine—a desalination process.
ten Holt WL, van Iperen CE, Schrijver G, et al: Severe hyponatremia during therapy with fluoxetine. Arch Intern Med 156:681, 1996.
Severe hyponatremia may be related to fluoxetine (Prozac) therapy.
Terzian C, Frye EB, Piotrowski ZH: Admission hyponatremia in the elderly: Factors influencing prognosis. J Gen Intern Med 9:89, 1994.

Admission hyponatremia occurred in 3.5% of patients and was a predictor of in-hospital mortality for elderly patients.

Tien R, Arieff AI, Kucharczyk W, et al: Hyponatremic encephalopathy: Is central pontine myelinolysis a component? Am J Med 92:513, 1992.
Disproves the association between hyponatremia and central pontine myelinolysis.

● ●

HYPERKALEMIA

Recommendations for hyperkalemia are from the medical literature.

1. In patients at risk for hyperkalemia or with clinical findings of hyperkalemia, measure serum potassium. Exclude artifactual hyperkalemia before proceeding with the work-up.

Hyperkalemia is an increased serum potassium concentration above 5.1 mEq/L (5.1 mmol/L). Normally, the serum potassium concentration is higher than the plasma concentration because of release of platelet potassium during clotting. The most important clinical features of hyperkalemia relate to alterations of cardiac excitability as manifested in the electrocardiogram and depression of neuromuscular activity. Causes of hyperkalemia include excessive intake of potassium, decreased excretion, and shifts of potassium from cells to extracellular fluid. Clinical features include cardiotoxic effects and depressive effects on skeletal muscle.

A serum potassium determination can be used to verify the presence of hyperkalemia. Serum or heparinized plasma can be used for potassium measurements, but avoid the use of potassium salts. If the sample is heparinized, promptly separate the serum or plasma from the cells. Artifactually high serum potassium concentrations can result from thrombocytosis, leukocytosis, hemolysis, fist clenching during phlebotomy (increase up to 10 to 20%), and allowing the serum to remain in contact with the clot for prolonged periods of time at room temperature.

Nondisease factors that alter plasma/serum potassium levels can be summarized as follows:

Factor	Effect	Mechanism
ACE inhibitor	↑	Suppresses aldosterone secretion
Cold storage temperature	↑	Inhibits glycolysis
Exercise	↑	Release from muscles
Fist clenching	↑	Release from muscles
Heparin therapy	↑	Suppresses aldosterone secretion
Hyperventilation, acute	↑ / ↓	Acute hyperventilation increases potassium. Afterwards it decreases.

Factor	Effect	Mechanism
Leukemia, acute myelogenous	↓ / ↑	Glycolysis lowers potassium. Afterwards, potassium increases.
Posture	↑ / ↓	Standing position higher than supine position
Pregnancy	↑	Undefined
Thombocytosis	↑	Release from platelets

Source: Gambino R: Nondisease factors that affect potassium levels. Lab Report Physicians 17:69, 1995.

2. Evaluate the test results.

The earliest electrocardiographic manifestation of hyperkalemia consists of peaked T waves, which occur when the serum level exceeds 6.5 mEq/L (6.5 mmol/L). Between 7 and 8 mEq/L (7 to 8 mmol/L) the PR interval is prolonged, followed by a loss of P waves and widening of the QRS complex. When the serum potassium concentration exceeds 8 to 10 mEq/L (8 to 10 mmol/L), a sine wave pattern can develop, and cardiac standstill can occur. In patients with hypothermia, hyperkalemia greater than 10 mEq/L (>10 mmol/L) is considered an index of irreversibility. Hyponatremia and acidosis can potentiate the adverse effects of hyperkalemia on the heart.

3. Interpret test results in the context of clinical findings.

Certain drugs such as antineoplastic agents, heparin, pentamidine, and potassium-sparing diuretics (triamterene, spironolactone) can cause an increased serum potassium concentration. Other causes of hyperkalemia include **excessive intake,** especially in patients with renal insufficiency; **increased cellular release of potassium** such as with metabolic acidosis, trauma, massive blood transfusion, burns, rhabdomyolysis, hemolysis, lysis of tumor tissue, drug usage (succinylcholine, digitalis, beta-blocking agents), hyperosmolality, insulin deficiency, hyperkalemic periodic paralysis, severe muscle disease, diabetic hyperglycemia, and hypothermia; and **decreased renal excretion of potassium** such as in acute oliguric renal failure, chronic renal failure, renal tubular disorders, Addison's disease, and hypoaldosteronism.

BIBLIOGRAPHY

Alappan R, Perazella MA, Buller GK: Hyperkalemia in hospitalized patients treated with trimethoprim-sulfamethoxazole. Ann Intern Med 124:316, 1996.
Standard-dose trimethoprim-sulfamethoxazole therapy used to treat various infections leads to an increase in serum potassium concentration.
Alvo M, Warnock DG: Hyperkalemia. West J Med 141:666, 1984.
Discussion of the diagnosis and management of hyperkalemia.

Beck LH, Kassirer JP: Serum electrolytes, serum osmolality, blood urea nitrogen, and serum creatinine. *In* Sox HC Jr (ed): Common Diagnostic Tests: Use and Interpretation, 2nd ed. Philadelphia, American College of Physicians, 1990, p 367.
American College of Physicians' guidelines for measuring serum potassium.

Don BR, Sebastian A, Cheitlin M, et al: Pseudohyperkalemia caused by fist clenching during phlebotomy. N Engl J Med 322:1290, 1990.
Another cause of pseudohyperkalemia.

Edner M, Ponikowski P, Jogestrand T: The effect of digoxin on the serum potassium concentration. Scand J Clin Lab Invest 53:187, 1993.
After rest, in the digitalized patient, the serum potassium may be increased as much as 0.8 mEq/L (0.8 mmol/L).

Greenberg S, Reiser IW, Chou S-Y, et al: Trimethoprim-sulfamethoxazole induces reversible hyperkalemia. Ann Intern Med 119:291, 1993.
Patients receiving high doses of trimethoprim-sulfamethoxazole require close monitoring of their serum potassium concentration, particularly 7 to 10 days after the start of therapy.

Kleyman TR, Roberts C, Ling BN: A mechanism for pentamidine-induced hyperkalemia: Inhibition of distal nephron sodium transport. Ann Intern Med 122:103, 1995.
Because pentamidine is eliminated through urinary excretion, this renal tubular effect provides a mechanism for pentamidine-induced hyperkalemia.

Laine EP, Nelson JM, George FW IV, et al: Hyperkalemia after massive blood transfusion. Lab Med 28:305, 1997.
Massive blood transfusion creates the potential for hyperkalemia.

Lutomski DM, Bower RH: The effect of thrombocytosis on serum potassium and phosphorus concentration. Am J Med Sci 307:255, 1994.
Thrombocytosis falsely elevates serum potassium and phosphorus.

Mäkelä K, Kairisto V, Peltola O, et al: Effect of platelet count on serum and plasma potassium: Evaluation using database information from two hospitals. Scand J Clin Lab Invest 55(Suppl 222):95, 1995.
Clinicians should be aware of the possibility of artifactual hyperkalemia in patients with increased platelet counts.

Oster JR, Singer I, Fishman LM: Heparin-induced aldosterone suppression and hyperkalemia. Am J Med 98:575, 1995.
Monitoring serum potassium periodically is recommended for patients receiving heparin for 3 or more days, with possible need to discontinue the heparin in cases of heparin-induced hyperkalemia.

Rutecki GW, Whittier FC: Hyperkalemia: How to identify—and correct—the underlying cause. Consultant 36:564, 1996.
Reviews the diagnosis and management of patients with hyperkalemia.

Schaller M-D, Fischer AP, Perret CH: Hyperkalemia: A prognostic factor during acute severe hypothermia. JAMA 264:1842, 1990.
In patients with severe hypothermia, hyperkalemia greater than 10 mEq/L (>10 mmol/L) is considered an index of irreversibility.

HYPOKALEMIA

Recommendations for hypokalemia are from the medical literature.

1. For patients at risk for hypokalemia or with clinical findings of hypokalemia, request measurement of serum potassium. Consider measuring serum magnesium and the 24-hour urinary excretion of potassium to document potassium depletion of renal origin.

Hypokalemia is a depressed serum potassium concentration, below 3.5 mEq/L (3.5 mmol/L). The normal serum potassium concentration is greater than the plasma concentration because of the release of platelet potassium during clotting. The most significant effects of hypokalemia relate to neuromuscular and electrocardiographic disturbances. The causes of hypokalemia include diuretic therapy, inadequate potassium intake, excessive renal loss, excessive gastrointestinal loss, and shifts from the extracellular fluid to the intracellular fluid. Clinical features include skeletal muscle weakness and paralysis and derangements in cardiac conduction. Recently, hypokalemia has been reported to cause tetany.

A serum potassium determination can be used to verify the presence of hypokalemia, and measurement of urinary potassium excretion is useful to determine the renal origin of hypokalemia. Hypomagnesemia is common in patients with hypokalemia and, unless corrected, impairs repletion of intracellular potassium.

The specimen collection and handling issues are the same as for hyperkalemia.

2. Evaluate the test results.

At serum potassium concentrations of 2 to 2.5 mEq/L (2 to 2.5 mmol/L), muscular weakness can occur. At lower values, areflexic paralysis can occur, with associated respiratory insufficiency and death. Electrocardiographic manifestations of hypokalemia include sagging of the ST segment, depression of the T wave, and elevation of the U wave. With marked hypokalemia, the T wave becomes progressively smaller, and the U wave shows increasing amplitude. In patients with digitalis, hypokalemia can precipitate serious arrhythmias.

3. Interpret test results in the context of clinical findings.

Certain drugs such as chloroquine overdose, the thiazides or loop diuretics, and theophylline can cause a decreased serum potassium concentration. Other causes of hypokalemia include **inadequate intake and excessive renal loss,** for example, from eating disorders, mineralocorticoid excess (primary or exogenous and licorice ingestion), Bartter's syndrome (secondary hyperaldosteronism related to increased renin with juxtaglomerular hyperplasia and hypokalemia); osmotic diuresis, chronic metabolic alkalosis, certain antibiotics (penicillin-like antibiotics, amphotericin B, gentamicin), renal tubular acidosis, acute leukemia, Liddle's syndrome (tubular disorder with hypokalemia, metabolic alkalosis, hypertension, and normal aldosterone), and magnesium depletion; **excessive gastrointestinal loss,** for example, from vomiting, diarrhea, secretory diarrhea, chronic laxative abuse, villous adenoma, fistulas, ureterosigmoidostomy, and inflammatory bowel disease; and **shifts from the extracellular fluid to the intracellular fluid,** for example, from acute alkalosis, hypokalemic periodic paralysis, ingestion of barium salts, insulin therapy, vitamin B_{12} therapy, epinephrine administration, thyrotoxicosis (rarely), and chronic metabolic alkalosis.

BIBLIOGRAPHY

Ault MJ, Geiderman J: Hypokalemia as a cause of tetany. West J Med 157:65, 1992.
Hypokalemia—a cause of tetany that has not previously been reported.

Beck LH, Kassirer JP: Serum electrolytes, serum osmolality, blood urea nitrogen, and serum creatinine. *In* Sox HC Jr (ed): Common Diagnostic Tests: Use and Interpretation, 2nd ed. Philadelphia, American College of Physicians, 1990, p 367.
American College of Physicians' guidelines for measuring serum potassium.

Clemessy J-L, Favier C, Borron SW, et al: Hypokalemia related to acute chloroquine ingestion. Lancet 346:877, 1995.
Plasma potassium levels were inversely related to clinical and laboratory indices of poisoning severity, including the amount of chloroquine ingested, blood chloroquine concentration, QRS duration and QT ratio on the electrocardiogram, and death.

Greenfeld D, Mickley D, Quinlan DM, et al: Hypokalemia in outpatients with eating disorders. Am J Psychiatry 152:60, 1995.
Hypokalemia is a recognized complication in patients with eating disorders.

Kantola IM, Tarssanen LT: Diagnosis of familial hypokalemic periodic paralysis: Role of the potassium exercise test. Neurology 42:2158, 1992.
Hypokalemia during an attack of hypotonic paralysis is diagnostic of familial hypokalemia periodic paralysis. A potassium exercise test may be a safe way to make the diagnosis.

Kaplan NM: How bad are diuretic-induced hypokalemia and hypercholesterolemia? Arch Intern Med 149:2649, 1989.
Believes that diuretic-induced hypokalemia may be harmful.

Kassirer JP, Kopelman RI: Case 2—Hypothesis triggering by an expert. *In* Learning Clinical Reasoning. Baltimore, Williams & Wilkins, 1991, p 53.
Discusses clinical reasoning in a patient with weakness secondary to hypokalemia.

Rutecki GW, Whittier FC: Hypokalemia: Clinical implications, consequences, and corrective measures. Consultant 36:124, 1996.
Reviews the diagnosis and management of patients with hypokalemia.

Schnaper HW, Freis ED, Friedman RG, et al: Potassium restoration in hypertensive patients made hypokalemic by hydrochlorothiazide. Arch Intern Med 149:2677, 1989.
Many patients taking 50 mg/day of hydrochlorothiazide require triamterene or supplementary potassium to maintain their serum potassium in the normal range.

Shannon M, Lovejoy FH Jr: Hypokalemia after theophylline intoxication: The effects of acute vs chronic poisoning. Arch Intern Med 149:2725, 1989.
Hypokalemia is common after theophylline intoxication.

Siegel D, Hulley SB, Black DM, et al: Diuretics, serum and intracellular electrolyte levels, and ventricular arrhythmias in hypertensive men. JAMA 267:1083, 1992.
Potassium concentrations should be carefully monitored during initiation of diuretic therapy.

Steigerwalt SP: Unraveling the causes of hypertension and hypokalemia. Hosp Pract 30:67, 1995.
The most common causes are diuretic therapy and primary aldosteronism.

Stein JH: Hypokalemia: Common and uncommon causes. Hosp Pract 23:55, 1988.
Reviews the differential diagnosis of hypokalemia.

Whang R, Whang DD, Ryan MP: Refractory potassium repletion: A consequence of magnesium deficiency. Arch Intern Med 152:40, 1992.
Serum magnesium should be measured routinely in patients with hypokalemia.

HYPERCALCEMIA

Recommendations for hypercalcemia are from the medical literature.

1. For patients at risk for hypercalcemia or with clinical findings of hypercalcemia, request at least three measurements of serum total

calcium, together with a complete blood count, serum albumin and globulins, phosphorus, magnesium, alkaline phosphatase, urea nitrogen, creatinine, electrolytes, a sensitive thyrotropin (S-TSH) test, and a 24-hour urinary calcium determination. In certain circumstances, measurement of serum ionized calcium may be helpful. Review the drug history for a possible hypercalcemic effect.

Before undertaking the differential diagnosis of hypercalcemia, artifactual causes of hypercalcemia should be excluded. If the serum calcium is truly high, the cause should be determined, keeping in mind that cancer and hyperparathyroidism are among the more common causes. Patients with hypercalcemia greater than 14 mg/dL (>3.50 mmol/L) need immediate, aggressive therapy.

After artifactual causes are excluded, the laboratory studies should be part of a thorough work-up that includes a careful history and physical examination, chest radiography, renal ultrasonography, and skeletal survey radiographs. Drugs such as vitamin D or antacids together with milk can cause hypercalcemia (milk-alkali syndrome).

In the past, patients with hyperparathyroidism usually were seen with clinical features of the disease before hypercalcemia was detected. With the advent of laboratory screening, the current typical presentation of patients with hyperparathyroidism is unexplained hypercalcemia. Although some experts believe that screening for hypercalcemia is valuable, others argue that there is no advantage in treating asymptomatic hyperparathyroidism and that screening with serum calcium measurements should be omitted. A recent study reports an unexpected decrease in the incidence of primary hyperparathyroidism.

Other causes of hypercalcemia that must be differentiated from hyperparathyroidism are shown in the table below:

Increased Gastrointestinal Absorption of Calcium	Increased Resorption of Bone	Increased Renal Resorption
Sarcoidosis	Cancer of bone*	Thiazide diuretics
Other granulomatous diseases		
Milk-alkali syndrome	Ectopic parathyroid hormone syndrome	Familial hypocalciuric hypercalcemia
Hypervitaminosis D	Hyperthyroidism	
	Paget's disease of bone	
	Immobilization	

*These are usually the osteolytic metastases of carcinoma of the breast, lung, and prostate or are multiple myeloma, acute leukemias, certain lymphomas, and Hodgkin's disease. Sometimes bone involvement is absent, and the hypercalcemia is induced by a parathyroid hormone–related humoral mediator.

Common causes for hypercalcemia are cancer and hyperparathyroidism. Most hospitalized patients with hypercalcemia have cancer, but most ambulatory patients have hyperparathyroidism, with only a few having cancer. Additional conditions associated with hypercalcemia include adrenal insufficiency; acromegaly; vitamin A intoxication; pheochromocytoma; the watery diarrhea, hypokalemia, achlorhydria syndrome; lithium therapy; and renal transplant.

Diurnal variation of serum calcium concentrations, although slight, makes a morning sample desirable. Remember that posture affects serum calcium levels. Because serum calcium is bound to albumin and albumin is higher in ambulatory than in recumbent patients, calcium levels are higher in ambulatory patients than in recumbent patients. Prolonged application of a tourniquet or muscular exercise of the limb chosen for venipuncture can artifactually increase the serum calcium concentration. Serum or heparinized plasma is a satisfactory sample, but do not allow prolonged contact with red blood cells because with time the cells become permeable to calcium. Using a cork stopper on the patient's sample can increase the calcium concentration because cork contains calcium.

Serum inorganic phosphorus concentration may be difficult to interpret unless the specimen is collected in the morning after an overnight fast (with no intravenous fluids). Under these conditions the reference range for adults is 2.7 to 4.5 mg/dL (0.87 to 1.45 mmol/L). The concentration is slightly higher before puberty and after gonadal failure.

Total calcium concentration in serum includes three forms: a protein-bound fraction (40%); a chelated fraction (10%); and an ionized, physiologically active fraction (50%). Serum measurements of total calcium are sometimes misleading because of changes in the relative proportions of these forms—especially among patients in intensive care units, in neonates, in patients undergoing liver and cardiac transplant surgery, and in patients with renal disease. In these patients determining serum ionized calcium concentrations may be helpful. Blood samples should be collected anaerobically and without venous stasis. If use of an anticoagulated specimen is necessary, use the smallest amount of heparin possible because heparin binds calcium and causes a decrease in the ionized calcium concentration. Ionized calcium should not be measured in specimens containing citrate or ethylenediaminetetraacetic acid.

2. Evaluate the tests and the results.

The accuracy and precision of present calcium methods are not good enough to distinguish normocalcemia sharply from borderline hypercalcemia—which is the reason that at least three measurements are recommended. Remember the effect of altered serum albumin values.

REFERENCE RANGE FOR IONIZED CALCIUM

Test	Specimen	Conventional Units	International Units
Calcium, ionized (iCa)	Serum, plasma, or whole blood (with heparin)	4.64–5.28 mg/dL	1.16–1.32 mmol/L

Serum total calcium measurements greater than 12 mg/dL (>2.99 mmol/L) are associated with toxicity (e.g., hypercalcemic coma), and medical therapy is indicated. Make certain that serum calcium is measured by an accurate and precise method. The reference method is atomic absorption. In addition, patients with mild hyperparathyroidism may have intermittent elevations. Thus, repeat measurements of serum calcium should be obtained. In questionable cases it may be useful to space the samples over several weeks or months.

The reference range for serum total calcium should be corrected for serum albumin concentration according to the ratio of 0.5 mg/dL (0.12 mmol/L) of serum calcium for every 1 g/dL (10 g/L) of serum albumin above or below the middle of the reference range. With an increase or decrease in albumin, other cations bound to albumin (e.g., magnesium and zinc) also increase or decrease.

Serum concentrations of phosphorus, alkaline phosphatase, urea nitrogen, creatinine, electrolytes, and magnesium outside the reference range favor a pathologic cause for an increased calcium value. Hypercalcemia may be caused by hyperlipoproteinemia or hyperproteinemia.

3. If hypercalcemia is documented by at least three serum calcium measurements and if drugs are not the cause, consider the differential diagnosis for hypercalcemia. If hyperparathyroidism is a serious consideration, measure immunoreactive parathyroid hormone.

Primary hyperparathyroidism can be diagnosed best by showing persistent hypercalcemia with an increased serum parathyroid hormone concentration. Patients with hypercalcemia from other causes such as malignancies and sarcoidosis have low-normal or decreased parathyroid hormone values. Recently the agent responsible for the humoral hypercalcemia of cancer was isolated: parathyroid hormone–related protein (PTHRP). In general, plasma PTHRP concentrations are not increased in patients with primary hyperparathyroidism, and plasma parathyroid hormone concentrations are not increased in the humoral hypercalcemia of cancer.

Severe hypercalcemia (>14 mg/dL [>3.49 mmol/L]) favors nonparathyroid causes, usually cancer. Milder serum calcium elevations are typically seen in patients with hyperparathyroidism; however, nonparathyroid causes may be responsible. A diagnostic rule of thumb is that hypercalcemia that lasts more than 1 year without signs of primary cancer (or another identifiable cause) is caused by parathyroid disease.

The ratio of serum chloride to phosphorus is helpful in differentiating hyperparathyroidism from other causes.

	Chloride Values	Phosphorus Measurement	Chloride: Phosphorus Ratio
Hyper- parathyroid patients	Higher; mean >107 mEq/L (>107 mmol/L)	Lower	32 to 80, 96% values higher than 33
Hyper- calcemia from other causes	Lower; mean 98 mEq/L (98 mmol/L)	Higher; mean 4.5 mg/dL (1.45 mmol/L)	18 to 32, 92% values lower than 30

If hypercalcemia is accompanied by an increased alkaline phosphatase level, the differential diagnosis includes hyperparathyroidism, hyperthyroidism, osteoblastic bone lesions, and malignancy. Alkaline phosphatase is not increased in multiple myeloma patients. A serum alkaline phosphatase value greater than twice the upper reference limit is unlikely to indicate uncomplicated primary hyperparathyroidism. A decreased serum alkaline phosphatase value may occur with hypervitaminosis D related to an increased phosphorus concentration.

Increased serum urea nitrogen and creatinine concentrations suggest the nephropathy of mild hyperparathyroidism.

Serum potassium values may be low in patients with hypercalcemia (32%), and potassium concentration varies inversely with calcium. Because patients with cancer have higher calcium values, these cancer patients have a higher prevalence of hypokalemia (52%).

A low urinary calcium concentration (usually <60 mg/24 hour [<1.50 mmol/24 hour]) is the diagnostic hallmark of familial hypocalciuric hypercalcemia, an autosomal dominant syndrome. The serum magnesium concentration may be increased. If a low urinary calcium value is found, this diagnosis should be considered, and family members should be screened for hypercalcemia.

4. If additional calcium measurements are normal and the increased calcium concentration can be explained on the basis of drug therapy, improper specimen collection and handling, or laboratory error, conclude that the patient does not have a pathologic cause of hypercalcemia.

5. In patients with hypercalcemia, the following blood test results may be increased:

- **Urea nitrogen, creatinine, and uric acid** secondary to nephropathy. Uric acid may be high in malignancy because of high cell turnover and proliferation.

- **Chloride.** Suggests hyperparathyroidism
- **Phosphorus** without renal failure suggests a nonparathyroid cause.
- **Serum transaminase and alkaline phosphatase** with granulomatous hepatitis (e.g., sarcoidosis)
- **Alkaline phosphatase,** often in malignancy and unlikely in primary hyperparathyroidism in the absence of osteitis fibrosa cystica. The Regan isoenzyme may occur in patients with carcinoma.
- **Hypergammaglobulinemia** favors sarcoidosis but has been seen in primary hyperparathyroidism.
- **Lactate dehydrogenase** caused by high malignant cell turnover and proliferation.

6. In patients with hypercalcemia, the following blood test results may be decreased:

- **Hemoglobin or hematocrit (and an increased erythrocyte sedimentation rate)** suggests a nonparathyroid cause, particularly malignancy, although these findings may occur in primary hyperparathyroidism.
- **Leukocytes.** Frequent in hyperparathyroidism.
- **Pco_2 and bicarbonate** because parathyroid hormone increases urinary bicarbonate excretion.
- **Serum magnesium** may occur in hyperparathyroidism.
- **Phosphorus** (when dietary phosphorus is adequate and the patient is not taking oral phosphate-binding agents) favors primary hyperparathyroidism but can occur in malignancy.

BIBLIOGRAPHY

Arvan DA: Hypercalcemia. *In* Panzer ER, Black ER, Griner PF (eds): Diagnostic Strategies for Common Medical Problems. Philadelphia, American College of Physicians, 1991, p 355.
Recommends strategies for the differential diagnosis of hypercalcemia.
Bilezikian JP: Management of acute hypercalcemia. N Engl J Med 326:1196, 1992.
Reviews the care of patients with hypercalcemia who require immediate treatment in the hospital.
Burtis WJ, Brady TG, Orloff JJ, et al: Immunochemical characterization of circulating parathyroid hormone–related protein in patients with humoral hypercalcemia of cancer. N Engl J Med 322:1106, 1990.
Describes the use of parathyroid hormone-related protein.
Consensus Development Conference Panel: Diagnosis and management of asymptomatic primary hyperparathyroidism: Consensus Development Conference statement. Ann Intern Med 114:593, 1991.
Establishes guidelines for diagnosing and treating asymptomatic patients with hyperparathyroidism.
Gökçe C, Gökçe O, Baydince C, et al: Use of random urine samples to estimate total urinary calcium and phosphate excretion. Arch Intern Med 151:1587, 1991.
Estimates of daily excretion of urinary calcium and phosphorus can be obtained by measuring random urinary calcium, phosphorus, and creatinine concentrations.
Gray TA, Paterson CR: The clinical value of ionized calcium assays. Ann Clin Biochem 25:210, 1988.
Reviews the use of ionized calcium measurements in patient care.

Greaves I, Grant AJ, Heath DA, et al: Hypercalcemia: Changing causes over the past 10 years. Br Med J 304:1284, 1992.
Although the incidence of symptomatic hypercalcemia in chronic renal failure is low, and only 2 of the 81 patients required parathyroidectomy, a need exists for more careful monitoring of calcium supplements in renal failure.

Heath H III: Primary hyperparathyroidism: Recent advances in pathogenesis, diagnosis, and management. Adv Intern Med 37:275, 1991.
Review of primary hyperparathyroidism from the Mayo Clinic.

Jacobus CH, Holick MF, Shao Q, et al: Hypervitaminosis D associated with drinking milk. N Engl J Med 326:1173, 1992.
Hypercalcemia may be caused by drinking milk that is excessively fortified with vitamin D.

Kassirer JP, Kopelman RI: Case 44—Watch and wait, or operate? *In* Learning Clinical Reasoning. Baltimore, Williams & Wilkins, 1991, p 222.
Discusses clinical reasoning in a patient with asymptomatic hyperparathyroidism.

Nikkilä MT, Saaristo JJ, Koivula TA: Clinical and biochemical features in primary hyperparathyroidism. Surgery 105:148, 1989.
Discusses biochemical findings in 61 surgical cases.

Ratcliffe WA, Hutchesson ACJ, Bundred NJ, et al: Role of assays for parathyroid hormone–related protein in investigation of hypercalcemia. Lancet 339:164, 1992.
Discusses the usefulness of parathyroid hormone–related protein to discover malignancy in cases of hypercalcemia.

Sorva A, Valvanne J, Tilvis RS: Serum ionized calcium and the prevalence of primary hyperparathyroidism in age cohorts of 75, 80, and 85 years. J Intern Med 231:309, 1992.
The mean ionized calcium remained unchanged, although the mean total calcium fell slightly with age.

Vassilopoulou-Sellin R, Newman BM, Taylor SH, et al: Incidence of hypercalcemia in patients with malignancy referred to a comprehensive cancer center. Cancer 71:1309, 1993.
In new cancer patients, the overall incidence of moderate and severe hypercalcemia was 1.1%.

Wermers RA, Khosla S, Atkinson EJ, et al: The rise and fall of primary hyperparathyroidism: A population-based study in Rochester, Minnesota, 1965–1992. Ann Intern Med 126:433, 1997.
The progressive decrease in the incidence of primary hyperparathyroidism is unexpected and suggests a significant change in the epidemiology of this disease.

Zahrani AA, Levine MA: Primary hyperparathyroidism. Lancet 349:1233, 1997.
Reviews the diagnosis and management of primary hyperparathyroidism.

HYPOCALCEMIA

Recommendations for hypocalcemia are from the medical literature.

1. For patients at risk for hypercalcemia or with clinical findings of hypocalcemia, request at least three measurements of serum calcium together with a complete blood count (CBC), serum albumin and globulin, magnesium, alkaline phosphatase, urea nitrogen, creatinine, and electrolytes. In certain circumstances, measurement of serum ionized calcium may be helpful.

Remember that certain drugs such as anticonvulsants, corticosteroids, diuretics, and laxatives may be associated with a low serum calcium concentration.

Measurements of albumin, phosphorus, and magnesium are useful to help to determine the cause of hypocalcemia. Serum urea nitrogen, creatinine, and electrolyte determinations help assess renal function, and a CBC and an alkaline phosphatase determination may provide valuable clues about the presence of malignancy.

See the discussion of hypercalcemia, which precedes this section, for specimen collection and handling issues.

2. Evaluate the tests.

See the discussion of hypercalcemia, which precedes this section, for testing issues.

3. If hypocalcemia is documented by at least three serum calcium measurements and drugs are not the cause, consider the differential diagnosis as follows:

Prior thyroid surgery is a common cause of a low serum calcium value secondary to hypoparathyroidism. If hypoparathyroidism is suspected, low ionized calcium and low parathyroid hormone values can confirm the diagnosis. Idiopathic hypoparathyroidism may also occur. In addition to a deficiency of parathyroid hormone, a low serum calcium level may be caused by failure of the kidneys to respond to normal amounts of parathyroid hormone, a condition known as **pseudohypoparathyroidism**. In a patient with either hypoparathyroidism or pseudohypoparathyroidism, the serum phosphorus level is high. Both **hypomagnesemia** and **hypermagnesemia** can impair parathyroid hormone secretion, causing hypocalcemia. **Renal failure** is perhaps the most common of all causes of hypocalcemia: The serum urea nitrogen, creatinine, and phosphorus levels are all increased. In patients with **intestinal malabsorption**, defective absorption of both calcium and vitamin D can occur, resulting in hypocalcemia. **Miscellaneous** causes of hypocalcemia include acute pancreatitis, osteoblastic metastatic bone disease, excessive transfusion with citrated blood, and rhabdomyolysis-induced renal failure. After parathyroid surgery, hypocalcemia may be caused by the hungry bone syndrome, in which remineralization of the skeleton causes hypocalcemia and hypophosphatemia, often with tetany, requiring vigorous, prolonged calcium and vitamin D therapy.

4. If hypocalcemia can be explained as an effect of drug therapy, improper specimen collection and handling, or laboratory error, conclude that the patient does not have a pathologic cause.

Hypocalcemia may be the result of a methodology problem, or it may be related to a low serum albumin level. Certain drugs such as phenytoin and other anticonvulsant medications have been implicated as a cause of vitamin D deficiency and borderline-low serum calcium values. It is important to identify these causes of hypocalcemia so that a needless search for some underlying disease or disorder can be averted.

BIBLIOGRAPHY

Brasier AR, Nussbaum SR: Hungry bone syndrome: Clinical and biochemical predictors
   of its occurrence after parathyroid surgery. Am J Med 84:654, 1988.
   After parathyroid surgery, remineralization of the skeleton may cause hypocalcemia.
Demeester-Mirkine N, Hooghe L, Van Geertruyden J, et al: Hypocalcemia after thyroidectomy. Arch Surg 127:854, 1992.
   *The fall in serum calcium was not related to preoperative thyroid function but was
   related to the extent of the thyroidectomy, with the greatest reduction after total
   thyroidectomy.*
Riancho JA, Arjona R, Valle R, et al: The clinical spectrum of hypocalcemia associated
   with bone metastases. J Intern Med 226:449, 1989.
   *Osteoblastic metastatic bone disease, particularly from prostate cancer, may cause
   hypocalcemia.*

HYPERPHOSPHATEMIA

Recommendations for hyperphosphatemia are from the medical literature.

1. For patients at risk for hyperphosphatemia, request a determination of serum phosphorus. Consider obtaining measurements of serum calcium, glucose, urea nitrogen, and creatinine and a urinalysis.

Hyperphosphatemia is an elevated serum phosphorus concentration, above 4.5 mg/dL (1.45 mmol/L). When severe, hyperphosphatemia can contribute to the acidosis of uremia, further reduce the concentration of ionized calcium in the extracellular fluid, and cause metastatic calcification in soft tissues. The most common cause is renal insufficiency. Hyperphosphatemia produces no direct clinical symptoms.

A serum phosphorus determination can be used to verify the presence of hyperphosphatemia. Hypocalcemia may be a clue to hypoparathyroidism, hyperglycemia a clue to acromegaly, and urea nitrogen and creatinine values and urinalysis indications of renal insufficiency.

Use of serum or heparinized plasma is satisfactory for testing. The patient **should be fasting** because postprandial phosphorylation of glucose decreases serum phosphorus. Collection of the specimen after an overnight fast is ideal. Thrombocytosis can elevate serum phosphorus as well as potassium. Hemolysis and prolonged contact with the clot should be avoided because they increase serum phosphorus.

2. Evaluate the test results.

Hyperphosphatemia can indirectly produce tetany by lowering serum calcium levels. With rapid elevations of serum phosphorus, hypocalcemia and tetany can occur with a serum phosphorus concentration as low as 6 mg/dL (1.94 mmol/L), a concentration that, if reached more slowly, has no detectable effect on serum calcium levels.

3. Interpret test results in the context of clinical findings.

Certain drugs such as steroids and thiazides can increase the serum phosphate concentration. If truly **large amounts of phosphate** are administered orally, parenterally, or rectally, hyperphosphatemia can occur, even in the presence of normal renal function. **Other causes of hyperphosphatemia** include increased tubular reabsorption (hypoparathyroidism, pseudohypoparathyroidism, acromegaly, hyperthyroidism, tumoral calcinosis), transcellular shifts (acidosis), cell lysis (rhabdomyolysis, hemolysis, chemotherapy, malignant pyrexia), and miscellaneous factors (e.g., familial intermittent hyperphosphatemia).

BIBLIOGRAPHY

Lutomski DM, Bower RH: The effect of thrombocytosis on serum potassium and phosphorus concentration. Am J Med Sci 307:255, 1994.
 Thrombocytosis falsely elevates serum potassium and phosphorus.
Scott MG: Inorganic phosphorus: Review of methods. Chicago, American Society of Clinical Pathologists, Core Analyte Vol 8, No 5, 1992.
 Discusses causes of hyperphosphatemia.
Yu GC, Lee DBN: Clinical disorders of phosphorus metabolism. West J Med 147:569, 1987.
 Discusses the diagnosis and management of hyperphosphatemia.

HYPOPHOSPHATEMIA

Recommendations for hypophosphatemia are from the medical literature.

1. For patients at risk for hypophosphatemia or with clinical findings of hypophosphatemia, request a serum phosphorus measurement. Consider obtaining a complete blood count (CBC), serum glucose, urea nitrogen, creatinine, calcium, and creatine kinase determinations, liver function tests, and a urinalysis.

Hypophosphatemia is a decreased serum phosphorus concentration below 2.7 mg/dL (0.87 mmol/L). The clinical features are produced by a deficiency of phosphorus for key metabolic functions, including the integrity of cell membranes, the structure of nucleic acids, a second messenger in endocrinologic functions (cAMP, cGMP), the release of oxygen by hemoglobin (2,3-DPG), and the buffering of urine. Causes include decreased intake of phosphate, impaired absorption of phosphate, excessive renal loss of phosphate, and a shift of phosphate into cells and bone. The diagnosis of hypophosphatemia and its cause depends on obtaining appropriate tests in the context of the clinical findings. These findings include red cell dysfunction and hemolysis, leukocyte dysfunction, platelet dysfunction, weakness, congestive cardiomyopathy, rhabdomyolysis, central nervous system dysfunction, and possible hepatic dysfunction.

If the serum phosphorus is decreased, be alert to clinical findings suggestive of anemia, thrombocytopenia, susceptibility to infection, hypoglycemia, hepatic dysfunction, renal dysfunction, and neuromuscular and central nervous system problems. To help sort out these issues, request a CBC, serum glucose, urea nitrogen, creatinine, and creatine kinase, as well as liver function tests and a urinalysis.

Specimen collection and handling are the same as for hyperphosphatemia.

2. Evaluate the test results.

It is unusual for hypophosphatemia to cause metabolic disturbances at concentrations greater than 1.5 mg/dL (>0.48 mmol/L). If you decide to treat with parenteral phosphate, be careful because hyperphosphatemia can result and ionized calcium can fall, producing tetany or convulsions. In addition, metastatic calcification of soft tissues can occur.

3. Interpret test results in the context of clinical findings.

Certain drugs such as steroids, diuretics, and insulin can decrease serum phosphorus. Decreased phosphate intake can occur with **vomiting** and **prolonged nasogastric suction**. Other causes include **impaired phosphate absorption** with drugs (aluminum- and magnesium-containing antacids), malabsorption, vitamin D deficiency, and alcoholism; **excessive renal loss of phosphate** such as in patients with hyperparathyroidism, renal tubular disorders, acidosis, and severe trauma; and **intracellular shifts of phosphate** such as in patients with carbohydrate loading, poorly controlled diabetes mellitus, hyperalimentation, respiratory alkalosis, rapid tumor growth, the nutritional recovery syndrome, recovery phase of burns, treatment of respiratory failure (severe asthma and obstructive pulmonary disease), and the hungry bone syndrome (hypocalcemia and hypophosphatemia caused by bone remineralization after parathyroid surgery).

BIBLIOGRAPHY

Brasier AR, Nussbaum SR: Hungry bone syndrome: Clinical and biochemical predictors of its occurrence after parathyroid surgery. Am J Med 84:654, 1988.
Hypophosphatemia can occur after parathyroid surgery.
Daily WH, Tonnesen AS, Allen SJ: Hypophosphatemia: Incidence, etiology, and prevention in the trauma patient. Crit Care Med 18:1210, 1990.
Severe hypophosphatemia occurs frequently after severe trauma, probably because of urinary loss.
Laaban J-P, Grateau G, Psychoyos I, et al: Hypophosphatemia induced by mechanical ventilation in patients with chronic obstructive pulmonary disease. Crit Care Med 17:1115, 1989.
After starting mechanical ventilation, patients with acute respiratory failure should be monitored to detect hypophosphatemia.
Laaban J-P, Waked M, Laromiguiere M, et al: Hypophosphatemia complicating management of acute severe asthma. Ann Intern Med 112:68, 1990.
After starting therapy, patients with acute severe asthma should be monitored to detect hypophosphatemia.
Scott MG: Inorganic phosphorus: Review of methods. Chicago, American Society of Clinical Pathologists, Core Analyte Vol 8, No 5, 1992.
Discusses causes of hypophosphatemia.

Singhal PC, Kumar A, Desroches L, et al: Prevalence and predictors of rhabdomyolysis in patients with hypophosphatemia. Am J Med 92:458, 1992.

Knochel JP: Hypophosphatemia and rhabdomyolysis. Am J Med 92:455, 1992.
Clinical study and editorial that describe the common occurrence of rhabdomyolysis in hypophosphatemia patients.

Yu GC, Lee DBN: Clinical disorders of phosphorus metabolism. West J Med 147:569, 1987.
Discusses the diagnosis and management of hypophosphatemia.

Zaloga GP: Hypophosphatemia in COPD: How serious—And what to do? J Crit Illness 7:364, 1992.
Patients with COPD are vulnerable to hypophosphatemia.

Zazzo J-F, Troché G, Ruel P, et al: High incidence of hypophosphatemia in surgical intensive care patients: Efficacy of phosphorus therapy on myocardial infarction. Intensive Care Med 21:826, 1995.
Hypophosphatemia is common in surgical intensive care patients and is associated with a higher mortality.

HYPERMAGNESEMIA

Recommendations for hypermagnesemia are from the medical literature.

1. In patients at risk for hypermagnesemia or with clinical findings of hypermagnesemia, measure serum magnesium, urea nitrogen, creatinine, calcium, and potassium.

Hypermagnesemia is an elevation of the serum magnesium concentration above 2.1 mEq/L (1.05 mmol/L). The magnesium ion exerts a depressive effect on the neuromuscular junction, and the clinical manifestations of hypermagnesemia are related to toxic effects on the central nervous and cardiovascular systems. Hypermagnesemia occurs in patients with renal insufficiency who ingest excessive amounts of magnesium, such as in magnesium-containing antacids. It can result from parenteral administration of magnesium, such as in the treatment of acute hypertension. Life-threatening hypermagnesemia due to laxative abuse has been described. Clinical manifestations include hypotension and cardiac arrhythmias. The cardiotoxicity of magnesium is aggravated by hypocalcemia, hyperkalemia, acidosis, digitalis therapy, and renal insufficiency (beyond its effect on the magnesium level).

In the context of other electrolyte disorders, physicians should consider hypermagnesemia, which can be detected or verified by a serum magnesium determination. Measurements of calcium and potassium can be helpful because of the synergistic effects of hypocalcemia and hyperkalemia. Serum urea nitrogen and creatinine determinations are useful to assess renal function. For magnesium measurements, use serum or heparinized plasma.

2. Evaluate the test results.

The cardiovascular effects of magnesium usually begin at values greater than 10 mEq/L (>5 mmol/L) and consist of peripheral vasodilation with hypotension, depression of the cardiac conduction system, bradyarrhythmias, and cardiac arrest in asystole, with more serious effects at higher levels (e.g., asystole at levels >25 mEq/L [>12.50

mmol/L]). Occasionally patients develop cardiotoxicity at 4.5 to 5.5 mEq/L (2.25 to 2.75 mmol/L).

3. Interpret test results in the context of clinical findings.

Certain drugs such as magnesium-containing medications can increase the serum magnesium concentration. Another common cause of hypermagnesemia is **renal insufficiency. Miscellaneous causes** of mild hypermagnesemia include Addison's disease, diabetic ketoacidosis, hypothyroidism, pituitary dwarfism, lithium therapy, viral hepatitis, and the milk-alkali syndrome.

BIBLIOGRAPHY

Kassirer JP, Kopelman RI: Case 33—Post hoc, ergo propter hoc. *In* Learning Clinical Reasoning. Baltimore, Williams & Wilkins, 1991, p 180.
  Discusses clinical reasoning in a patient with flaccid quadriplegia secondary to hypermagnesemia.
Qureshi TI, Melonakos TK: Acute hypermagnesemia after laxative use. Ann Emerg Med 28:552, 1996.
  The patient consumed 50 grams of Epsom salts diluted with water about 6 hours before admission.
Reinhart RA: Magnesium metabolism: A review with special reference to the relationship between intracellular content and serum levels. Arch Intern Med 148:2415, 1988.
  Discusses the diagnosis and management of hypermagnesemia.
Trehan S, Rutecki GW, Whittier FC: Magnesium disorders: What to do when homeostasis goes awry. Consultant 36:2, 1996.
  Discusses the detection and management of hypermagnesemia and hypomagnesemia.
Varsou A, Papadimitiou JC, Koch TR, et al: Occurrence of abnormal serum magnesium concentrations in uremic and nonuremic patients treated with digoxin. Lab Med 21:226, 1990.
  Patients taking digoxin may develop abnormal serum magnesium values.
Whang R, Ryder KW: Frequency of hypomagnesemia and hypermagnesemia: Requested vs routine. JAMA 263:3063, 1990.
  Hypermagnesemia frequently is not suspected by physicians.

HYPOMAGNESEMIA

Recommendations for hypomagnesemia are from the medical literature.

1. For patients at risk for hypomagnesemia or with clinical findings of hypomagnesemia, request measurements of serum magnesium, calcium, and potassium.

Hypomagnesemia is a depression of the serum magnesium concentration to below 1.3 mEq/L (0.65 mmol/L). It is more common than hypermagnesemia and usually occurs as a component of a more complex deficiency state. Therefore, look for other deficiencies, such as hypokalemia and hypocalcemia. Low levels of magnesium ions cause hyperirritability of nerves and muscles with manifestations in the neuromuscular, cardiovascular, and gastrointestinal systems. Causes of hypomagnesemia include decreased absorption from dietary sources, increased loss from the body, and internal redistributions. Clinical manifestations include lethargy, weakness, irritability, short attention span, fainting, convulsions, and Chvostek's and Trousseau's signs. There may be anorexia, nausea, vomiting, paralytic ileus, and cardiac arrhythmias. Hypomagnesemia has been observed in patients with delayed healing of stasis ulcers and wounds.

In the context of other electrolyte disorders, physicians should consider hypomagnesemia, which can be detected or verified by a serum magnesium determination. Measurements of calcium and potassium can be helpful because hypocalcemia and hypokalemia frequently accompany hypomagnesemia. The hypocalcemia and hypokalemia are resistant to treatment unless the hypomagnesemia is corrected first. Routine determinations of serum magnesium are unnecessary in patients with uncomplicated hypertension who are receiving triamterene-containing diuretics or low-dose (50 mg/day or less) hydrochlorothiazide. For magnesium measurements, use serum or heparinized serum.

2. Evaluate the test results.

Clinical findings increase in number and severity as the serum magnesium level becomes progressively decreased. Values of 1.2 mEq/L (0.60 mmol/L) or lower are associated with weakness, irritability, tetany, and convulsions.

3. Interpret test results in the context of clinical findings.

Certain drugs such as diuretics may be associated with hypomagnesemia. Other causes include **decreased absorption from dietary sources** such as with a low magnesium diet, inhibition of absorption by ethanol, malabsorption, uremia, and a selective defect in magnesium absorption (rare); **increased magnesium loss** such as with gastrointestinal disorders (diarrhea) and renal disorders (tubular defects); and **internal redistribution of magnesium** such as with acute pancreatitis and increased loss into bone.

BIBLIOGRAPHY

Kroenke K, Wood DR, Hanley JF: The value of serum magnesium determination in hypertensive patients receiving diuretics. Arch Intern Med 147:1553, 1987.
It is not necessary to measure serum magnesium routinely in patients receiving low-dose hydrochlorothiazide.
Lum G: Hypomagnesemia in acute and chronic care patient populations. Am J Clin Pathol 97:827, 1992.
The prevalence of hypomagnesemia in hospitalized patients depends on the type of patient population, with significantly higher prevalence in acute medical and surgical patients than in chronic care patients.
Madias JE, Sheth K, Choudry MA, et al: Admission serum magnesium level does not predict the hospital outcome of patients with acute myocardial infarction. Arch Intern Med 156:1701, 1996.
Hypomagnesemia is seen in approximately one fourth of patients with myocardial infarction, is not linked to hypokalemia, has some relationship to preadmission use of

diuretic agents, is associated with early presentation to the hospital, and is not a predictor of increased morbidity or mortality.

Reinhart RA: Magnesium metabolism: A review with special reference to the relationship between intracellular content and serum levels. Arch Intern Med 148:2415, 1988.
Discusses the diagnosis and management of hypomagnesemia.

Rubeiz GJ, Thill-Baharozian M, Hardie D, et al: Association of hypomagnesemia and mortality in acutely ill medical patients. Crit Care Med 21:203, 1993.
Hypomagnesemia in acutely ill patients is an independent risk factor for an increased mortality rate.

Shechter M, Hod H, Marks N, et al: Beneficial effect of magnesium sulfate in acute myocardial infarction. Am J Cardiol 66:271, 1990.
Cardioprotective effect of adequate magnesium deserves additional study.

Tosiello L: Hypomagnesemia and diabetes mellitus: A review of clinical implications. Arch Intern Med 156:1143, 1996.
Reviews a long list of causes of hypomagnesemia, including poor diabetic control and insulin resistance.

Trehan S, Rutecki GW, Whittier FC: Magnesium disorders: What to do when homeostasis goes awry. Consultant 36:2485, 1996.
Reviews the detection and management of hypermagnesemia and hypomagnesemia.

Varsou A, Papadimitious JC, Koch TR, et al: Occurrence of abnormal serum magnesium concentrations in uremic and nonuremic patients treated with digoxin. Lab Med 21:226, 1990.
Patients receiving digoxin therapy frequently develop hypomagnesemia.

Whang R, Ryder KW: Frequency of hypomagnesemia and hypermagnesemia: Requested vs routine. JAMA 263:3063, 1990.
Hypomagnesemia frequently is not suspected by physicians.

GENERAL BIBLIOGRAPHY

Bakerman P, Strausbauch P: ABC's of Interpretive Laboratory Data, 3rd ed. Myrtle Beach, SC, Interpretive Laboratory Data, Inc, 1994.

Bennett JC, Plum F (eds): Cecil Textbook of Medicine, 20th ed. Philadelphia, WB Saunders, 1996.

Branch WT Jr (ed): Office Practice of Medicine, 2nd ed. Philadelphia, WB Saunders, 1987.

Cogan MG: Fluid and Electrolytes: Physiology and Pathophysiology. Norwalk, CT, Appleton & Lange, 1991.

Cotran RS, Kumar V, Robbins SL: Robbins Pathologic Basis of Disease, 5th ed. Philadelphia, WB Saunders, 1994.

Dale DC, Federman DD (eds): Scientific American Medicine. New York, Scientific American, Inc, 1978–1997.

Friedman RB, Young DS: Effects of Disease on Clinical Laboratory Tests, 3rd ed. Washington, DC, American Association for Clinical Chemistry Press, 1997.

Henry JB (ed): Clinical Diagnosis and Management by Laboratory Methods, 19th ed. Philadelphia, WB Saunders, 1996.

Hoffman R, Benz EJ Jr, Shattil SJ, et al (eds): Hematology: Basic Principles and Practice. New York, Churchill Livingstone, 1991.

Howanitz JH, Howanitz PJ (eds): Laboratory Medicine: Test Selection and Interpretation. New York, Churchill Livingstone, 1991.

Kjeldsberg CR (ed): Practical Diagnosis of Hematologic Disorders, 2nd ed. Chicago, American Society of Clinical Pathologists Press, 1995.

Lippert H, Lehmann HP: SI Units in Medicine. Baltimore, Urban & Schwarzenberg, 1978.

Lott JA, Wolf PL: Clinical Enzymology: A Case-Oriented Approach. New York, Field, Rich & Associates, 1986.

Ravel R: Clinical Laboratory Medicine: Clinical Application of Laboratory Data, 6th ed. St. Louis, Mosby–Year Book, 1995.

Speicher CE: The Right Test: A Physician's Guide to Laboratory Medicine, 1st & 2nd ed. Philadelphia, WB Saunders, 1990, 1993.

Speicher CE, Smith JW Jr: Choosing Effective Laboratory Tests. Philadelphia, WB Saunders, 1983.

Statland BE: Clinical Decision Levels for Lab Tests. Oradell, NJ, Medical Economics Books, 1983.

Tietz NW (ed): Clinical Guide to Laboratory Tests, 3rd ed. Philadelphia, WB Saunders, 1995.

Tietz NW, Conn RB, Pruden RL (eds): Applied Laboratory Medicine. Philadelphia, WB Saunders, 1992.

United States Preventive Services Task Force: Guide to Clinical Preventive Services, 2nd ed. Baltimore, Williams & Wilkins, 1996.

Wallach J: Interpretation of Diagnostic Tests, 6th ed. Boston, Little, Brown & Co, 1996.

Watts NB, Keffer JH: Practical Endocrinology, 4th ed. Philadelphia, Lea & Febiger, 1989.

Wilson JD, Braunwald E, Isselbacher KJ, et al (eds): Harrison's Principles of Internal Medicine, 12th ed. New York, McGraw-Hill, 1991.

Young DS: Effects of Drugs on Clinical Laboratory Tests, 4th ed. Washington, DC, American Association for Clinical Chemistry Press, 1995.

Index

Note: Page numbers in *italics* refer to illustrations; page numbers followed by t refer to tables.

A

Abdominal pain, 183–187
  in appendicitis, 184
  in cholecystitis, 185
  in dyspepsia, 185–186, *186*
  in pancreatitis, 184–185
  in porphyria, 187
  laboratory tests for, 183–184
Abuse, alcohol, 80–85. See also *Alcohol abuse.*
  drug, 88–90. See also *Drug abuse.*
Acid-base disorder(s), 308–310
  acidosis as, 309t, 309–310
  alkalosis as, 309
  classification of, 305–306
  mixed, 310
  simple, 309–310
Acidosis, metabolic, 310
  primary uncompensated, 308t
  pure, 309t
  respiratory, 309–310
Acquired immunodeficiency syndrome (AIDS), 99–103
  abnormal blood tests in, 102–103
  CD4 lymphocyte counts in, 101, 102t
  CNS disorders in, 103
  ELISA test for, 100–101
  plasma HIV-1 RNA concentration in, 101
  Western blot assay for, 100
Activated partial thromboplastin time (APTT), in bleeding disorders, 300
  prolonged, in platelet disorders, 301t–302t
Acute myocardial infarction. See *Myocardial infarction.*
Acute renal failure, 249–251
ADH (antidiuretic hormone), low levels of, 313
  normal levels of, 312–313
Adolescent(s), serum cholesterol in, classification of, 59t

Adrenal insufficiency, 273–275, 274t
Aeroallogen panel, 162
Aeroallogen screening test, 162
AIDS. See *Acquired immunodeficiency syndrome (AIDS).*
Alanine aminotransferase (ALT), in cirrhosis, 227
  in liver disease, 204
  in viral hepatitis, 212
Albumin, urine dipstick test for, 239
Alcohol, blood, estimation of, 85
Alcohol abuse, 80–85
  CAGE questionnaire in, 80, 82t, 82–83
  tests for, 81
  U.S. National Council of Alcoholism criteria for, 83t
Alcoholic hepatitis, 217–218. See also *Hepatitis* entries.
Alcoholism, and liver disease, 292
  definition of, 80
Alcohol-related disorder(s), levels of, 81t
Alder-Reilly anomaly, 278
Alkaline phosphatase (ALP), abnormal levels of, 43–45
  in alcohol abuse, 84
  in cholestasis, 205
  in liver disease, 205
  in prostate cancer, 76
Alkalosis, metabolic, 309
  primary uncompensated, 308t
  respiratory, 309
Allergic rhinitis, 161–163
  evaluation of tests for, 162–163
Allergy, food, 118t
ALP. See *Alkaline phosphatase (ALP).*
ALT. See *Alanine aminotransferase (ALT).*
Ambulatory (outpatient) setting, common medical problems in, 9t–10t
American Cancer Society recommendations, for early detection of cancer in asymptomatic people, 95t–96t